Mechanisms and Machine Science

Volume 48

Series editor

Marco Ceccarelli
LARM: Laboratory of Robotics and Mechatronics
DICeM: University of Cassino and South Latium
Via Di Biasio 43, 03043 Cassino (Fr), Italy
e-mail: ceccarelli@unicas.it

More information about this series at http://www.springer.com/series/8779

Manfred Husty · Michael Hofbaur
Editors

New Trends in Medical and Service Robots

Design, Analysis and Control

Springer

Editors
Manfred Husty
Unit Geometry and CAD
University of Innsbruck
Innsbruck
Austria

Michael Hofbaur
Department of Robotics
Joanneum Research
Klagenfurt, Kärnten
Austria

ISSN 2211-0984 ISSN 2211-0992 (electronic)
Mechanisms and Machine Science
ISBN 978-3-319-59971-7 ISBN 978-3-319-59972-4 (eBook)
DOI 10.1007/978-3-319-59972-4

Library of Congress Control Number: 2017943221

Printed on acid-free paper

This Springer imprint is published by Springer Nature
The registered company is Springer International Publishing AG
The registered company address is: Gewerbestrasse 11, 6330 Cham, Switzerland

Preface

Nowadays, medical and service robotics have become a major part in the field of robotics. Medical robotics, in particular, benefits from theoretical and technological advances and the increased acceptance as supporting technology for rehabilitation, surgery and other services that serve our society. Furthermore, medical robots represent the economically most important subclass in the service robotics domain. There is an ongoing demand on new devices for a wide spectrum of applications ranging from robotic devices for keyhole surgery, devices for camera navigation, surgical assistance robots, rehabilitation devices, medical transportation systems, sanitation and disinfection robots, robots that work within an MRI scanner to the application of robots in the treatment of autistic children.

MeSRob2016 was the fifth edition of this series of conferences starting in 2012 in Cluj-Napoca, Romania, followed by the second workshop MeSRob2013 organized by Institute "Mihailo Pupin" in Belgrade, Serbia, the third MeSRoB2014, in Lausanne, Switzerland organized by EPFL and the fourth MeSRob2015 was held in Nantes, France, organized by IRCCyN. The next MeSRob workshop will be in Cassino, Italy in 2018.

MeSRob2106 has covered a wide range from the issues mentioned above, but has also gone beyond these topics. Examples contained in the book are the design of high-precision devices for biopsy or the motion analysis of the left ventricle for the design of a cardiovascular mock-loop. There are also several contributions dealing with gait analysis and the design of exoskeletons. Furthermore, new rehabilitation robots are presented and analyzed in a couple of papers. But there are also some interesting less mainstream papers dealing with robot–child interaction, force balancing mechanisms or devices that are inspired by biology.

These contributions are provided as a collection of 23 papers that were selected by the Scientific Committee from the papers that have been presented during MeSRob2016. All presented papers had also been selected on the basis of a peer-review process. We would therefore like to express our gratitude to the authors, who provided the valuable content, the reviewers and Scientific Committee for their contribution to ensure the scientific quality of MeSRob'2016 and the organizing committee and support staff for managing this successful scientific meeting. We are further grateful to IFToMM, the University of Innsbruck and JOANNEUM RESEARCH Forschungsgesellschaft mbH for their support of MeSRob2016.

We are also grateful to Nathalie Jacobs, Anneke Pot and the staff of Springer for their excellent editorial support.

Innsbruck, Austria — Manfred Husty
Klagenfurt am Wörthersee, Austria — Michael Hofbaur

Contents

Design of a Needle Insertion Module for Robotic Assisted Transperineal Prostate Biopsy

C. Vaida, I. Birlescu, N. Plitea, N. Crisan and D. Pisla

Abstract The paper presents the design of a needle insertion module for robotic assisted transperineal prostate biopsy, using a commercially available biopsy gun. The module is designed to be used as an end-effector for different robotic systems suitable for this medical task. The geometric and kinematic parameters of the insertion module are presented in correlation with a set of experimental data that supplied critical inputs for the solution development.

Keywords Needle insertion module · Transperineal prostate biopsy · Transrectal ultrasound · Biopsy gun

1 Introduction

Prostate cancer is the most commonly diagnosed form of cancer among men, and one of the leading causes for cancer-related deaths in both Europe and USA, with over 220,000 cases predicted and over 25,000 fatalities for 2015 in USA [1, 2]. Diagnosis and treatment methods for this pathology usually consist of: prostate specific antigen (PSA) analysis and biopsy which serve as a diagnosis method and brachytherapy (i.e. radioactive seed placement inside the tumor volume) for

C. Vaida · I. Birlescu (✉) · N. Plitea · D. Pisla
CESTER, Technical University of Cluj-Napoca, Cluj-Napoca, Romania
e-mail: iosif.birlescu@mep.ucluj.ro

C. Vaida
e-mail: calin.vaida@mep.ucluj.ro

N. Plitea
e-mail: nicolae.plitea@mep.ucluj.ro

D. Pisla
e-mail: doina.pisla@mep.ucluj.ro

N. Crisan
University of Medicine and Pharmacy, Craiova, Romania
e-mail: drnicolaecrisan@gmail.com

M. Husty and M. Hofbaur (eds.), *New Trends in Medical and Service Robots*,
Mechanisms and Machine Science 48, DOI 10.1007/978-3-319-59972-4_1

therapy. Prostate needle interventions use specialized needles: on one hand, for biopsy the needle is designed for sampling tissue from the prostate gland; on the other hand, for brachytherapy the needle is designed to deliver the radioactive seeds within the tumor volume.

With the advance in the medical robotics since the end of twentieth century more and more solutions for needle placement are found in the literature [3, 4]. The motivation for robotic assisted needle placement, guided with different methods of medical imaging, lies in the fact that robots can exceed the human limitations (e.g. accuracy, undesired movement, natural tremor) [4, 5]. Currently, three medical imaging methods exist for robotic assisted needle placement, each with distinct advantages and disadvantages [5]: transrectal ultrasonography (TRUS), computerized tomography (CT), and magnetic resonance (MR) imaging. TRUS is the "golden standard" imaging method for prostate biopsy due to the fact that is cost effective and widely available. However, TRUS offers limited precision, with biopsy sensitivity between 60 and 85% [5] and sometimes the patient needs to be re-biopsied due to false negative results [5]. CT and MR imaging solves the precision limitations of TRUS due to high tissue contrast and high volumetric resolution. However, both CT and MR methods have their limitations: the ionizing radiation dose received by the patient and/or clinician during the procedure duration for CT guided needle placement, and robot design challenges for MR guided interventions (i.e. due to the high magnetic field magnetic components are prohibited, and metal components should be used with increased care since they introduce noise in the MR image) [4, 5].

Increased effort was made in the past 30 years in the scientific community to develop reliable robotic models for prostate interventions [4]. From all the proposed models in the literature, only a few are selected to highlight the current state of the art in robotic assisted needle placement with applications in prostate biopsy.

Li et al. presented a robotic model with 6 DoF (3 Cartesian DoF for needle position, and 3 DoF for needle driving module) for transperineal prostate biopsy [6]. The robot is MRI compatible, is designed to use standard biopsy needles, and offers needle rotation in the insertion stage. Krieger et al. developed a series of APT-MRI (Access to Prostate Tissue under MRI guidance) robotic systems designed for transrectal biopsy. APT-I and APT-II contains a manually actuated 3 DoF needle guidance module (2 DoF for the needle translation and rotation, and 1 DoF for the needle insertion) [7, 8]. In contrast with the manually actuated needle guiding approach from APT I and APT II, the needle guiding module from APT-III is designed with 2 motor actuated DoF for needle position and manually (1 DoF) needle insertion [9]. Staianovici et al. developed MrBot, a fully actuated MRI compatible robot with 4 DoF for transperineal prostate interventions. MrBot uses pneumatic stepper actuators designed for MRI compatibility [10]. Fichtinger et al. presented a robotic structure with 6 DoF designed for transperineal prostate biopsy under CT guidance [11]. All the above mentioned robotic systems, with their associated needle insertion modules, have their distinct characteristics; however none of them are designed for automatically needle insertion and firing of a biopsy gun after the insertion. To our best knowledge there are no modules that are able to perform this operation using commercially available biopsy guns. The study in this paper is focused on developing a fully actuated needle guiding module with 2 DoF (1 DoF for needle insertion/retraction, and 1 DoF for gun firing) for transperineal prostate biopsy using the BARD™ Monopty 22 mm biopsy gun [12]. The needle guiding module is designed to be integrated into the BIO-PROS1 parallel structure presented in [13, 14], to perform automated transperineal prostate biopsy guided by TRUS imaging).

2 Clinical Characteristics

Prostate cancer is a progressive disease with metastatic risk correlated with the tumor size. Research shows that metastasis can only appear in tumors with volume greater than 4 mL [9, 15]. A tumor volume of 0.5 mL was proposed for clinical relevance for prostate cancer [9]. Assuming a tumor volume of 0.5 mL, with a spherical shape, the resulted tumor diameter will be 9.8 mm [9]. Krieger et al. reports in [5] that a needle placement target accuracy of 5 mm or better is desired for prostate biopsies guided with MR imaging.

The prostate gland is about 40 $\times$ 30 $\times$ 30 mm in size, and it is localized under the bladder, completely surrounding the proximal part of urethra. Depending on the thickness of the subcutaneous tissue the prostate is localized at 70 $\pm$ 20 mm behind the perineum tissue [9].

The most common used screening method for prostate cancer is the prostate-specific antigen test (PSA), which measures the blood concentration of PSA to estimate the likelihood of prostate cancer. However this method alone can't accurately determine the presence of prostate cancer. Therefore a biopsy is required (usually 12–18 cores are removed) if the PSA levels are higher than normal, to determine the cancer presence and the degree of its extension [9].

The current "golden standard" for prostate biopsy is the TRUS guided needle biopsy i.e. the biopsy needle is inserted in the gland trough the wall of the rectum. An alternative way for prostate biopsy is the transperineal approach, i.e. the needle is inserted in the gland through the perineum tissue. The disadvantage of this approach, in comparison with the transrectal biopsy, is the longer needle insertion path, and more patient discomfort. However, the transperineal approach offers some advantages that determined the scientific community to explore this method: (i) it eliminates the risk of infection (that is up to 5%) present in TRUS biopsy; (ii) it eliminates other possible TRUS complications (acute urinary retention and clot retention), (iii) it provides the sampling possibility of the entire prostate volume (the apex being impossible to reach transrectally) [16].

The needle guiding module described in this study is designed to work, guided by the BIO-PROS-1 parallel robotic structure [13, 14, 17]. BIO-PROS-1 has two parallel modules, one for the needle guidance and one for the TRUS probe guidance [13, 14, 17]. Designed to be used for transperineal prostate biopsy, the BIO-PROS - 1 robotic system has to synchronize the two robotic arms, positioning the TRUS probe always below the needle guiding device. The TRUS probe will be inserted inside the patient through the rectum while the needle will be inserted through the perineum, the two entry points being located at a distance between 30 and 50 mm apart on the vertical axis, depending on the size of the patient. The structure, presented in Fig. 1 consists of two modules connected together: the first is a parallel module with 3 DOF with three active joints (q_1, q_2, q_3) which are translational along axes parallel with the OY (q_1), respectively OZ (q_2, q_3) of the fixed frame of the robot, generating the positioning of the mobile platform with constant orientation in space. The second module is a 3 DOF module working in cylindrical coordinates, having two active translational joints (q_4, q_5). The mobile platforms of the two modules are connected using two Cardan joints. The robotic arm which drives the needle insertion module has a similar configuration of the modules as the first arm, but with both modules placed on the same side of the robotic system (Fig. 1).

A protocol for automated prostate biopsy is presented in [6], and it is extended in this paper (Fig. 2) for transperineal prostate biopsy under TRUS guidance:

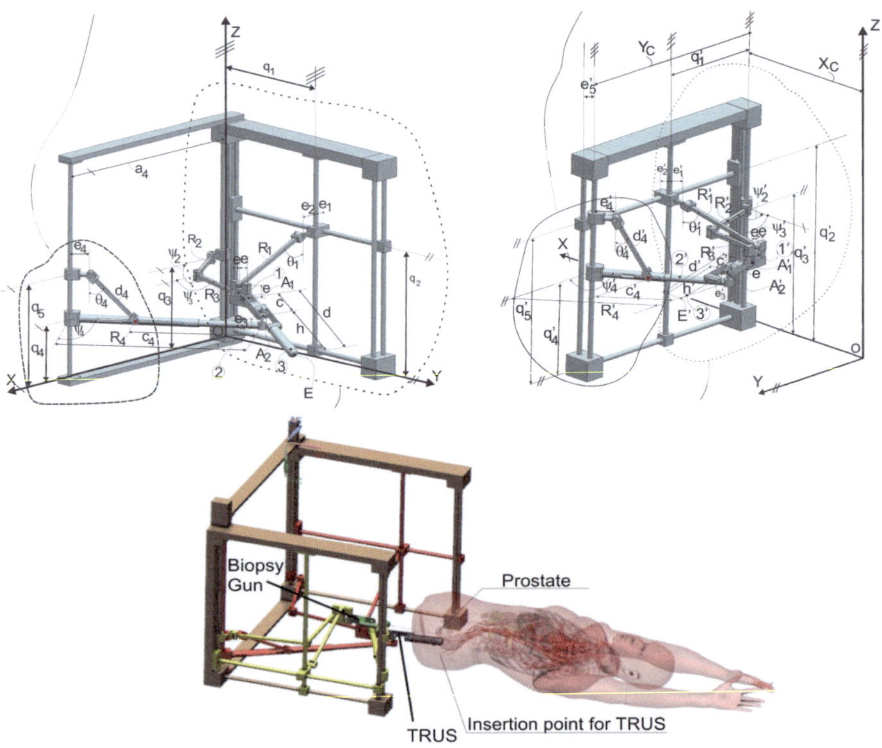

Fig. 1 BIO-PROS 1: TRUST guiding module on the *top left*; needle insertion module on the *top right*; virtual model within medical environment [14]

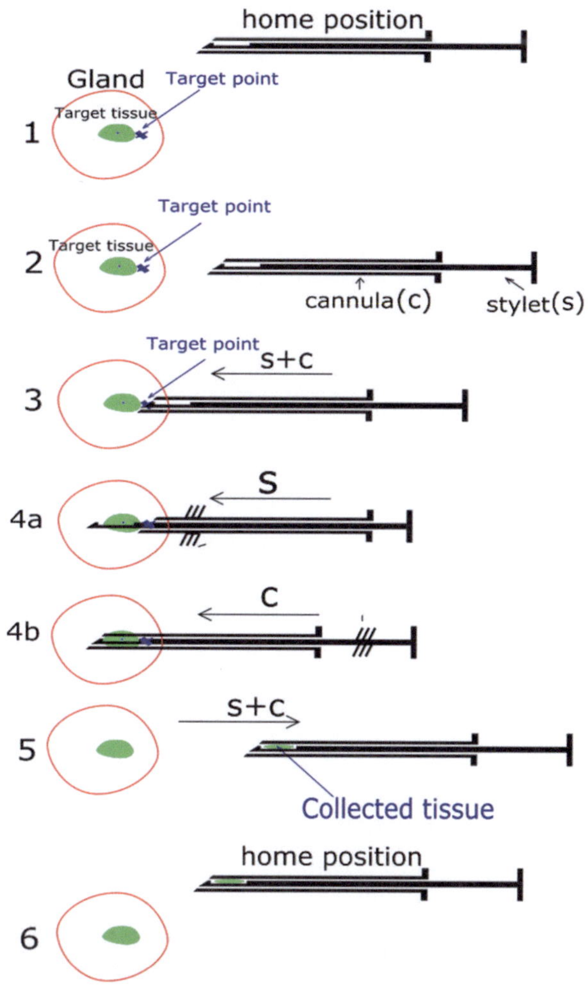

Fig. 2 Protocol for robotic assisted prostate biopsy using a biopsy gun

1. The robot (BIO-PROS-1) is initialized and the module is moved in home position.
2. The robot positions the module to a predefined needle position and orientation, i.e. the module is moved from the home position and the needle is aligned with the insertion point.
3. The needle is inserted through the perineum tissue, on a linear trajectory, into the prostate gland until the target point is reached.
4. The biopsy gun is fired leading to a quick actuation of the stylet (a) followed by quick actuation of the cannula (b) in order to capture the target tissue inside the needle (see Fig. 2).

5. The needle is retracted from the patient (linear trajectory).
6. The module is moved back to the home position

After the biopsy is completed, following the above mentioned protocol, the biopsy gun is removed from the guiding module, the tissue is collected, the biopsy gun is placed back on the module, and the procedure is repeated until all the tissue samples are collected.

3 Model Design

The needle insertion module (subject to a patent [18]) is designed to work with the BIO-PROS-1 parallel structure but it can be adapted with minimal modifications to work with any robot which can perform the necessary motions for the transperineal biopsy of the prostate (even a robotic arm for instance [19]). For transperineal prostate biopsy the patient is placed in a gynecologic position, therefore the TRUS probe will operate under the biopsy gun. By taking this into consideration, the needle insertion module should be designed with increase care on using components in its lower part, to avoid collisions with the TRUS probe. Therefore the actuator is fixed on top of the module and the translation mechanism on the side, as it is described further in this section.

The needle insertion module works with the BARD Monopty 22 mm biopsy gun (Fig. 3), which contains a biopsy needle with the back side encapsulated into a plastic handle with a rotating sleeve that is used to load the gun, and a circular button behind the handle to fire the biopsy gun. The gun loading procedure is done in a sequence having two steps: by rotating the sleeve counter-clockwise about 180° the needle cannula gets retracted by about 18 mm (after this step the biopsied tissue is collected from the needle), and next, by rotating the sleeve counter-clockwise another 180° the stylet is retracted by 18 mm. The gun loading sequence is performed manually by the clinician, which does not impose any disadvantage since the biopsied tissue has to be collected from the gun anyway.

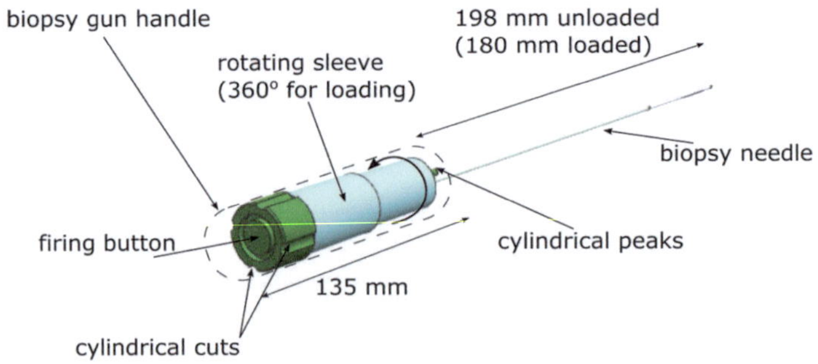

Fig. 3 CAD illustration of the biopsy gun

Referring to the robot characteristics and the operating specifications above mentioned, designing a needle insertion module to work with the BARD Monopty 22 mm biopsy gun is feasible. The module should have three main components namely: a platform that is linked with the robot, a mobile (relative to the fixed platform) support that holds the biopsy gun, and a needle tip holder.

The linkage between the fixed platform and the biopsy gun support is described in Fig. 4. The Cartesian coordinate system is fixed on the platform of the module into a point desired for the connection with the BIO-PROS-1 parallel robot (this will make it easy to relate the needle insertion module to the robot coordinate system). Therefore the center of the chosen coordinate system and the center of the universal joint from the frontal part of the end effector (for the biopsy needle) are equivalent (see Fig. 4). The needle axis is parallel to the OX axis and lies in the XOZ plane at distance d_{needle}. The linkage between the platform and the mobile support is created via two parallel passive cylindrical joints (using the shaft (1) from the support and the bushings (2) from the platform). This will ensure the translation motion that will insert the needle on the linear trajectory inside the patient body.

The shaft length (l_{shaft}) and the tube length (l_{tube}) permit a total translation (l_{trans}) of the support (and needle):

$$0 \leq |l_{trans}| \leq l_{shaft} - l_{tube} \tag{1}$$

As the shafts slide through the bushings l_{trans} varies, i.e. if the shafts are translated along X′ and X″ axes (parallel to OX) allowing the motion in both directions, i.e. the insertion and retraction of the needle.

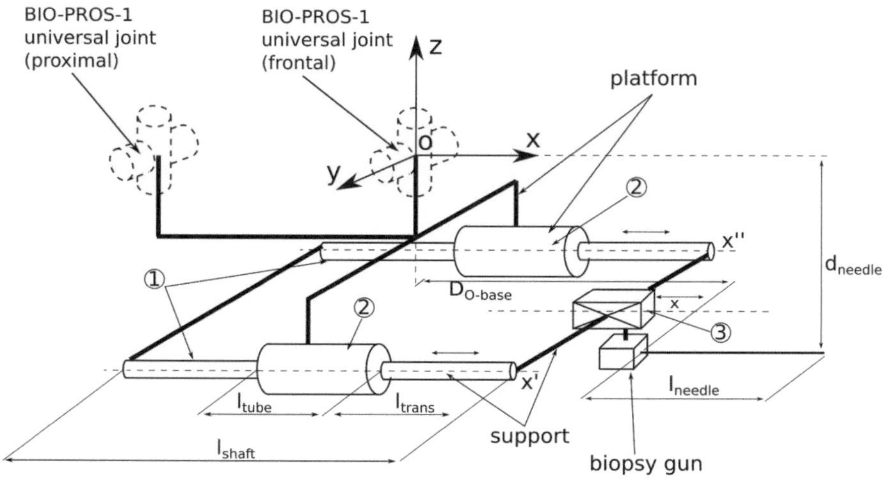

Fig. 4 Conceptual scheme of the needle insertion module

The needle tip has the coordinates:

$$\begin{pmatrix} x_{nt} \\ y_{nt} \\ z_{nt} \end{pmatrix} = \begin{pmatrix} x_{nt} \\ 0 \\ d_{needle} \end{pmatrix} \tag{2}$$

where x_{nt} can be determined as following:

$$x_{nt} = l_{needle} + l_{trans} + d_{st} \tag{3}$$

where d_{st} is the distance in along the X axis from the origin O and the proximal part of the needle when translation is minimum (i.e. zero in our case) and it can be computed from:

$$d_{st} = d_{O-base} - l_{trans} \tag{4}$$

where $d_{O\text{-}nbase}$ is the distance (X coordinate) from O to the needle base (the proximal part). Finally the needle tip coordinates are obtained:

$$\begin{pmatrix} x_{nt} \\ y_{nt} \\ z_{nt} \end{pmatrix} = \begin{pmatrix} l_{needle} + l_{trans} + d_{st} \\ 0 \\ d_{needle} \end{pmatrix} \tag{5}$$

The linear motion is obtained through the active prismatic joint (3) which is actuated along the Xt axis (parallel to OX) using a screw/nut mechanism.

The CAD design of the needle insertion module and its components, developed in Siemens NX, are presented in Fig. 5. The biopsy gun support has a fixed part (4) and a revolving part (5) (around R axis parallel to OX) to allow an open/close sequence to place and fix the biopsy gun. The pistol is placed into the mobile part (5) of the support and then the support is closed by pushing it up against the fixed part (4) and locking the two parts together via a screw mechanism (6). The biopsy gun handle has a design with four cylindrical partially cuts in the back side and two cylindrical peaks in the front side (see Fig. 3). The support design takes advantage of these geometric features, and with a back cover (7), it ensures a reliable fixed position of the pistol when the support is closed. On the left and right side of the support there are cylindrical shafts (1), which create cylindrical joints with the fixed platform. On the top there is a platform (8) (parallel to XOZ plane) with a carving in which a ball nut (3) is fixed to create the translation mechanism. The firing mechanism is simply a spindle drive (9) fixed into a support (10) placed and fixed behind the back cover (7) of the fixed support part (4).

The platform (11) (lying on a plane parallel to OXZ) is connected with the pistol support via two cylinder tubes (2) which in combination with the cylindrical shafts (1) from the support creates two parallel cylindrical joints. The translation motion of the support relative with the fixed platform is made with a rotating ball screw (12) (connected with the nut (3)) rotated by the motor (13) through a gear

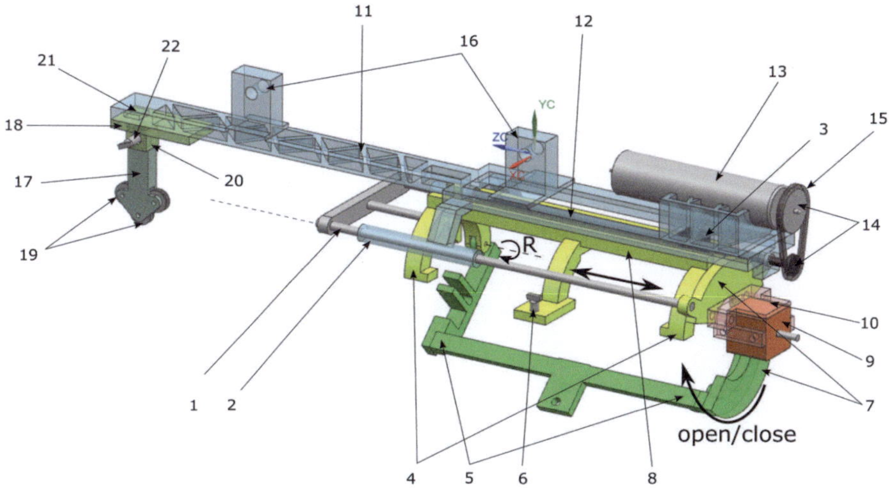

Fig. 5 CAD illustration of the needle insertion module with its highlighted components

mechanism with two cogwheels (14) and a rubber belt (15). Two extensions (16) are fixed to the platform, in the same plane, to connect the needle insertion module with the BIO-PROS-1 parallel robot.

The needle tip holder (17) is connected in the frontal part of the fixed platform (11) via a sliding sledge (18). The holder has a mechanism designed with three grooved wheels (19) with spinning axes parallel with OY. The sledge purpose is to allow the motion of the holder along an axis parallel to the needle axis, motion that is needed when the clinician mounts the gun into the support. I.e. the holder must be moved away from the gun when the pistol is being mounted, and moved back after the support is closed so the needle goes through the holder. The holder is removable from the sledge for sterilization related issues. The holder (17) is fixed into its plug (20) using a magnet (21) for exact positioning and a screw (22) for stiffness. The needle holder is fixed relative to the insertion point, and the biopsy needle slides through it in the insertion stage. The wheel mechanism reduces friction in comparison with a fixed needle holding mechanism, which helps especially on the pistol firing stage when the needle velocities are high. The space between the wheels is 1.6 mm i.e. the mechanism is designed for the standard 1.6 mm diameter biopsy needles found within the Monopty 22 mm biopsy gun.

For a needle insertion correlated with the clinical specifications presented in Sect. 2, the length of the cylindrical shafts is chosen 175 mm while the length of the cylindrical counterparts from the platform is 60 mm. This offers a total of 115 mm translation of the needle tip, which allows certain flexibility in determining the needle distance relative to the insertion point, and allows the reach of the target point from various needle positions and orientations.

The total mass of the needle insertion module is:

$$m_{\text{module}} = m_{fix} + m_{move} \tag{6}$$

where m_{fix} is the mass of the parts that are not actuated by the modules motor (platform, needle holder, motor), and m_{move} is the mass of the motor actuated parts (support, biopsy gun, firing mechanism).

The formula needed to calculate the thrust generated when torque is applied is:

$$F_a = \frac{2\pi \cdot \eta 1 \cdot T}{Ph} \tag{7}$$

With:

F_a Thrust generated by the torque (N);
Ph Feed screw lead (mm);
$\eta 1$ Positive efficiency of the feed screw (%);
T Driving torque (N mm).

F_a can be viewed as the frictional resistance on the guided surface (i.e. friction inside the cylindrical joints of the module):

$$F_a = \mu \cdot m_{move} \cdot g \tag{8}$$

Assuming perfect surface contact in the cylindrical joints, and taking into account the tissue resistance on needle insertion, using Eq. (7) the net thrust when torque is applied is defined as:

$$F_{total} = F_a + F_{tissue} \tag{9}$$

where F_{tissue} = tissue resistance.

The torque needed to maintain a linear motion (constant velocity) of the biopsy gun in the insertion stage is:

$$T = F_{total} \cdot \frac{Ph}{2\pi \cdot \eta 1} \tag{10}$$

The torque needed to accelerate the needle has to be computed by accounting all the moments of inertia of the rotating parts:

$$T_{acc} = J \cdot \dot{\omega} \tag{11}$$

where:

J total moment of inertia (kg m^2)
$\dot{\omega}$ angular acceleration (rad s^{-2})

The total moment of inertia is calculated from:

$$J = m_{move} \cdot \left(\frac{P}{2 \cdot \pi}\right)^2 + J_s + J_a + J_b \tag{12}$$

where:

J_s moment of inertia of the screw
J_a moment of inertia of the gear attached to the screw
J_b moment of inertia of the gear attached to the motor shaft

$$J_a = J_b = m_{pul} \cdot d^2 \cdot \frac{1}{8} \tag{13}$$

where:

m_{pul} mass of the pulleys from the gear (10 g)
d outer diameter of the pulleys (15 mm)

The angular acceleration can be calculated from:

$$\dot{\omega} = \frac{d(2 \cdot \pi \cdot N)}{dt} \tag{14}$$

with:
N number of rotations per sec.

The tissue resistance was experimentally determined using ex vivo animal tissue (pig leg) as a test sample (Fig. 6). The needle was inserted into the tissue using the ZWICK/ROELL testing equipment that has a 24 bit measured-value resolution and an acquisition rate of 2 kHz. The reactive force was continuously registered. The results obtained from 5 experimental trials, as well as the mean of those trials are presented in Fig. 6 for biopsy needle insertion, with and without skin incision. The point of insertion was carefully selected not to be closer than 5 mm than the previous insertion point to avoid following a needle path that was already used, therefore measuring lower forces since the tissue was already penetrated. However with this approach it is easy to observe the variations in the force curve since the needle, most likely, penetrated trough different tissue (fat, muscle etc.) for every experimental trial. The velocity during needle insertion was 10 mm/s and the force was registered for 8 s. This leaves a variable interval of depth length of about 70 mm. As illustrated in Fig. 7, the resulted tissue resistance to needle insertion was in less than 10 N.

The experimental results validated also a medical variation of the transperineal procedure performed by specialists from the European Institute of Oncology, Italy, which perform a small incision in the perineum skin and insert the needle in a cone shape through a single port, rather than using parallel trajectories [20]. With this approach, where a skin incision was performed, the resistance force of the tissue has

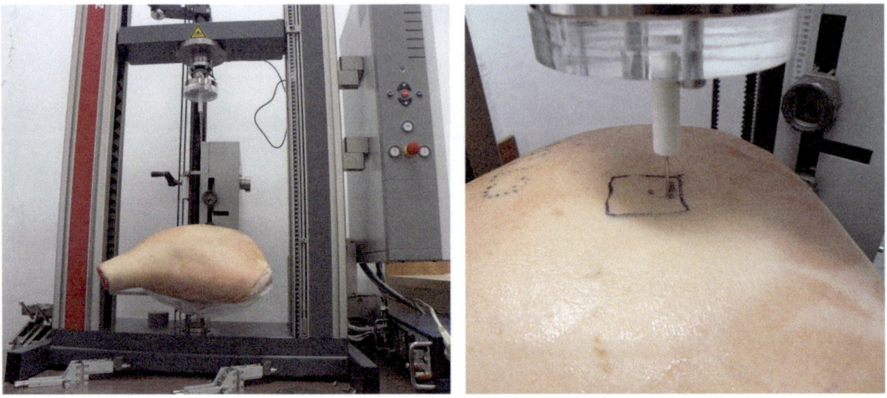

Fig. 6 Tissue resistance on needle insertion experimental setup. Overview on the *left*; close view on *right*

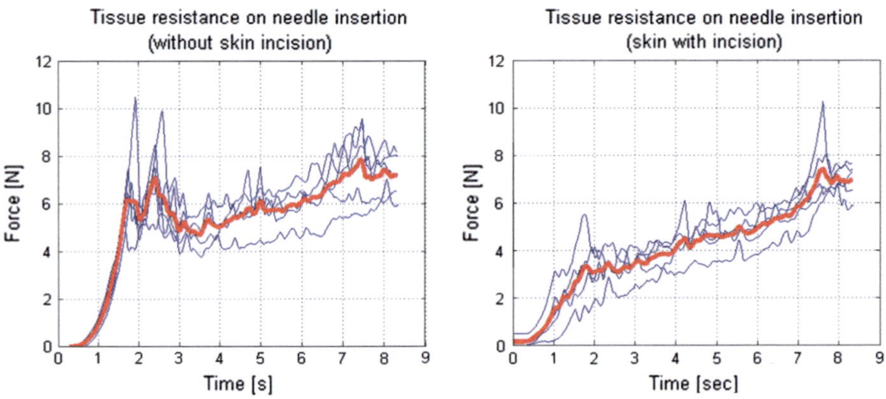

Fig. 7 Reported tissue resistance for needle insertion using ex vivo animal tissue without skin incision (*on the left*) and with skin incision (*on the right*)

a more linear evolution, eliminating the spike which appear when the skin is penetrated which leads to an increased accuracy due to the elimination of the needle deflection. This approach eliminates the use of a guiding template making the manual needle insertion somewhat more difficult, but using a robotic arm for the needle guidance this drawback is eliminated. Simulation using Siemens NX™ software showed a mass of the mobile parts of the needle insertion module ≈175 g (using Al 5086). The biopsy gun mass is ≈50 g, and by considering the nut and the spindle drive masses, the total moving mass of the module is ≈240 g. The friction coefficient in the cylindrical joints is 0.04 (steel to Teflon since Teflon bushings are used inside the joints). By using Eq. (9) the torque value required for needle insertion (at constant velocity) of ≈0.0017 Nm is obtained. Using Eqs. (11–14), with the screw moment of inertia $\approx 0.0285 \times 10^{-6}$ (kg m^2), the pulleys moments of inertia $\approx 0.2813 \times 10^{-6}$, the required needle velocity = 10 mm s^{-1} and acceleration = 10 mm s^{-2} (thus the acceleration time is 1 s), and finally the rotational velocity 10 rot s^{-1}, the extra torque required for accelerating motion is obtained 37.52×10^{-6} Nm.

The force needed to fire the biopsy gun was experimentally determined by pressing the loaded biopsy gun firing button against a force sensor FSR® from Interlink Electronics™, while the data was acquired using National Instruments™ hardware (NI USB-6210) and MatLab™ software (Fig. 8). The experimental bench was developed inside CESTER research center. Output data from 31 experimental trials showed a normal distribution with a mean of 2.689 V (at gun firing instance) and a standard deviation of 0.11. The force sensor was calibrated using standardized weights to determine the characteristic curve that describes volt to force conversion (Fig. 8). Out of this curve, a force of 7.84 N resulted to be de mean value at the gun firing instance.

An electromagnet or a spindle drive that offers a force of 10 N is recommended since it gives an extra ≈25% interval to ensure the gun firing. In the selection of the actuation solution weight is a critical parameter which has to be minimized.

Following the above results (calculated and experimentally determined) the proposed actuators (motor and spindle drive) for the needle insertion module and the screw/nut mechanism are the following:

- The Spindle Drive GP 6 S Ø6 mm from Maxon Motor™; max continuous force of 10 N, max intermittent force 18 N, with a mass of 4 g.
- The motor, ECX SPEED 8M Ø8 mm, and the planetary gearhead GPX 8 Ø8 mm from Maxon Motor™; offer continuous torque of 0.008 Nm and a maximum intermittent torque of 0.012 Nm with a mass of 9 g.
- The ball screw and the ball nut from THK, screw model MDK 0401-3 with its afferent nut. The mechanism has the lead of 1 mm, efficiency of 0.95 and it works well at a rotating speed of 600 RPM. The mass of the screw is 10.15 g while the mass of the nut is 10 g.

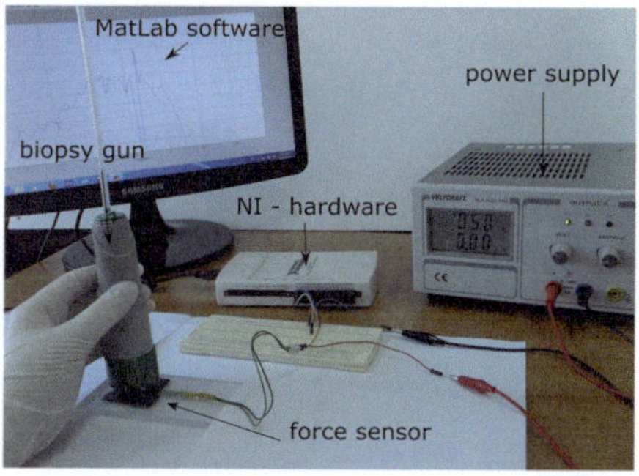

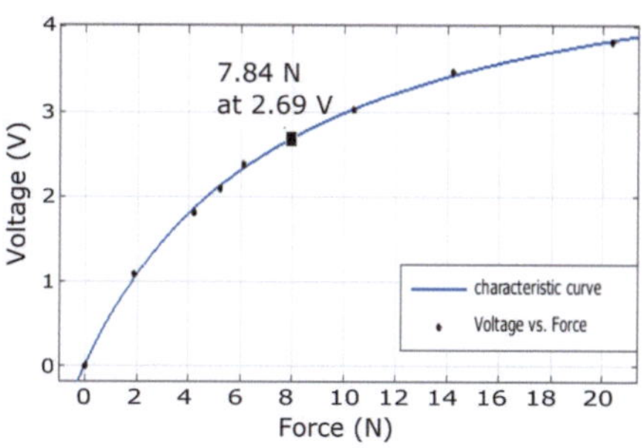

Fig. 8 Experimental setup for the gun firing needed force (*left*). Voltage to force characteristic curve of the force sensor (*right*)

The total mass of the needle insertion module with the biopsy gun mounted is around 560 g. The compact solution proposed for the needle insertion module makes this device suitable for a wide variety of biopsy procedures, extending its utilization to other organs as well: liver, kidneys, breast, and thyroid. The overall size makes this device also capable of performing CT-Sim guided biopsies, working as the end-effector of a robotic arm which works inside the gantry of the imaging device, such the PARA-BRACHYROB robot [21]. The modular design allows, with minimal changes its conversion towards another biopsy gun, imposing as a single restriction the presence of the release mechanism at the end of the proximal head of the medical instrument.

4 Conclusions

This paper presents a needle insertion module for transperineal prostate biopsy designed for the BIO-PROS-1 parallel robot. The module has 2 DoF, one for needle insertion/retraction, and another for gun firing and its parameters reflect its intended purpose. I.e. the total linear translation of the needle allows the reach of the entire prostate gland volume from various points of insertion and needle orientations, while the force provided by the actuators is sufficient for a reliable needle insertion and biopsy gun firing.

Further research is proposed to optimize the needle insertion module (mostly to increase the needle placement accuracy). These optimizations can be either architectural (e.g. placing the needle holder on the correct position by measuring the axial stress along the needle to determine where the needle is more likely to bend in the insertion stage) or structural (e.g. reducing various components mass to move the center of mass on the needle axis). These optimizations are intended to reduce the needle deflection, therefore, as specified, increasing the needle target accuracy.

Acknowledgements This paper was realized within the Partnership Programme in priority domains—PN-II, which runs with the financial support of MEN-UEFISCDI through the Project no. 59/2015, code PN-II-RU-TE-2014-4-0992—ACCURATE and Project no. 247/2014, code PN-II-PT-PCCA-2013-4-0647—ROBOCORE.

References

1. Siegel, R., Miller, K.: Cancer statistics. CA Cancer J. Clin. **65**, 5–29 (2015)
2. Ferlay, J., Steliarova-Foucher, E.: Cancer incidence and mortality patterns in Europe: estimates for 40 countries in 2012. Eur. J. Cancer **49**, 1374–1403 (2013)
3. Tarun, K.P. et al: AAPM and GEC-ESTRO guidelines for image-guided robotic brachytherapy: report of Task Group 192. Am. Assoc. Phys. Med. (2014)
4. Stoianovici, D., et al.: "MRI Stealth" robot for prostate interventions. Minim. Invasive Allied Technol. **16**(4), 241–248 (2007)

5. Kriger, A., et al.: Design of a novel MRI compatible manipulator for image guided prostate interventions. IEEE Trans. Biomed. Eng. **52**(2), 306–313 (2005)
6. Gang, Li, et al.: A fully actuated robotic assistant for MRI-guided prostate biopsy and brachytherapy. Proc. SPIE Int. Soc. Opt. Eng. **12**(8671), 867117 (2013)
7. Krieger, A., et al.: Design of a novel MRI compatible manipulator for image guided prostate interventions. IEEE Trans. Biomed. Eng. **52**(2), 306–313 (2005)
8. Krieger, A., et al.: An MRI-compatible robotic system with hybrid tracking for MRI-guided prostate intervention. IEEE Trans. Biomed. Eng. **58**(11), 3049–3060 (2011). doi:10.1109/TBME.2011.2134096
9. Krieger, A., et al.: Development and evaluation of an actuated MRI-compatible robotic system for MRI-guided prostate intervention. IEEE ASME Trans. Mechatron. **18**(1), 273–284 (2012). Epub 2011 Oct 17
10. Stoianovici, D. et al.: "MRI Stealth" robot for prostate interventions. Minim. Invasive Ther. Allied Technol. **16**(4), 241–248 (2007) [Erratum in: Minim. Invasive Ther. Allied Technol. 2007;16(6):370]
11. Fichtinger, G., et al.: System for robotically assisted prostate biopsy and therapy with intraoperative CT guidance. Acad. Radiol. **9**(1), 60–74 (2002)
12. C.R. Bard Inc. http://www.bardbiopsy.com/products/monopty.php. Accessed 30 Jan 2016.
13. Plitea, N., Pisla, D., Vaida, C., Gherman, B., Tucan, P., Govor, C., Covaciu, F.: Family of innovative parallel robots for transperineal prostate biopsy. Patent pending: A/00191/13.03.2015
14. Pisla, D., et al.: On the kinematics of an innovative parallel robotic system for transperineal prostate biopsy. In: 14th World Congress in Mechanism and Machine Science, Taipei, Taiwan, pp. 25–30 (2015)
15. Tokuda, J., et al.: Preclinical evaluation of an MRI-compatible pneumatic robot for angulated needle placement in transperineal prostate interventions. Int. J. Comput. Assist. Radiol. Surg. **7**(6), 949–957 (2012)
16. Huang, S., et al.: Significant impact of transperineal template biopsy of the prostate at a single tertiary institution. Urol. Ann. **7**(4), 428–432 (2015).
17. Pisla, D., et al.: Graphical simulation system for functional analysis of a parallel robot for transperineal prostate biopsy. Appl. Mech. Mater. **823**, 101–106. ISSN 1662-7482.
18. Vaida, C., Birlescu, I., Gherman, B., Tucan, P., Plitea, N., Pisla, D.: Automated medical instrument used for robotic assisted biopsy. Patent pending: A/00936/29.11.2016
19. Tarnita, D., Marghitu, D.: Analysis of a hand arm system. Robot. Comput.-Integr. Manuf. **29**(6), 493–501 (2013)
20. Cobelli, O., et al.: Predicting pathological features at radical prostatectomy in patients with prostate cancer eligible for active surveillance by multiparametric magnetic resonance imaging. PLoS ONE **10**(10), e0139696. doi:10.1371/journal.pone.0139696
21. Vaida, C., Pisla, D., Schadlbauer, J., Husty, M., Plitea, N.: Kinematic Analysis of an Innovative Medical Parallel Robot using Study parameters, New Trends in Medical and Service Robots: Human Centered Analysis, Control and Design (2016) (in press).

Motion Analysis of the Left Ventricle of a Human Heart for Realization in a Cardiovascular Mock-Loop

S. Kurtenbach, F. Wieja, I. Müller, M. Neidlin, S.J. Sonntag, A. Goetzenich, N. Hatam, P. Bruns, F. Chuembou Pekam, M. de la Fuente Klein, K. Radermacher, C. Hopmann, R. Autschbach, U. Steinseifer, M. Hüsing and B. Corves

Abstract Within the further development of a special mechanical representation of the human circulatory system the CVELoop at the Department of Cardiovascular Engineering at RWTH Aachen University, a contractive MockHeart was developed. This MockHeart simulates a healthy heart in the CVELoop. In opposition to all previous cardiovascular system simulators, the left ventricle is externally driven by several cam mechanisms. These cam mechanisms provide the necessary power to create the pressure-volume-work for the fluid circulation but also the important time dependent radial contraction, which is the most influential degree of Freedom in the human heart. The aim is to produce a MockHeart providing valid boundary

S. Kurtenbach (✉) · F. Wieja · M. Hüsing · B. Corves
Department of Mechanism Theory and Dynamics of Machines (IGM),
RWTH Aachen University, Aachen, Germany
e-mail: kurtenbach@igm.rwth-aachen.de

F. Wieja
e-mail: wieja@igm.rwth-aachen.de

M. Hüsing
e-mail: huesing@igm.rwth-aachen.de

B. Corves
e-mail: corves@igm.rwth-aachen.de

I. Müller · M. Neidlin · S.J. Sonntag · U. Steinseifer
Department of Cardiovascular Engineering (CVE), RWTH Aachen University,
Aachen, Germany
e-mail: mueller@ame.rwth-aachen.de

M. Neidlin
e-mail: neidlin@ame.rwth-aachen.de

S.J. Sonntag
e-mail: sonntag@ame.rwth-aachen.de

U. Steinseifer
e-mail: steinseifer@ame.rwth-aachen.de

M. Husty and M. Hofbaur (eds.), *New Trends in Medical and Service Robots*,
Mechanisms and Machine Science 48, DOI 10.1007/978-3-319-59972-4_2

conditions for the connected VAD (Ventricular Assist Device). The systematic approach of the development of the mechanism is performed based on an accurate measurement of the kinematic properties of a healthy human heart at RWTH Aachen University with the speckle tracking echocardiography-procedure.

Keywords MockHeart · CVELoop · Left ventricle · Left ventricular assist device (LVAD)

1 Introduction

Realistic simulators for the cardiovascular system provide the opportunity to perform in examinations under laboratory conditions ahead of testing and researching ventricular support systems in living organisms. That way, animal experiments, which still provide the most meaningful test results, can be reduced [1]. Since this reduces costs in most cases as well as time expense and efforts during the development of a cardiac support system, numerous different cardiovascular simulators have been developed. The fact that animal experiments are not always viable and ethically questionable contributes to the effort of developing new systems. So far, it was not possible to reproduce every single part of the cardiovascular system realistically [2]. The models, which have been developed up to this point, not only

P. Bruns · C. Hopmann
Institute of Plastics Processing (IKV) in Industry and the Skilled Crafts
at RWTH Aachen Universit, RWTH Aachen University, Aachen, Germany
e-mail: philipp.bruns@ikv.rwth-aachen.de

C. Hopmann
e-mail: Christian.hopmann@ikv.rwth-aachen.de

F. Chuembou Pekam · M. de la Fuente Klein · K. Radermacher
RWTH Aachen University, Aachen, Germany
e-mail: chuembou@hia.rwth-aachen.de

M. de la Fuente Klein
e-mail: fuente@hia.rwth-aachen.de

K. Radermacher
e-mail: Radermacher@hia.rwth-aachen.de

A. Goetzenich · N. Hatam · R. Autschbach
Clinic for Thoracic and Cardiovascular Surgery (THG), RWTH Aachen University, Aachen, Germany
e-mail: agoetzenich@ukaachen.de

N. Hatam
e-mail: nhatam@ukaachen.de

R. Autschbach
e-mail: rautschbach@ukaachen.de

differ in the number of simulated parts of the cardiovascular system, but also in their specific execution [2].

Basically, the number of actuators that have been implemented for the simulation of ventricles distinguish between three main categories: single-chamber-system, double-chamber-system and multi-chamber-system. Single-chamber-systems, usually controlled using a pneumatic drive, yield cost-efficient results due to their simple design. Their general goal is to simulate the pressure-volume-work of a native heart [3–9]. They are capable of reproducing the contraction of a human ventricle considering the Frank-Starling-mechanism; however they do not involve the systematic effects of the pulmonary circulation [2]. As an example the independently developed simulators by Colacino et al. [10] and Ferrari et al. [11] should be mentioned. Double-chamber-systems with two ventricles or alternatively one ventricle and one atrium can be used to develop further aspects of the circulatory systems [2]. This is exemplified by the cardiovascular simulator CVELoop by the Department of cardiovascular at RWTH Aachen University [12–14].

Weak spot of the double-chamber-systems is the poor illustration of the interaction between the atrium and the ventricle as well as the interaction between the ventricle and the artery in both the systemic and pulmonary circulation. Multi-chamber-systems that usually consist of four chambers are capable of replicating the diastolic and systolic pressure as well as the flow rate. However, until the development of the cardiovascular simulator by Ruiz et al. [2] they were not suited to depict the filling phase of the chambers reliably. Ruiz considered the cause to be the use of multiphase motors and pneumatic drives. Multiphase motors in particular are unsuitable for the emulation of pathophysiologic conditions, because of their disadvantages according to controlling possibilities. Pneumatic drives admittedly are able to illustrate the contraction phase realistically by injecting air into a flexible membrane, but they also generate a vacuum due to the necessary ventilation during the diastole. This limits the simulation of the faster and slower filling phases [2].

Since the native cardiovascular system and therefore basically the function of the heart cannot be illustrated by the controlling of multiphase motors or pneumatic drives, there is a demand for a suitable drive concept for ventricles simulated through flexible membranes.

The goal of the following concept is not just to provide the necessary pressure-volume-work for the fluid circulation, but rather in particular to realize the significant radial contraction of the human left ventricle realistically, so that the cardiovascular simulator yields valid test conditions for the connected cardiac support system. In order to realize this radial movement of the left ventricle, an unevenly transmitting mechanism is developed using methods commonly utilized in mechanical engineering.

2 Contraction of the Human Heart

The contraction of the left ventricle happens through the excitation of the heart muscle cells, which are constructed in a unique pattern. Their structure through the three layers of the myocardium results in a complex deformation of the left ventricle during contraction [4, 7]. The heart starts contracting along the longitudinal axis and the wall of the ventricle thickens radially. The valve plane moves towards the cardiac apex and the additional shift of the valve plane facilitates the ejection of blood into the aorta. At the same time this movement generates a pull into the atrium in favor of the blood flow from the pulmonary vein. During diastole the valve plane moves back. Besides the aforementioned radial contraction and the axial movement, the contraction also causes an opposed torsion between the base and apex of the heart. Figuratively speaking, the left ventricle is "wrung out". During the relaxation phase the torsion regresses. Its movement between base and apex facilitates the inflow of blood into the ventricle. In addition to that, the contraction of the atrium contributes to the filling of the ventricle during diastole [15–17].

2.1 The Radial Contraction

The foundation for the development of a mechanism is the result of an extensive study on the radial contractions of a healthy grown heart at the medical center of RWTH Aachen University. The study has been performed with the aid of the Speckle tracking echocardiography (STE) using the software 4D LV Function™ by TomTec Imaging Systems GmbH. STE is a three-dimensional parametric ultrasound measuring procedure that, compared to the conventional two-dimensional echocardiography, should enable an, as far as possible, examiner independent, objective and quantitative analysis of the "myocardial functions" [18]. With the aid of this parametric method it is possible, depending on the problem, to analyze tissue velocity and deformation rate as well as forms of contractions and even derived parameters. That way the myocardial radial strain, which describes the contraction, or deformation respectively, relative to a reference length or reference point in radial direction, can be determined [18]. This determination takes place in the center transverse sectional plane of the left ventricle (Fig. 1).

Figure 1 displays the followed pixels in the end-systolic and end-diastolic condition. The shortening of endocardial pixels to lines by steps of 5° was monitored using the software mentioned above. The measuring was executed, beginning in the end-diastolic state, in steps of 34 ms of a 893 ms long cardiac cycle.

The radial path of motion of the examined pixels on one beam is shown as an example in Fig. 2 by reference to the 135° line. The radial back-and-forth motion follows the typical phases of a cardiac cycle [17, 19]. One cardiac cycle consists of

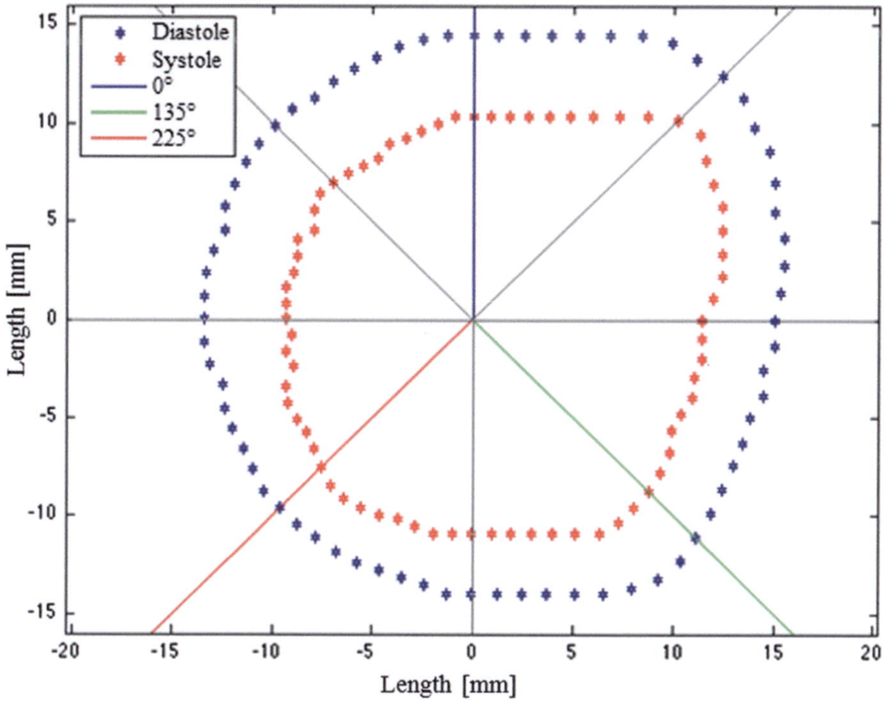

Fig. 1 Determined measurement data from the end-systole and end-diastole

the systole with the tension and ejection phase as well as the diastole with the relaxation and filling phase.

Based on the end-diastolic condition the ascertained pixels stagnate initially for about 120 ms. During this isovolumetric tension phase the ventricular pressure of about 4–6 mmHg increases to about 80 mmHg [19]. Since the mitral valve as well as the aortic valve is closed, the tensioning takes place under constant volume. Once the intraventricular pressure exceeds the pressure of the aorta (about 80 mmHg) the aortic valve opens and blood flows into the aorta. This marks the beginning ejection phase that lasts for about 200 ms. As soon as the intraventricular pressure falls below the pressure of the aorta, the aortic valve closes and the ejection of blood comes to a stop. This is followed by a relaxation phase that lasts about 70 ms. During this phase, the pressure of the ventricle under constant volume decreases further. Once it falls below the pressure of the left atrium, the mitral valve opens and the filling phase begins. The volume of the ventricle increases steadily until the ventricular pressure equals the atrium pressure when the valve opens. Towards the end of the diastolic filling, the atrium excited by sinoatrial node cells contracts, which causes the ventricular pressure to increase slightly and the volume to grow until the end-diastolic filling volume is reached and the cardiac cycle begins all over

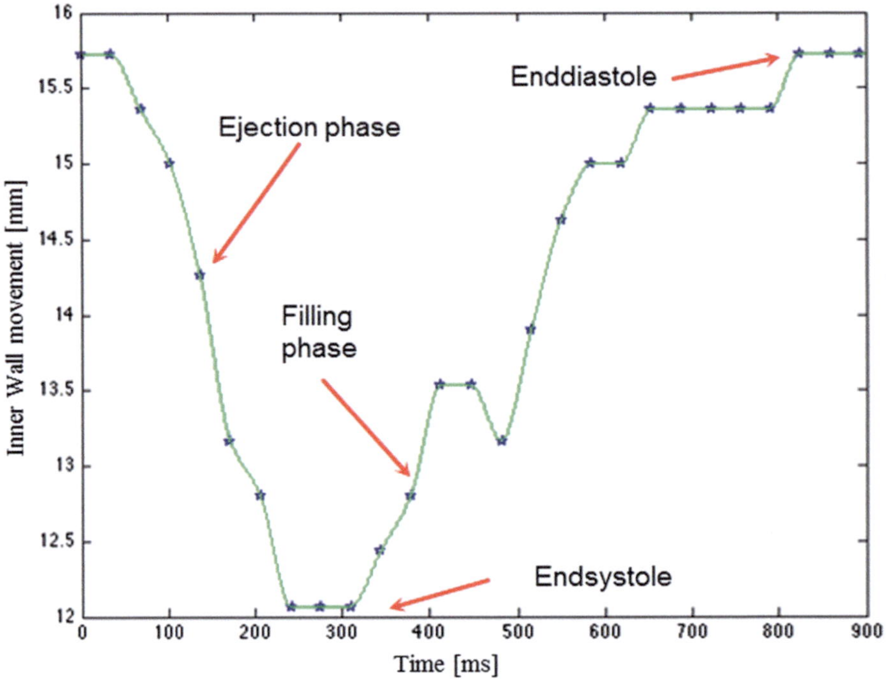

Fig. 2 The radial movement of the 135° line

again [17, 19]. During the diastole the heart itself is supplied with blood through the coronary vessels [17].

The radial path of movement of the pixels on all examined lines does not coincide temporally. As an example, Fig. 3 shows the path of movement of three different lines. During the plateau phase of the action potential, every cell of the working myocardium is absolutely refractory and within that time not excitable again. As soon as the myocardia cells polarize towards negative potentials, action potentials can be triggered again [19, 20]. These are initially short-lived and in between neighboring cells they are only transmitted slowly. For a short while during this phase the excitability of the working myocardium is inhomogeneous [20].

The left ventricle of the heart fulfills its function by temporally contracting single muscle cells and therefore neither a superposition of single twitches nor muscle cramps can occur [20]. As part of a motion study by Alkhadi et al. [21] the following images originated from a computer tomographic examination (Fig. 4).

In three transversal sections parallel to the valve plane the end-systolic (top) and the end-diastolic (bottom) conditions have been determined. Here as well the irregular and temporally shifted radial contractions of single muscle cells of the left ventricle are visible. While the intraventricular area in the end-diastolic state in

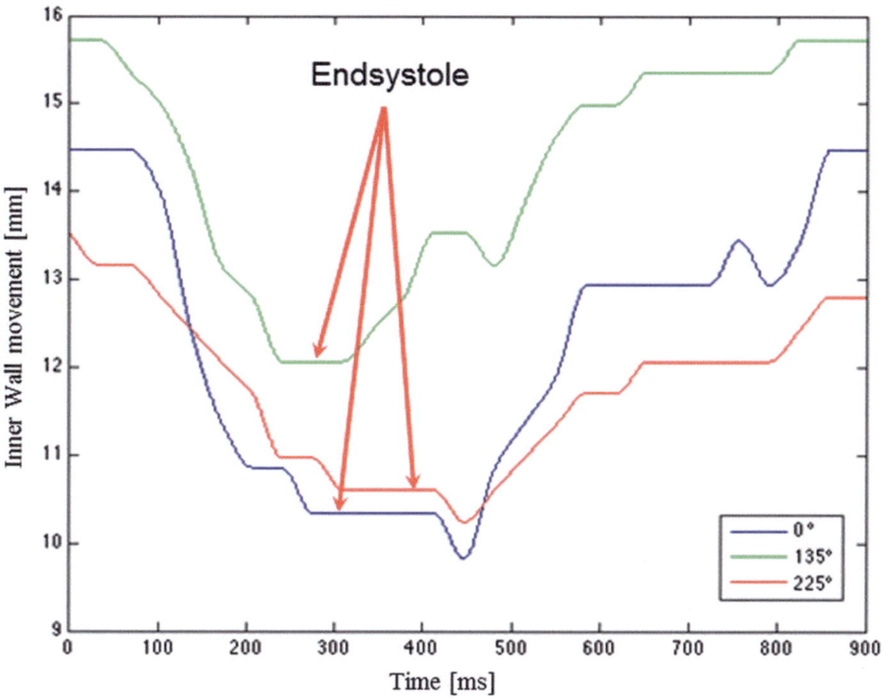

Fig. 3 The inner wall movement compared for three different beams

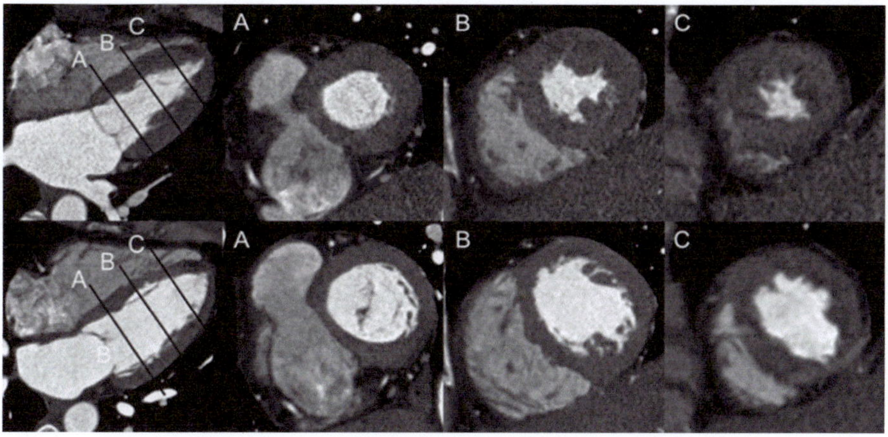

Fig. 4 Transversal sections of the left ventricle during heart contractions

Fig. 4 is approximately elliptical, it resembles a circle in the end-systolic state. The increase in thickness of >5 mm as well as the characteristic relief in the inside of the ventricle is also obvious [21].

3 Structural and Dimensional Synthesis

In order to realize the contraction motion of the left ventricle and its fluid-mechanical properties realistically, a suitable mechanism following the VDI-guideline 2221 has been developed. In doing so, the steps planning, structural synthesis, dimensional synthesis and the preliminary design of the mechanism have been completed [22, 23].

The radial contractions of the left ventricle (LV) are realized through a mechanism that has a ring structure and is mounted horizontally to the flexible main chamber. The dynamic motion of the mechanism is controlled by a drive. Several pressure forces caused by the mechanism, which externally act onto the main chamber, cause the pulsating cyclical contractions of the MockHeart. The evenly distributed pressure forces acting onto the main chamber overcome the inner pressure of the chamber, which is equal to intraventricular pressure. The amount of blood extruded by the MockHeart during this process equals the stroke volume of the left ventricle.

During the structural synthesis, planar structures have been developed that can ensure the guidance of work components according to the provided measurement data. These structures are based on quadrinomial and six-membered kinematic chains. The systematic variation of joint types, frames or arrangement of the mechanism elements to one another lead to kinematic structures, that allow different designs and movement patterns of posterior mechanisms. The solution field generated using construction technology approaches and is expanded using heuristic methods and techniques from analogy observation. The results of the structural synthesis are a multitude of planar ring structures that are composed of basic kinematic structures. After an evaluation of the ring structures, those structures, which are either rigid or do not enable a parallel guide due to their arrangement, were eliminated. Additionally the structures that cannot be controlled using a drive were disqualified. The structures shown in Fig. 5 are pursued further in the subsequent dimensional synthesis.

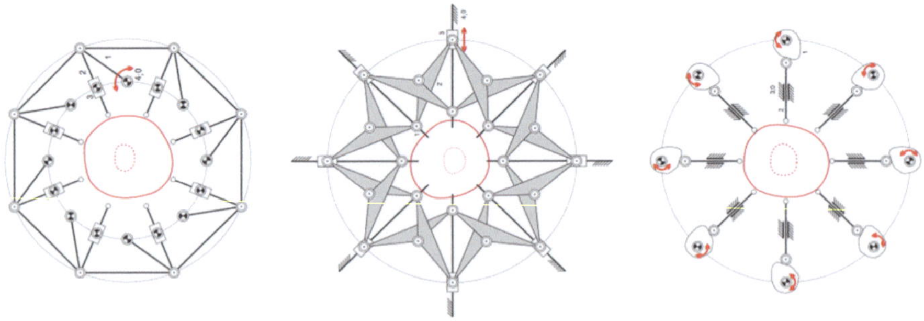

Fig. 5 Kinematic structures to be pursued further

The first ring structure consists of basic crankshafts and it is controlled by a rotary driven component. The second structure is composed of basic crossing over linkages and is driven linearly by a thrust component. In contrast, the third structure is composed of basic cam mechanisms in their original form with roller tappets mounted centrically. During the design phase, the main kinematic dimensions of the pursued kinematic structures have been determined.

The basic dimensions of the mechanism elements of both crank mechanisms were both determined using the three-pose-synthesis, whereas the preset of three positions on a trajectory is sufficient [23]. The selection of the positions, which correspond with the positions of the LV in the end positions of the diastole and systole and also an additional position in between, ensures that the entire radial movement of the simulated LV can be reproduced on one beam.

The basic dimensions of the basic mechanism elements of the crank mechanism were determined using the zero-order transfer function of the radial motion as well as the approximation method by Flocke [23]. The transfer function of the single cam elements were predefined through the measurement results of the previous echocardiographic examination at discrete positions. One cardiac cycle, beginning with the systole, is passed through within 893.63 ms and corresponds with one revolution of the cam. The radial distance covered by the point, which matches the output motion of the roller tappet, amounts to an average of 4–6 mm. The discrete measurement results need to be interpolated in a way that the measuring points are reproduced exactly and high-quality operating characteristics of the cam mechanism are aspired. These high-quality operating characteristics feature a minimization of harmful oscillatory phenomena, a reduced noise emission and a decrease of wear. Furthermore, shocks and jolts are avoided. Since the cyclical excitation of the human cardiac muscle is equivalent to a sinus rhythm, the periodic measurement data can be interpolated most conveniently through an approximation with trigonometric functions.

The basic dimension of the respective cam discs were eventually selected in a way that all discs can be fixed to a circle, which does not fall below the minimum transmission angle and at the same time ensures the same length for all roller tappets.

4 Evaluation

The mechanism based on the pursued mechanism design must not only enable the radial back-and-forth motion of the simulated left ventricle, but also transfer the force, that is necessary to drive out the fluid.

After the structural and dimensional synthesis, a last comparative evaluation of the mechanism designs is performed to decide which concept is suited for the realization of the radial movements and therefore should be pursued.

The crank mechanism, which is easy to manufacture, can enable the radial movement through three given positions. However, neither their transmission can be changed nor a correct time response for the temporal contractions of the single muscle cells of the simulated left ventricle can be realized through a required drive. Furthermore, it is not possible to generate the necessary even pressure force with the aid of their output link. Even though the necessary force can be generated at the drive, there is loss of energy due to the arrangement of the elements and the resulting division of the acting forces into their radial and tangential components towards the MockHeart. The loss of energy can be amplified by prismatic joints liable to wear and potential tolerances in the bearing of both mechanisms. That is why the energy provided at the drive component cannot generate the same force in radial direction at the eight interfaces to realize the necessary pressure force. In contrast, the designed cam mechanism can realize the zero-order transfer function at the 24 predefined discrete positions exactly. Besides the radial contractions required for the fluid circulation during the ejection and the filling phase, a further contraction, necessary for self-sufficiency of the heart, is realized. However, this contraction is not relevant to the provided pressure-volume-work within the cardiovascular simulator. Through the selection of trigonometric transfer functions jolts and shocks of the cam mechanism are avoided and the operability is enabled. Besides the radial contractions, the synchronously controlled cam mechanism also generates the even pressure force, necessary for the pressure-volume-work of the MockHeart, provided that a contraction of the simulated left atrium facilitates the opening of the atrioventricular valve as well as the following filling of the ventricle. In order to realize the pressure-volume-work as well as the radial movement of a potential pathological heart, cam discs can easily be dismantled or exchanged to suit the problem. Since the cam mechanism has crucial advantages compared to the crank mechanism, the following cardiovascular simulator CVELoop is controlled using a cam mechanism.

5 Design

The scaled rough design of the cam mechanism is mainly geared to the kinematic main dimensions attained during the dimensional synthesis.

The simple structure is composed of a basic frame, a round base plate and eight basic cam mechanisms mounted to the frame in their original form including a roller tappet. By selecting an evenly transmitted drive concept, the eight basic cam mechanisms can be controlled synchronously using only one drive application. The function of synchronous controls can be realized by using belt drives or even gear pairs. Thus, an identical force is induced into every one of the eight cam mechanisms, which simultaneously provides a basis for an even radial movement of the MockHeart. For the purposes of this project this drive concept has been chosen due to the space saving installation. The rough design of the cam mechanism is displayed in Fig. 6.

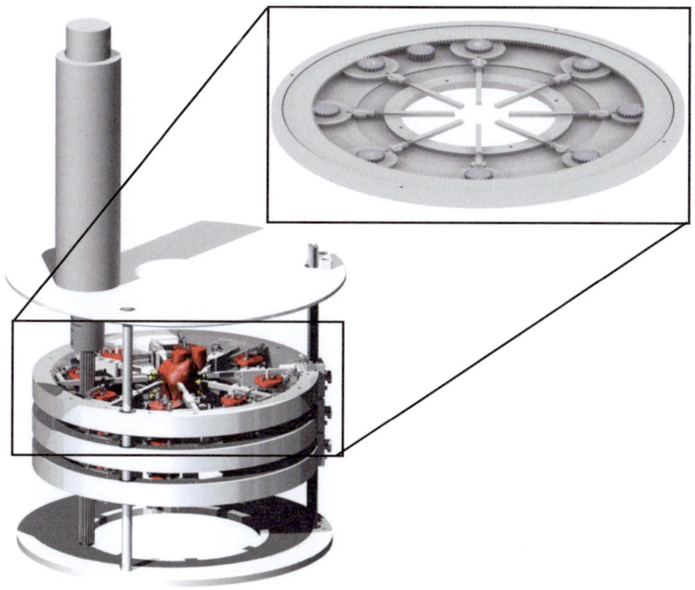

Fig. 6 Prototype with the three levels and a single level with eight cam mechanisms

6 Conclusions

As part of the further development of the cardiovascular simulator CVELoop at the Department of cardiovascular engineering of RWTH Aachen University a contractive MockHeart, which simulates the healthy heart of a human in the cardiovascular system, has been developed. In contrast to the numerous already developed simulators, the main component of the simulator is controlled by a mechanism. Starting from a healthy heart it is the long-term goal to simulate pathophysiological conditions and to develop and dimension VADs for these conditions.

The mechanism must not only enable the radial back-and-forth movement of the simulated left ventricle, but also transmit the force that is necessary for the ejection of the fluid.

The crank mechanisms, which are easy to manufacture, offer a realization of the radial movement through three predefined positions, however neither the transmission can be changed nor a correct time response through a required drive can be enabled. In addition to that, they cannot generate the necessary even pressure force, required for the fluid circulation, with their output components. On the other hand, the designed cam mechanisms can realize the zero-order transfer function at the 24 predefined discrete positions exactly. Besides the radial contractions, the synchronously controlled cam mechanism generates the even pressure force necessary for the pressure-volume-work of the MockHeart.

7 Outlook

A concept for the points of intersection between the output components of the cam mechanism and the MockHeart has to be acquired over the further course of the development. In doing so, it is important to consider that the silicone bags of the MockHeart deform evenly and without any “dents”.

In order to realize the radial movements in multiple transverse intersecting planes as well as the pressure-volume-work and the radial movements of a possible pathological heart, the determination of further radial strains through the Speckle-Tracking-echocardiography-method is necessary.

Furthermore, the installation of multiple mechanisms in the horizontal planes on top of each other needs to be facilitated. For example, these can be connected to each other through a shaft going through the cam disc pivot points, because hereby the mechanisms can be controlled dependently on each other using only one drive.

For a simulated holistic movement of the left ventricle an axial movement and a torsion need to be enabled aside from the radial movement. However, the cam mechanism cannot enable any torsion. In contrast, an axial movement is possible using Oldham or Schmidt clutches to connect the jointly driven shafts of the cam mechanisms, which are arranged on top of each other.

Moreover, it is important to take into account that the cam mechanisms connected to one another only enable the movement and fluid-mechanical properties of the left ventricle. In further work steps towards realization of the natively generated pressure-volume-work of the left heart, additional concepts for the realization of the contraction of the atrium as well as the fluid-mechanical properties of the left heart and the underlying simulated blood vessels need to be developed.

Acknowledgements The project MockHeart was funded by the Excellence Initiative of the German federal and state governments.

References

1. Pantalos, G.M., Ionan, C.: Expanded pediatric cardiovascular simulator for research and training. ASAIO J. **56**, S. 67–72 (2012). ISSN 0162-1432
2. Ruiz, P., Rezaienia, M.A.: In vitro cardiovascular system emulator (bioreactor) for the simulation of normal and diseased conditions with and without mechanical circulatory support. Int. J. Artif. Organs **37**, S. 549–560 (2013). ISSN 1525-1594
3. Beneken, J.: A mathematical approach to cardiovascular function, the uncontrolled human system. Ph.D. thesis, University of Utrecht, The Netherlands (1965)
4. Kozarski, M., et al.: A hybrid mock circulatory system: development and testing of an electro-hydraulic impedance simulator. Int. J. Artif. Organs **26**, S. 53–63 (2003). ISSN 0391-3988
5. Kozarski, M., et al.: A new hybrid electro-numerical model of the left ventricle. Comput. Biol. Med. **38**, S. 979–989 (2008). ISSN 0010-4825

6. Piedimento, F., et al.: A new elastance-based artificial ventricle for mock circulatory systems: analysis of interaction with a closed-loop hydraulic circulation. Int. J. Artif. Organs **29**, S. 505–505 (2006). ISSN 0391-3988
7. Robinson, D.: Quantitative analysis of cardiac loop for the evaluation of left, right, and biventricular assist devices. ASAIO J. **29**, S. 207–221 (1965). ISSN 0162-1432
8. Suga, H., Sagawa K., Shoukas A.A.: Load independence of the instantaneous pressure-volume ratio of the canine left ventricle and effects of epinephrine and heart rate on the ratio. Circ. Res. **32**, S. 314–322 (1973). ISSN 1524-4571
9. Suga, H., Sagawa, K.: Instantaneous pressure-volume relationships and their ratio in the excised supported canine left ventricle. Circ. Res. **35**, S. 117–126 (1974). ISSN 1524-4571
10. Colacino, F.M., et al.: A modified elastance model to control mock ventricles in real-time: numerical and experimental validation. ASAIO J. **54**, S. 563–573 (2008). ISSN 0162-1432
11. Ferrari, G., et al.: A hybrid mock circulatory system: testing a prototype under physiologic and pathological conditions. ASAIO J. **48**, S. 487–494 (2002). ISSN 0162-1432
12. Lehr- und Forschungsgebiet für Kardiovaskuläre Technik: Kreislaufsimulator CVELoop (2015). www.ame.hia.rwth-aachen.de/index.php?id=919
13. Jansen-Park, S.H., Müller, I., Miesel, D., Lommel, M., Sonntag, S.J., Steinseifer, U.: An anatomical mock heart circulation loop with contracting silicone ventricles and an anatomical aorta. Int. J. Artif. Organs **38**(7), 376 (2015)
14. Jansen-Park, S.H., Mahmood, M.N., Müller, I., Turnhoff, L.K., Schmitz-Rode, T., Steinseifer, U., Sonntag, S.J.: Effects of interaction between ventricular assist device assistance and autoregulated mock circulation including frank–starling mechanism and baroreflex. Artif. Organs (2015)
15. Jiang, K., Yu, X.: Quantification of regional myocardial wall motion by cardiovascular magnetic resonance. Quant. Imaging Med. Surg. **4**, S. 345–357 (2014). ISSN 2223-4292
16. Esch, B.T., Warburton, D.E.R.: Left ventricular torsion and recoil: implications for exercise performance and cardiovascular disease. J. Appl. Physiol. **106**, S. 362–369 (2009). ISSN 8750-7587
17. Schmidt, R.F., et al.: Physiologie des Menschen, mit Pathophysiologie. Springer, Berlin, Heidelberg (2011)
18. Butz, T., Trappe, H.-J.: Möglichkeiten und Grenzen der myokardialen Strain-Analyse mittels Speckle-Tracking-Echokardiografie. Kardiologie update **8**, S. 193–200 (2012). ISSN 1611-6534
19. Gekle, M., et al.: Taschenlehrbuch Physiologie. Georg Thieme Verlag, Stuttgart (2010)
20. Pape, H.-C., et al.: Physiologie. Georg Thieme Verlag, Stuttgart (2014)
21. Alkhadi, H., et al.: Praxisbuch Herz-CT. Springer Medizin, Heidelberg (2009)
22. Verein Deutscher Ingenieure: VDI 2221:1993-05, Methodik zum Entwickeln und Konstruieren technischer Systeme und Produkte. Beuth Verlag, Berlin (1993)
23. Kerle, H., Corves, B., Hüsing, M.: Getriebetechnik, Grundlagen, Entwicklung und Anwendung ungleichmäßig übersetzender Getriebe. Vieweg+Teubner Verlag/Springer Fachmedien Wiesbaden GmbH, Wiesbaden (2012)

Improved Design of a Gait Rehabilitation Robot

C.J. Stolle, C.A. Nelson, J.M. Burnfield and T.W. Buster

Abstract Gait therapy is important to a person's recovery following spinal cord or brain injury, stroke, lower extremity surgery, as well as with many chronic conditions (e.g., Parkinson's disease or multiple sclerosis). Although some affordable equipment for adult gait rehabilitation exists, such equipment for adaptive gait rehabilitation across the spectrum of pediatric sizes is not commercially available. This paper presents design improvements for a new pediatric gait rehabilitation machine intended to address this technology gap. The design is in the style of elliptical machines but is synthesized to emulate the normal kinematic demands of walking. It includes a 7-bar linkage for each foot, a chain/sprocket coupling for left/right synchronization, and motorized speed control.

Keywords Gait rehabilitation · Pediatric gait · Robotic rehabilitation · Kinematic synthesis

1 Introduction

Gait rehabilitation typically constitutes part of the therapy needed following spinal cord injury, brain injury, or other conditions affecting motor coordination. For adults, various forms of therapy are available, including treadmill training with partial body-weight support [1], robotic guidance of the legs [2], and assistive

C.J. Stolle · C.A. Nelson (✉)
University of Nebraska-Lincoln, Lincoln, USA
e-mail: cnelson5@unl.edu

C.J. Stolle
e-mail: cale.stolle@huskers.unl.edu

J.M. Burnfield · T.W. Buster
Madonna Rehabilitation Hospital, Lincoln, USA
e-mail: jburnfield@madonna.org

T.W. Buster
e-mail: tbuster@madonna.org

M. Husty and M. Hofbaur (eds.), *New Trends in Medical and Service Robots*,
Mechanisms and Machine Science 48, DOI 10.1007/978-3-319-59972-4_3

elliptical machines [3–6]. These therapeutic approaches all have different advantages, but with limited exceptions [3] they are very costly either based on the equipment or personnel needed. Furthermore, affordable therapies for pediatric patients [7] are very limited, in part because the equipment is designed for specific ranges of motion (or step length), and pediatric patients can have step lengths which vary more than can be accommodated by typical equipment. Therefore, there is a need for gait therapy devices which are adaptable to the full spectrum of step lengths while remaining affordable for widespread clinical adoption.

A pediatric gait training device was recently proposed [8] to fill this need. A device was constructed comprising carriages riding on two pivoting rails, as shown in Fig. 1. The carriages propelled the foot through a gait-like motion. To model the motion of the toe, the carriages slid along the rail as the rail pivoted on a central axle. To model the motion of the heel, which in turn drives the angle and motion of the rest of the foot, the back of the carriage rolled along another rail that translated vertically. The forward and backward sliding of the carriages was controlled by a pair of identical four-bar linkages. The pivoting of the rails was controlled by cams, and the timing of all these elements of motion was synchronized using timing belts. A line diagram of power transmission in the robot design is shown in Fig. 2.

The initial design proved overly complex for practical implementation and suffered from excessive frictional losses due to the large number of mechanical interconnections. In this paper we present a new design for scale-adaptable robotic gait rehabilitation. The original design is assessed and critically evaluated in terms of the original design goals. Emphases were made on assessing any modifications and their impact on scaling and overall foot trajectory. From this assessment, a new design was proposed and implemented.

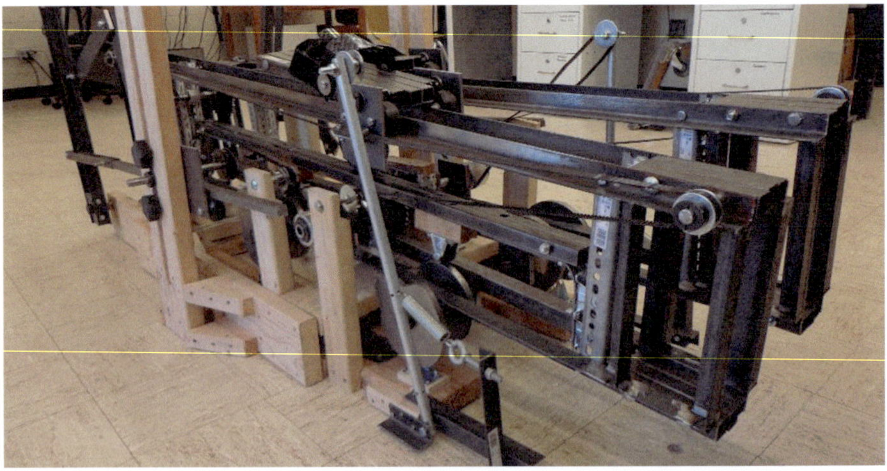

Fig. 1 Initial prototype of gait rehabilitation robot (as in [8])

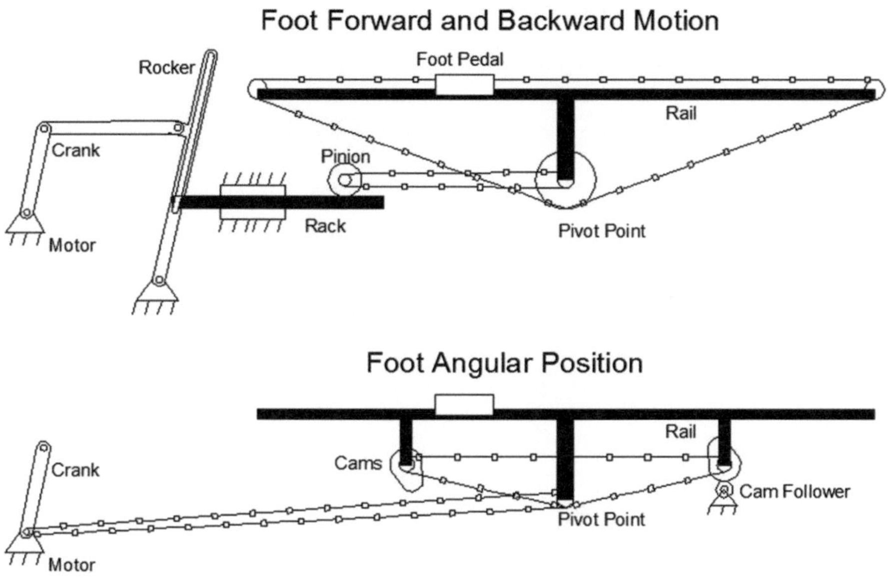

Fig. 2 Power transmission in gait rehabilitation robot (as in [8])

2 Design Requirements

The initial design needed to be simplified in order to be functional. The primary design goals were assessed.

- The robot must propel the foot through a gait-like trajectory. The trajectory does not have to be exact, but significantly closer to walking mechanics compared with other low-cost gait-simulating machines.
- The robot must have scalable output so that pediatric and adult patients are able to use it.

Secondary design goals were also reviewed:

- Small footprint
- Comfortable for the patient
- Smooth and easy to operate
- Cost efficient

While most of these goals were achieved in the original design, the greatest deficiency of the design was in smoothness and ease of operation. It was determined that in order to achieve improved performance in this regard, and simultaneously reduce cost and complexity, some modest decreases in satisfaction of the other requirements may be acceptable.

3 Initial Design

An initial design was constructed according to the design goals listed above, and is detailed in [8]. We summarize here some of its design features for comparison.

3.1 Motion Scaling

The design needed to accommodate various stride lengths of users. Ideally, the scaling would be perfectly linear. This would provide consistency of foot path shape as the stride length is changed from short to large. The scaling mechanism must be fairly robust and reliable at each scaling value in order to function properly.

There are multiple ways of achieving scalable motion using mechanisms. By using a four-bar linkage with variable link lengths, the output could be manipulated to produce the same trajectory shape. However, since all four links would have to be simultaneously adjusted to maintain proportions, this was not pursued as a scaling mechanism. Similar issues were present if using a pantograph. Attempts at Cartesian parametrization also proved difficult. These options are explained in more detail in [8].

One approach is to parametrize the motion path in polar coordinates. This expresses the path as a function of angular displacement, with radius as the primary variable. When scaling such a curve, the angular position remains the same while the radial distance scales. This allows the scaling problem to be limited to one independent variable. The polar parametrization can be realized through a slider on a pivoting rail where the pivot serves as the fixed point about which trajectories are scaled.

The initial design utilized a carriage travelling on top of the rail, where the rail was pivoted about a central axis. The forward and backward motion of the carriage was controlled by the rocker of a four-bar linkage. The rocker contained a slot to allow for a wheel to travel inside of it. The lateral deflection of the wheel was lengthened by increasing the distance between the pivot point and the wheel's axle. Since the relationship between radius and distance are linear at fixed angular deflections, this would provide an even, smooth scaling for the system.

The follower wheel was attached to a gear rack which was constrained to only move horizontally, as shown in Fig. 3. The rack meshed with a pinion to convert the horizontal oscillatory motion to a rotary motion. The rotary motion was transmitted to a belt to drive the foot carriage, which converted it back to a linear motion. This chain of conversions allowed the carriages to be positioned anywhere relative to the follower wheel on the rocker.

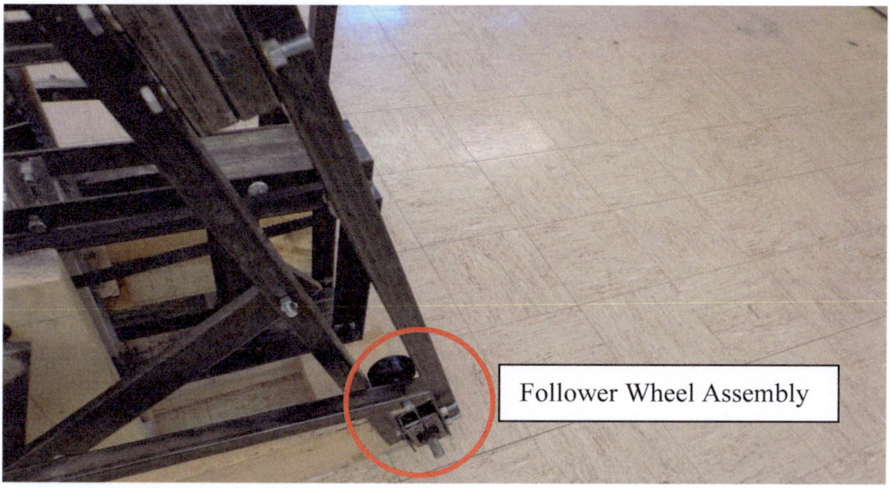

Fig. 3 Rocker and follower wheel

3.2 Gait-Like Motion

The main purpose of this design effort was to develop a robot that replicated the motion of the foot during a normal gait cycle. The expectation was that this would help to drive a normal gait pattern in rehabilitation patients using the machine. This could be realized by fully constraining the foot motion to match the foot trajectory of a sample gait path at both the metatarsal and heel positions, as shown in Fig. 4. Both the metatarsal and heel trajectories were measured relative to the forward motion of the individual as determined by the position of the hip. The trajectories were measured using motion-tracking software and an infrared camera system.

As stated in Sect. 3.1, it was determined that the foot trajectory would be traced with a crank-slider mechanism. However, neither the metatarsal nor heel trajectories would be feasible to model with a crank-slider system using a polar coordinate system because conversion of the trajectories shown in Fig. 4 resulted in angular accelerations that were excessive for an actual mechanism. A sample of the radial and angular accelerations for the metatarsal trajectory, with the pivot point of the rail located in front of the furthest forward point of the toe, is shown in Fig. 5.

To model human gait patterns, a projected point on the foot had to travel through a trajectory that could be modeled in polar coordinates and realized as a crank-slider system. This was determined by interpolating the trajectory of a point on the foot using the X and Y position of the metatarsal and heel points. A 2-dimensional profile was generated as a function of the position of the foot based on the heel and metatarsal trajectories. This assumed the connection between the heel and metatarsal was rigid. Based on this analysis, it was determined that a point on the foot located slightly in front of the toe has a self-intersecting trajectory with tangency

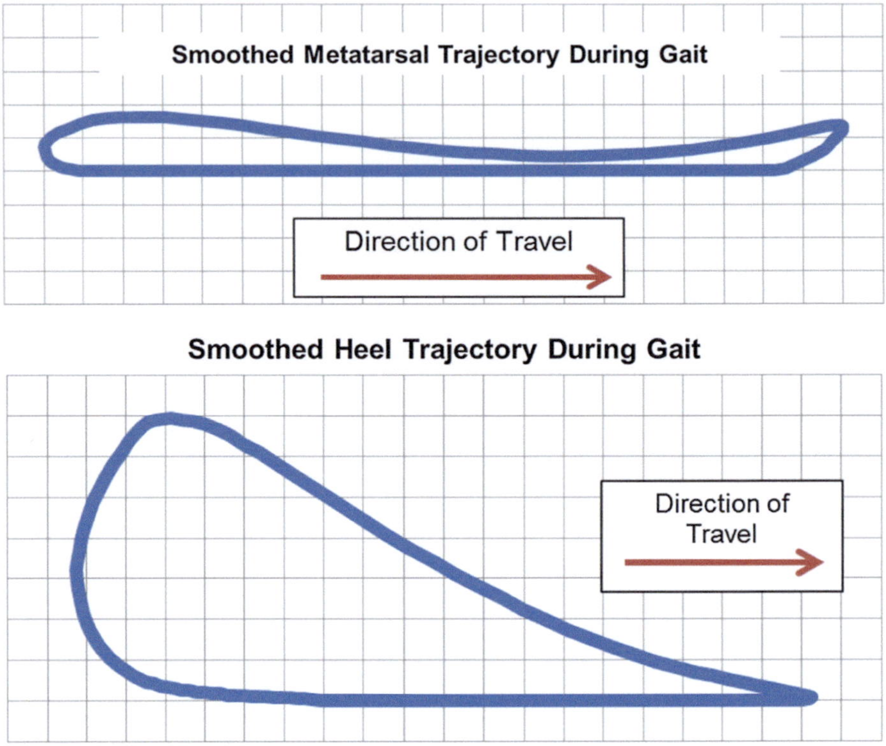

Fig. 4 Sample metatarsal and heel trajectories during gait

near the middle of the trajectory, as shown in Fig. 6. This intersection minimizes the rail motion while providing biomechanically accurate motion of one point on the foot.

3.3 Path Generation

For the initial design [8], the trajectory was recreated using a pivoted rail. Since the crank-slider trajectory experienced relatively small angular deflection (reaching a maximum value of 9.6° and a minimum value of −3.5° relative to horizontal), cams were chosen to drive the pivoting motion of the rail. A four-bar linkage was used to drive the forward and backward motion of the slider carriage.

The maximum speed of the machine was chosen to be approximately one stride (one left and one right step) per second. Treating the rail as a cam-follower, acceleration analysis indicated that the rail would "hop" due to downward accelerations exceeding the gravitation constant. To reduce vibrations in the system, the

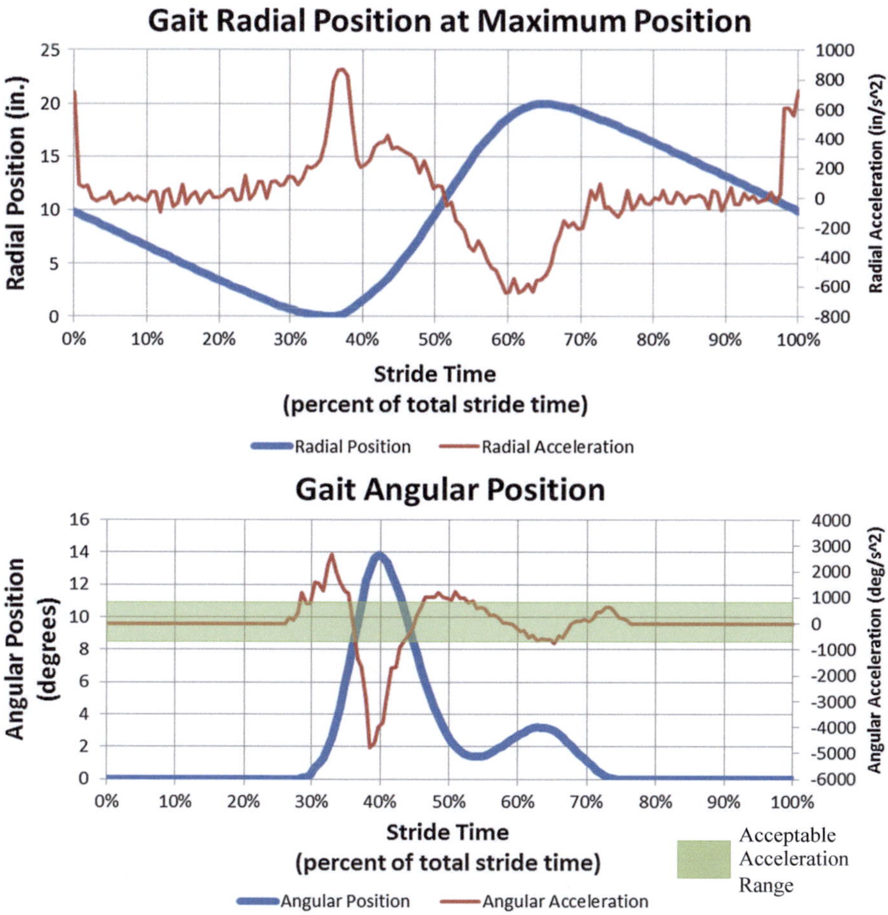

Fig. 5 Radial and angular position and acceleration of gait cycle

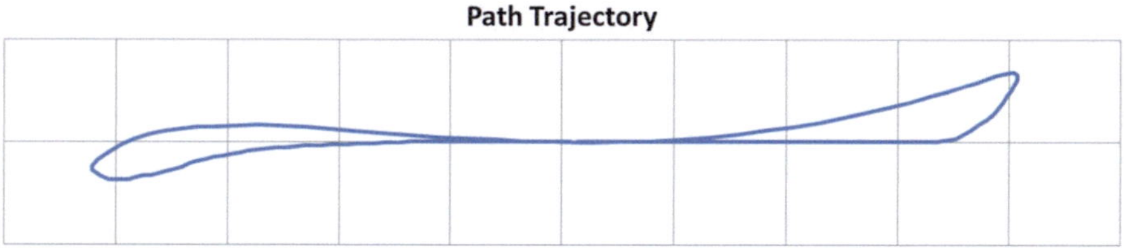

Fig. 6 Crank-slider compatible path trajectory

cam profile was manually adjusted to limit accelerations to 330 in/s^2. The velocity and displacement of the end of the path was adjusted accordingly with the new acceleration profile.

The rail and carriage configuration and the angular position described in Fig. 6 only constrained a point on the foot in front of the toe. In order to fully constrain the foot, a design feature was created that incorporated a secondary motion-constrained point on the foot pedal. It was decided that secondary cams would drive the vertical motion of a bar extended across the length of the pivoting rail. A wheel connected to the rear of the foot carriage would follow the bar and constrain the rise and fall of the heel. Similar to the toe cam profile, the heel cam profile was acceleration-limited to 330 in/s^2.

4 Shortcomings of Initial Design

As mentioned previously, the initial design did not function properly. The mechanism did not move under human power as intended.

4.1 Deficiencies in the Initial Motion Scaling Design

After construction, the system proved impractical due to the excessive force required to drive it. The frictional losses at the rack and pinion and at other mechanical interconnections were significant, making the conversion between linear and rotary motion inefficient. Attempting to directly connect the follower wheel to the carriage required significantly more constraint on the follower wheel, and this jammed the system. This occurred because the follower wheel was poorly constrained and the connection with the rocker of the four-bar linkage was not sufficiently precise.

While methods could have been employed to significantly strengthen the constraints on the follower wheel, it would not have decreased the power losses at the pinion. Furthermore, tooth contact in the spur-type pinion-rack mesh was noisy and was anticipated to create a poor user experience.

4.2 Limitations of Initial Path Generation Design

While the accelerations of the cam were slightly below the gravitational constant, the cams produced large forces on the rail. Furthermore, the somewhat severe profile of the cam meant that the cam follower experienced questionable pressure angles, causing the device to be difficult to drive without significant torque.

The axle driving the heel was also integrally linked to the rest of the system. The high accelerations experienced by the heel required high torque to overcome the steep cam slopes. The combination of these two sets of cams was ultimately too much for the system to drive, and caused the system to seize.

5 Description of Revised Design

Following the failure of the first design, the goals of the design were reevaluated and used to create a new robot. The new robot had to have significantly improved power transmission over the initial design, and the motion scaling and path generation would need to be changed.

The new design consisted of a seven-bar linkage with an additional cam constraint. A crank-rocker four-bar linkage formed the foundation of the design. A block slid along the rocker, and could be fixed in place with a pin. The block was attached to a bar that connected to a carriage. The block and bar assembly is shown in Fig. 7. This carriage carried the off-axis loading from the linkage and transmitted it into longitudinal motion along a pivoting rail. With cams driving the angular displacement of the pivoting rails, and the cam rotation coupled to the crank of the four-bar, this forms a cam-constrained seven-bar linkage with one DOF. The schematic of the robot and the line diagram for power transmission is shown in Fig. 8. A picture of the assembled robot is shown in Fig. 9.

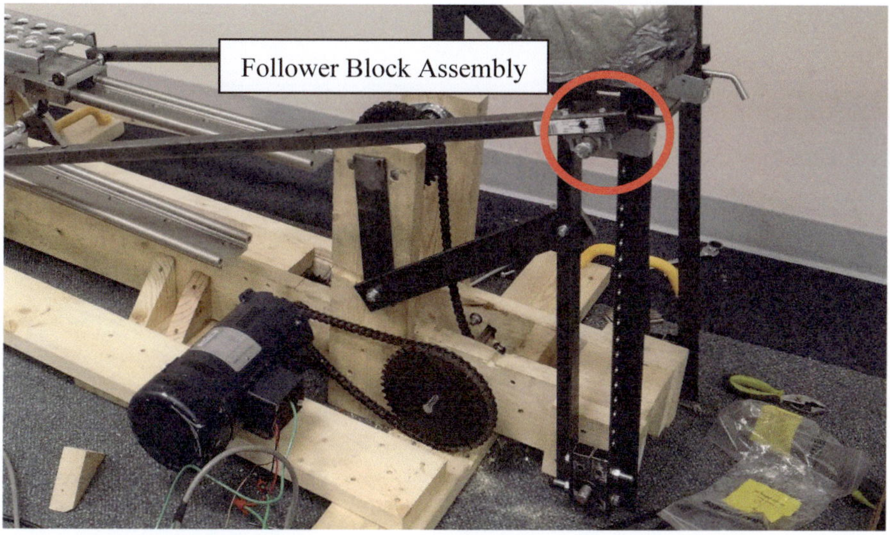

Fig. 7 Follower block assembly on crank-rocker

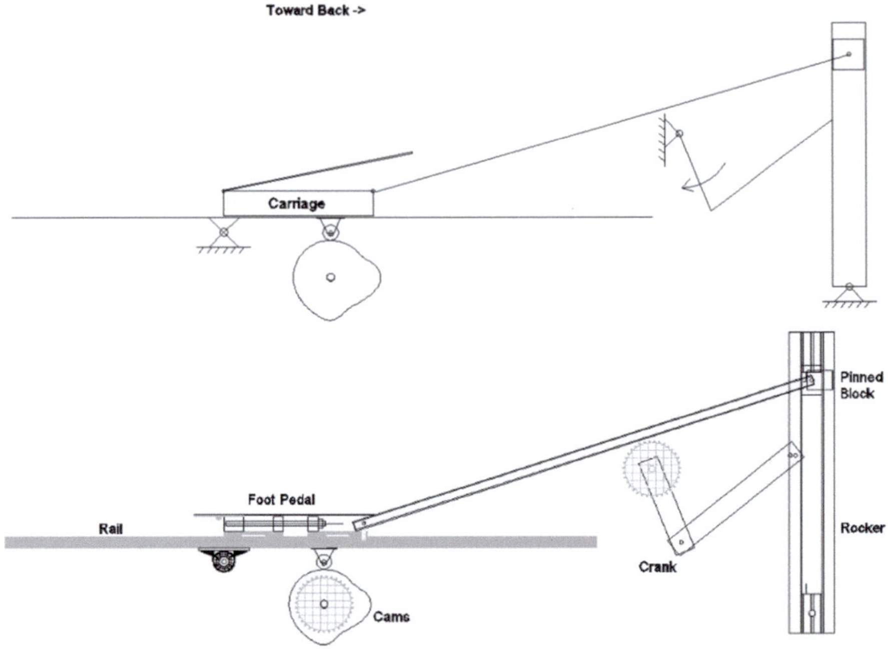

Fig. 8 Revised design schematic diagram and component models

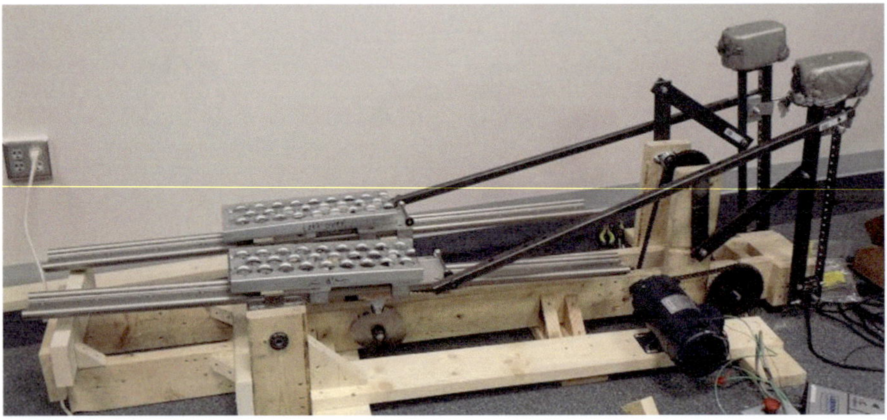

Fig. 9 Prototype based on revised design

5.1 Improved Motion Scaling Design

Unfortunately, as per the first design, it would not be possible to have a well-constrained follower wheel and connection linkage to the carriage while maintaining perfect scaling at every length along the rocker. Thus, a significantly simplified connection between the rocker and the carriage was designed. A block was pinned into position on the rocker arm, as shown in Fig. 7. A linkage connected the pinned block rigidly to the carriage. One drawback of this design was that changing the position of the pinned block in the rocker changed the distance between the block and the centerline of the rail, meaning that the carriage would trace an inaccurate trajectory. To compensate for this, the connection between the pinned block and the carriage was adjustable. After setting the block at the desired height along the rocker (which would, in turn, regulate the stride length of the robot), the link between carriages was adjusted so that the foot pedal was aligned correctly with the pivot point to achieve the correct trajectory.

5.2 Improved Path Generation Design

During the terminal stance and pre-swing phases of a normal gait cycle, the heel naturally rises, enabling the body to pivot over the forefoot [9]. Then, during initial swing, the toes and forefoot begin to elevate to ensure foot clearance. By mid-swing, as the tibia achieves a vertical position, the toes and heel align parallel to the ground allowing only a minimal threshold for foot clearance. By terminal swing, the toes are again elevated relative to the heel as the foot prepares for a heel first initial contact. This implies that it is desirable to avoid constraining the heel, as it naturally lifts during the latter half of stance, and the slope of the rail during early swing phase is such that the heel would be slightly elevated. Thus, it was decided that the prescriptive constraint of heel motion would be removed from the design requirements.

The cam profiles experienced excessive accelerations in the initial design. Thus, the cam profiles were reduced to further limit the accelerations. For the new design, the cams were limited to a peak acceleration of 220 in/s^2. The desired profile, initial design accelerations, and second design accelerations are shown in Fig. 10.

The peak angular displacement values and the times at which they occur in the gait cycle are important to the performance of the robot. Peak times and displacements from the desired toe trajectory, the initial design, and the revised design are compared in Table 1. Overall, based on the data presented in the table, the new design showed slightly reduced fidelity to typical walking biomechanics compared to the first design. However, the increase in system stability and overall performance and usability were significant.

While the first design used large, bulky rails, removing the heel constraint allowed the rails to become significantly thinner and lighter in the revised design. It was decided that standard linear motion bearings would be used for this design, which would significantly reduce the time and effort required to construct the foot-pedal carriages while ensuring quality and weight capacity.

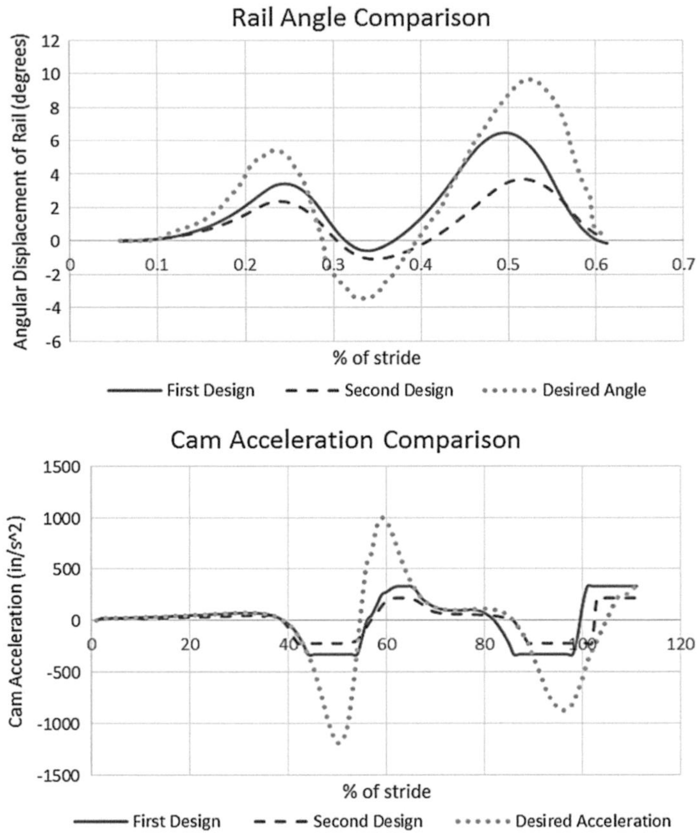

Fig. 10 Rail angular displacement and acceleration comparison

Table 1 Peak timing (% gait cycle) and angular displacements (°) of toe trajectory

	Peak description	1st positive peak	Negative peak	2nd positive peak
Peak times (% gait cycle)	Old profile	24.5	33.9	49.6
	New profile	24.0	34.7	51.7
	Desired profile	24.5	32.8	52.5
Peak angle (°)	Old profile	3.42	−0.57	6.46
	New profile	2.36	−1.09	3.66
	Desired profile	5.19	−3.47	9.69

The same four-bar linkage and rocker were used on the new design. It was determined that, due to the oscillatory nature of the foot strides, the machine became stuck at the toggle positions of the crank and coupler. These positions coincided with the maximum and minimum stride positions of the carriages, which are points at which it is difficult (and feels unnatural) to apply forces from the feet to the pedals to drive the system. Thus, a motor was installed to ensure the robot moved smoothly through these toggle positions and generated overall motion consistent with normal human gait; this is also consistent with our goal of using this system for rehabilitation (patients will typically require motorized assistance). Synchronization of the 4-bar linkages and cams is achieved using a chain and sprockets as opposed to the timing belts in the initial design. The design schematic is shown in Fig. 8, and the constructed machine is shown in Fig. 9.

6 Conclusions

Based on development of a pediatric gait therapy device, analysis of the design showed that there were several inadequacies. The cam shapes had excessively large accelerations, which translated to significant torque on the system. The connections to the carriages driving the sliding motion were inefficient. The mechanisms to constrain the heel motion during a gait cycle were excessive. These issues were resolved by simplifying the design and changing the cam profiles, leading to a redesigned gait rehabilitation robot. Preliminary testing of the new prototype system shows greatly improved performance. Future work will include testing the system with human subjects to assess the benefits of the system for gait rehabilitation.

References

1. Dodd, K.J., Foley, S.: Partial body-weight-supported treadmill training can improve walking in children with cerebral palsy: a clinical controlled trial. Dev. Med. Child Neurol. **49**(2), 101–105 (2007)
2. Hidler, J., Wisman, W., Neckel, N.: Kinematic trajectories while walking within the Lokomat robotic gait-orthosis. Clin. Biomech. **23**(10), 1251–1259 (2008)
3. Nelson, C.A., Burnfield, J.M., Shu, Y., Buster, T. W., Taylor, A.P., Graham, A.: Modified elliptical machine motor-drive design for assistive gait rehabilitation. J. Med. Devices **5**(2), 021001–021001-7 (2011)
4. Burnfield, J.M., Shu, Y., Buster, T.W., Taylor, A., Nelson, C.A.: Impact of elliptical trainer ergonomic modifications on perceptions of safety, comfort, workout and usability by individuals with physical disabilities and chronic conditions. Phys. Ther. **91**(11), 1604–1617 (2011)
5. Burnfield, J.M., Irons, S.L., Buster, T.W., Taylor, A.P., Hildner, G.A., Shu, Y.: Comparative analysis of speed's impact on muscle demands during partial body weight support motor-assisted elliptical training. Gait Posture **39**(1), 314–320 (2014)
6. Burnfield, J.M., Shu, Y., Buster, T.W., Taylor, A.P.: Similarity of joint kinematics and muscle demands between elliptical training and walking: implications for practice. Phys. Ther. **90**(2), 289–305 (2010)

7. Meyer-Heim, A., Borggraefe, I., Ammann-Reiffer, C., Berweck, S., Sennhauser, F.H., Colombo, G., Knecht, B., Heinen, F.: Feasibility of robotic-assisted locomotor training in children with central gait impairment. Dev. Med. Child Neurol. **49**, 900–906 (2007)
8. Stolle, C.J., Nelson, C.A., Burnfield, J.M., Buster, T.W.: Synthesis of a rehabilitation mechanism replicating normal gait. In: Proceedings of the 14th World Congress in Mechanism and Machine Science, Taipei, Taiwan, pp. 25–30, Oct 2015 (2015)
9. Perry, J., Burnfield, J.M.: Gait Analysis, Normal and Pathologic Function, 2nd edn. Slack, Thorofare, NJ (2010)

The Role of Technology in the Implementation and Learning of Minimally-Invasive Surgery

N. Crişan, I. Andraş and I. Coman

Abstract The assimilation of the surgical techniques by the resident doctors should not affect patients' safety. Practicing certain surgical gestures in a repetitive manner allows a better understanding of the technique and the correct acquisition of the manual skills. The use of simulators as a part of the training programs has considerably reduced the number of surgical errors and has improved the operative time and the quality of robotic and laparoscopic surgical procedures. The latest technologies, like 3D vision, next generation instruments, the use of intraoperative imaging have enabled the development of minimally-invasive surgery, so that a number of laparoscopic and robotic procedures have become the standard of care. Our objective was to evaluate the manner in which the latest technologies influence the development of minimally invasive surgery (laparoscopic and robotic). Also, we assessed the main parameters that influence the learning curve of these two types of minimally invasive approach. We observed that the use of the robotic platform during the learning curve allows the performance of laparoscopic procedures with the same accuracy, but with much lower costs.

Keywords Robotic surgery · Laparoscopic surgery · Surgical simulators · Learning curve

N. Crişan · I. Andraş (✉) · I. Coman
Urology Department, Clinical Municipal Hospital,
University of Medicine and Pharmacy "Iuliu Haţieganu", Cluj-Napoca, Romania
e-mail: dr.iuliaandras@gmail.com

N. Crişan
e-mail: drnicolaecrisan@gmail.com

I. Coman
e-mail: jcoman@yahoo.com

M. Husty and M. Hofbaur (eds.), *New Trends in Medical and Service Robots*,
Mechanisms and Machine Science 48, DOI 10.1007/978-3-319-59972-4_4

1 Introduction

The assimilation of the surgical techniques by the resident doctors should not affect patients' safety. In fact, the learning of a surgical technique is the capacity of one doctor to reproduce in a correct and timely manner a surgical intervention. The possibility of practicing certain surgical gestures in a repetitive manner will only allow a better understanding of the technique and the correct acquisition of the manual skills.

In this aspect several concepts have been developed that will allow the repetition of certain surgical gestures and acquisition of the needed surgical skills. This way, the training programs, modern technology (medical robots, flexible instruments, 3D imaging, intraoperative imaging) and the simulators' use have the purpose to reduce the learning curve by practicing, repeating and acquiring the surgical techniques. There are two different situations in the learning process:

- The resident doctors have a double learning curve, one of the surgical technique and one of the surgical approach (robotic and laparoscopic)
- The doctors with open surgery experience, who are already aware of the surgical technique and will only have to acquire knowledge regarding the surgical approach (laparoscopic or robotic)

After the introduction of the robotic surgery in the clinical practice, the majority of the surgeons have crossed directly from the open surgery to the robotic one [1]. In these robotic centers some interventions (radical prostatectomy, partial nephrectomy, hysterectomy) have been subsequently performed exclusively using the robotic approach. This way young doctors have had the opportunity to learn a number of surgical procedures directly by robotic approach. An identical situation was seen in laparoscopy, this approach being exclusively used for certain surgical interventions as cholecystectomy or radical nephrectomy [22].

Our objective was to evaluate the manner in which the latest technologies influence the development of minimally invasive surgery (laparoscopic and robotic). Also, we assessed the main parameters that influence the learning curve of these two types of minimally invasive approach.

2 Impact of Advances in Technology on Surgical Procedures

Minimally invasive approach (laparoscopic, robotic, single site or by natural orifices) has completely changed the surgical armamentarium in recent years. Patients have smaller or no skin incisions, a faster recovery, lower post-operative pain, lower blood loss, a shorter hospital length of stay, a more rapid social reintegration and an improved quality of life. For the surgeons, the technical advances in minimally invasive surgery have led to an enhanced visualization of the anatomical structures, improved dexterity, tremor filtering and the possibility of performing very precise procedures. But all these come with important costs for the healthcare system, thus limiting their availability. As a result, the most widespread minimally invasive surgical technique is laparoscopy.

Laparoscopy implies the insertion of surgical instruments into the abdominal cavity through small incisions (up to 12 mm). Despite all the advantages of a minimally invasive approach, laparoscopy poses some challenges with regard to the lack of depth perception and tactile feedback, a steep learning curve and physical burdens to the surgeon, like inadequate ergonomy, muscular fatigue and exhaustion. A number of techniques have been developed in order to overcome these challenges: the 3D endoscope, next generation instruments and the intra-operative fluorescence and imaging.

2.1 The 3D Visualization

Classic laparoscopy was initiated at the end of 1980s and is based on a 2 dimensional (2D) image displayed on a monitor, which gives a lack of depth perception, so the surgeon performs the tasks using visual indicators to judge instrument position and depth. This fact can be a considerable challenge, especially when performing very complex surgical steps that require precision and dexterity, like lymphadenectomy, urethro-vesical anastomosis after radical prostatectomy or anastomosis between urethra and neobladder after radical cystectomy. New systems that try to overcome these limitations have upgraded to the 3 dimensional (3D) stereoscopic vision. The first 3D systems were still rudimentary, using the technique of active optic shuttering of alternating high-frequency signals emanating from a 3D screen and causing eye strain, headache, dizziness, disorientation, physical discomfort and poor visualization. Newer 3D systems use passive micropolarization technology and are believed to limit surgeon fatigue, by providing superior depth perception and resolution [37].

The 3D visualization offers three types of advantages: for challenging procedures, for the learning curve and for the ergonomy of the surgeon.

2.1.1 Advantages for Challenging Procedures

Several studies have confirmed the superiority of 3D over the 2D laparoscopy, concluding that the 3D vision simplifies complicated procedures [8], improves orientation in the abdominal cavity and reduces the operative time [40]. Also, the 3D imaging improves the measures of performance, regardless the surgeon's previous laparoscopic experience [31], enabling the surgeon to approach difficult procedures earlier during the learning curve.

One of the most demanding and complex procedures in urology is radical cystectomy with pelvic lymphadenectomy with/without neobladder construction (the complete removal of the urinary bladder, the prostate and the pelvic lymph nodes in patients with muscle-invasive, non-metastatic bladder cancer). This surgery poses some challenges because it requires a precise dissection of major blood vessels and inside the deep pelvis, which restricts the movements of the instruments. The surgeon must dissect the virtual space between the bladder, prostate and the rectum and around the major blood vessels, maintaining the balance between the oncological results (the complete removal of the tumor) and the possibility of digestive tract or vascular complications. The use of 3D imaging for performing radical cystectomy has been shown to reduce the total operative time and the duration of pelvic lymph node dissection in comparison with 2D, without altering the results in terms of blood loss, postoperative complications, hospital length of stay or total costs of the procedure [38].

Another urologic procedure that has an important impact on the patient's quality of life is radical prostatectomy and urinary incontinence is one of the functional complications that are associated with this surgery. Laparoscopic 3D approach has shown shorter operative time, reduced blood loss and higher early continence rates in comparison with 2D vision [6].

2.1.2 Advantages for the Learning Curve

The 2D video systems and the instruments with fewer degrees of freedom slow down the learning curve of the surgeons. In order to facilitate the training, robotization of laparoscopic instruments and interface and 3D vision become crucial [20].

When comparing subjects with various experience in laparoscopy, 3D visualization was associated with a shorter time to completion of the tasks and improved task precision for peg transfer, pattern cutting and suturing/knot tying in comparison with a 2D system [37]. Also, when comparing subjects with standard laparoscopic experience in performing tasks using daVinci robot, the 3D vision shows a significant improvement in performance times and error rates in comparison with 2D vision, independent of the ergonomic advantages of the robotic system [10].

2.1.3 Advantages for the Ergonomy of the Surgeon

Although it has shown an improvement in patient outcomes and quality of life, laparoscopic surgery associates a greater amount of stress, muscular fatigue, discomfort and exhaustion for the surgeon [36], due to the need of performing repetitive and precise movements in a restricted space with ergonomically inadequate instruments. The 3D technology enables the surgeon to have depth awareness and a better visualization of the operative field, thus being able to perform complex surgeries with a more accurate technique. Subjects with no experience in laparoscopy showed an improvement in the operative time and the number of mistakes made when using 3D visualization. Also, this system seems to increase the accuracy and execution speed for the most complex surgical steps. As a result, the 3D vision is considered to ensure a lower mental workload, with a considerable difference in frustration, when compared with 2D in subjects with no experience in laparoscopy [15].

2.2 *Next Generation Instruments*

Minimally invasive surgery ensures smaller skin incisions, improved cosmetics, reduced post-operative pain and shorter recovery time. Single-site surgery aims to enhance these advantages by positioning all the instruments through a solitary port. But a number of challenges arise from this approach, due to the coaxial access of the instruments through the incision, reduced triangulation, reduced range of motion and instrument collision [16].

Several technical advances have been made in order to overcome these challenges, leading to the development of articulated or magnetic instruments and endoscopes.

2.2.1 Articulated Instruments

Articulated instruments seek to restore triangulation by rotating through 360° and articulating by up to 80° at their effector end. Using this type of instruments in conventional laparoscopy has been shown to improve performance in novices and to allow experts to maintain their performance [25]. On the other hand, the use of articulated instruments in single-site surgery has not demonstrated so far the superiority over straight instruments. The only significant improvement in surgeon performance was shown in the peg-transfer task when using a combination of one straight and one articulated instrument [12].

2.2.2 Magnetic Instruments

Irrespective of the type of minimally invasive approach, single-site or natural orifices surgery, the movement of the instruments is restrained by the access port. Investigation of possibilities of removing these constraints, led to the development of magnetically driven instruments. These instruments are formed of an external (outside the abdominal wall) and an internal unit (inside the abdominal wall), which interact by transferring the mechanical power from the driving magnet to the driven one, thus performing the surgery. The surgical devices have the advantage to be fully inserted into the abdominal cavity, achieve access to all abdominal quadrants, without the conventional rigid link connection with the external unit. The power and torque is transmitted from the external unit across the abdominal wall through magnetic linkage. This concept of magnetic instruments is still under investigation, but shows great potential so far to replace conventional abdominal surgery, taking the surgical robotics to the next level [21].

2.3 Intraoperative Imaging

Nowadays, patient safety and accuracy of the procedure have become the two main targets of surgical approach. Every technique has several limitations, whether it is laparoscopic or robotic-assisted. New imaging techniques have been implemented in order to enhance the surgeons' understanding of anatomical structures, like intraoperative ultrasound or near-infrared fluorescence.

Partial nephrectomy is a surgical technique that represents the removal of a kidney tumor with a minimal amount of healthy surrounding tissue, with the intent of preservation of the renal function. This technique is recommended for kidney tumors smaller than 4 cm and can be performed by minimally invasive approaches —laparoscopic or robotic. Robotic partial nephrectomy has shown important advantages in terms of learning curve and warm ischemia time (renal ischemia during tumor excision caused by the clamping of renal blood vessels) [7, 28]. Usually during the tumor excision, the ischemia time is necessary in order to ensure a lower blood loss and increased visualization of the surgical field. Studies have shown that prolonged ischemia time can impair the renal function, so zero-ischemia or selective ischemia partial nephrectomy (clamping only the arteries that supply blood to the part of the kidney where the tumor is located) have been recently developed. Moreover, the increasing experience in partial nephrectomy enables the use of this technique for more complex, endophytic tumors.

At the present time, partial nephrectomy poses two main challenges: to minimize the warm ischemia time by selective clamping and to ensure complete removal of endophytic tumors. Various imaging techniques can be used to assist these two surgical steps, and one of the most widely spread is intra-operative ultrasound. The use of a specific microbubble contrast substance with intra-operative ultrasound can enable the identification of renal microvasculature in real time, thus facilitating the identification of the tumor and selective arterial clamping, with a decreased risk of positive surgical margins and permanent loss of nephrons [3].

2.4 Fluorescence

Near-infrared fluorescence seems to have the greatest potential for entering the clinical practice in the near future, by offering an increased tissue visualization using widely available dyes like indocyanine green or methylene blue [33]. The near-infrared system is available for minimally invasive surgery techniques, both laparoscopic and robotic (since 2010), which can switch from white-light mode to near-infrared mode. The ability to merge these two modes into a single real-time image is still under development for the robotic system.

The physical and chemical characteristics of indocyanine green enables the possibility of better visualization of blood vessels, bile ducts, sentinel lymph nodes or lymphatic vessels [34]. As a result, the clinical applications of fluorescence in robotic surgery are [13]:

- ***recognition of vascular anatomy***—reduces the risk of iatrogenic damage, especially at the beginning of the learning curve; it ensures the identification of mesenteric arcades during intracorporeal ileal neobladder construction in order to preserve the blood supply [23]; also, it can be used to assist superselective clamping during partial nephrectomy, thus facilitating zero-ischemia technique and shortening the learning curve [9]
- ***evaluation of organ and tissue perfusion***—mostly used in general surgery in order to evaluate the microcirculation and viability of tissues, in an effort to early recognize ischemia of the stumps and to reduce the anastomotic leak and stricture rates [17]; to assess blood perfusion of the transplanted kidney [5]
- ***visualization of biliary anatomy*** during cholecystectomy, in order to prevent bile duct injuries [14]
- ***identification of lymph nodes***—with the purpose of excising only metastatic lymph nodes, providing an accurate staging and better oncologic outcomes, with decreasing complications [32]
- ***identification of specialized tissue***—for example, the nerves or nerve-bundles, in order to avoid iatrogenic damage and preserve their functionality [13]
- ***identification of lesions-based on vascular and metabolic pattern***—in order to preserve the organ and excise only the tumor: identification of renal tumors during partial nephrectomy (malignant lesions are hypofluorescent in comparison with normal tissue)[39]; identification of adrenal tumors (hypofluorescent) and performing partial adrenalectomy [24].

3 Learning Minimally-Invasive Surgery

3.1 Laparoscopy Learning Curve

Traditional laparoscopy learning curve is generally longer due to the 2D imaging, rigid instruments, a low degree of instruments movement, diminished tactile feedback, physiological tremor and reduced ergometry. Due to these limitations an increased number of complications have been encountered during the learning curve of a certain technique (urinary fistula in urology or the common biliary duct injury in general surgery). As well, the use of traditional laparoscopy is limited in complex cases that will require reconstructions or intracorporeal sutures (digestive surgery or intracorporeal urinary diversions). From the ergonomical point of view, traditional laparoscopy is more demanding using mainly the upper arms muscles (biceps and flexor carpi ulnaris). In the robotic surgery the trapezius muscle is mainly involved, but this phenomenon is mostly encountered in inexperienced doctors. These ergonomy differences lead to superior performance for the robotic surgeons [19].

3.2 Robotic Surgery Learning Curve

The robotic approach corrected the main disadvantages of the traditional laparoscopy. This way the 3D imaging is offering depth, the flexible instruments are offering a wide range of movements, there is no physiological tremor and the ergonomy is excellent. The patient is the main beneficiary of all the advantages offered by the robotic surgery: the blood loss, postoperative pain and the hospitalization period are considerably reduced compared to the traditional laparoscopy [30].

The robotic surgery advantages allow a shorter learning curve for the surgeons especially in the case of complex interventions (reconstructions and intracorporeal sutures) or stressful interventions (cardiovascular surgery).

The advantages offered by the robotic surgery in case of complex interventions have been evaluated in a study that included medical students with no previous laparoscopic, robotic or simulator experience. The subjects have done intracorporeal digestive sutures by traditional laparoscopic or robotic approach using three attempts. In the robotic group, the sutures have been done more rapidly compared to the laparoscopy group (460 vs. 600 s, $p < 0.0001$) and with a better quality, less errors and less vital organs injuries. The performances improved during the three robotic attempts but did not modify during the laparoscopy attempts. This fact suggests a more difficult learning curve for the traditional laparoscopy. The subjects practicing intracorporeal sutures complained of work overload and important psychological pressure [35].

On the other hand, the stress level during procedures is different for a beginner compared to an experienced surgeon. For a beginner, the stress level is lower in robotic compared to laparoscopic procedures [18]. For an experienced surgeon, the level of intraoperative stress is similar for both laparoscopic and robotic surgery. However cardiovascular adaptation (blood flow and vascular resistance) is better for the robotic surgeons compared to the ones in the traditional laparoscopy group. In highly stressful environment the robotic approach allows a more accurate performance with less errors. The performance of robotic interventions which associate a high level of stress offers better long term health results for the surgeons [27].

3.3 *The Role of Laparoscopy in the Robotic Surgery Learning Curve*

The implementation of robotic surgery can be achieved without previous laparoscopy experience, the leap from open surgery to robotics being possible. However the surgeons with previous laparoscopy experience acquire more rapidly the skills for the robotic surgery especially in the case of complex interventions (intracorporeal sutures). These observations are valid for all surgical specialties (urology, gynecology, general surgery or thoracic surgery) [26].

This way the previous experience in laparoscopy allows the surgeons to perform more rapidly. This phenomenon is valid as well for the surgeons crossing from robotic surgery to laparoscopy. The explanation for this phenomenon is that both approaches are based on the physical and cognitive elements. The physical elements are represented by the characteristics of these two surgical approaches (imaging, instruments, etc.). The cognitive elements once acquired in laparoscopy could be afterwards transferred to robotics and backwards. This cognitive aspect explains the more rapid learning curve in robotics for the surgeons with previous experience in laparoscopy and in laparoscopy for the robotic surgeons [4].

3.4 *The Role of Robotic Surgery in the Laparoscopy Learning Curve*

Using the robotic surgery platform during the laparoscopy learning curve could be very important for the surgical techniques acquisition.

A study which evaluated the laparoscopy learning process included gynecology resident doctors with and without previous surgical experience. Some of the doctors had been included in the laparoscopy training, which did not include the robotic platform, while another group used the robotic platform in the training. The learning curve included the following parameters: hands synchronization, cutting and sutures. The use of the robotic platform lead to >50% better performance for the junior doctors with no surgical experience as well as for the doctors with previous surgical experience [22].

3.5 *Simulators*

The robotic systems are composed of two parts:

- the console—used by the surgeon to generate tasks
- the robot—to deliver tasks

The console and robot activity could be reproduced with the help of simulators. There are two types of simulators:

- physics (mechanics)—the box type which can deliver tasks under video control (laparoscopy simulators)
- virtual—based on a computer which can generate a virtual reality (robotic simulators).

At the present, there are five different systems of robotic simulators (RoSS simulator, Simsurgery educational platform, ProMIS simulator, Mimic dV-Trainer system and daVinci Skill Simulator). These simulators are based on developing the eye-hand coordination capacity and the objective is tissue manipulation, dissection, sutures and performing knots [1]. The main role of these simulators is the acquisition of surgical skills during the training programs. The simulators offer as well the opportunity to evaluate and monitor the level of surgical skills acquisition [11].

Residents who have completed a training in laparoscopy performed more correctly the intracorporeal knots and sutures, have a reduced operating time and commit fewer errors [2]. Also, trainings conducted on virtual simulators lead to a reduced operative time and improved surgical performance compared to mechanical ones. Mechanical simulators require two people for performing the training compared to virtual simulators. The additional person is needed to control video quality and for evaluating training quality by offering feedback. For the virtual simulation, the evaluation is performed by the computer. However, mechanical simulators are much cheaper and offer the advantage of increased realism (e.g. tactile sensation present). Currently there is a concern for the construction of simulators that combine virtual reality and mechanical simulators [29].

4 Personal Experience

The experience of the Urology Department of the Cluj-Napoca Municipal Hospital includes open surgery, laparoscopy (since 1996) and robotics (since 2009). Implementing robotic surgery took place after a prior experience in laparoscopy for a senior surgeon and one inexperienced in laparoscopy junior surgeon. Previous training in laparoscopy allowed senior surgeon to perform urological robotic interventions of great difficulty: radical prostatectomy, partial nephrectomy, radical cystectomy with ileal intracorporeal neobladder. Since 2015 we started a program of three-dimensional laparoscopy and the main advantage is lower costs for laparoscopy (3D laparoscopy implementation costs represented ~5% of the costs of implementing robotics). For this purpose we evaluated how prior experience in robotic radical prostatectomy (250 cases) has influenced the adoption of 3D laparoscopic radical prostatectomy. Between March 2015 and January 2016 we performed 76 3D laparoscopic radical prostatectomies. The evaluated parameters were operative time, conversion rate, blood loss, transfusion rate and the duration of maintaining the catheter. Operative time was shorter for 3D laparoscopic surgery compared with the robotic one (132 vs. 210 min). Blood losses were comparable (mean blood loss 300 ml for both types of approach), but transfusion rate was higher for robotic radical prostatectomy (6 cases vs. 1 case). No cases of conversion were recorded in either group. The duration of preservation of the bladder catheter was 7 days for robotic radical prostatectomy and 14 days for 3D laparoscopy. The advantages for 3D laparoscopic approach are lower costs and reduced operative time. For the robotic approach the advantages are shorter need of drainage and bladder catheter and shorter hospital stay. Although the learning curve in laparoscopic radical prostatectomy is higher, prior experience in robotics and 3D image allowed a quick and safe implementation of this procedure.

5 Conclusion

The latest technologies, like 3D vision, next generation instruments, the use of intraoperative imaging have enabled the development of minimally-invasive surgery, so that a number of laparoscopic and robotic procedures have become the standard of care. The use of simulators as a part of the training programs have considerably reduced the number of surgical errors and have improved the operative time and the quality of robotic and laparoscopic surgical procedures. The use of the robotic platform during the learning curve allows the performance of laparoscopic procedures with the same accuracy, but with much lower costs.

Acknowledgements This paper was realized within the Partnership Programme in priority domains—PN-II, which runs with the financial support of MEN-UEFISCDI, Project no. 247/2014.

References

1. Abboudi, H., Khan, M.S., Aboumarzouk, O., Guru, K.A., Challacombe, B., Dasgupta, P., Ahmed, K.: Current status of validation for robotic surgery simulators—a systematic review. BJU Int. **111**(2), 194–205 (2013)
2. Al-Kadi, A.S., Donnon, T.: Using simulation to improve the cognitive and psychomotor skills of novice students in advanced laparoscopic surgery: a meta-analysis. Med. Teach. **35** (Suppl 1), S47–55 (2013).
3. Alenezi, A.N., Karim, O.: Role of intra-operative contrast-enhanced ultrasound (CEUS) in robotic-assisted nephron-sparing surgery. J. Robot. Surg. **9**(1), 1–10 (2015)
4. Angell, J., Gomez, M.S., Baig, M.M., Abaza, R.: Contribution of laparoscopic training to robotic proficiency. J. Endourol. **27**(8), 1027–1031 (2013)
5. Arichi, N., Mitsui, Y., Ogawa, K., Nagami, T., Nakamura, S., Hiraoka, T., et al.: Intraoperative fluorescence vascular imaging using indocyanine green for assessment of transplanted kidney perfusion. Transp. Proc. **46**, 342–345 (2014)
6. Aykan, S., Singhal, P., Nguyen, D.P., Yigit, A., Tuken, M., Yakut, E., et al.: Perioperative, pathologic, and early continence outcomes comparing three-dimensional and two-dimensional

display systems for laparoscopic radical prostatectomy–a retrospective, single-surgeon study. J. Endourol. **28**(5), 539–543 (2014)
7. Benway, B.M., Bhayani, S.B., Rogers, C.G., Dulabon, L.M., Patel, M.N., Lipkin, M., et al.: Robot assisted partial nephrectomy versus laparoscopic partial nephrectomy for renal tumors: a multi-institutional analysis of perioperative outcomes. J. Urol. **182**, 866–872 (2009)
8. Birkett, D.H., Josephs, L.G., Ese-McDonald, J.: A new 3-D laparoscope in gastrointestinal surgery. Surg. Endosc. **8**, 1448–1451 (1994)
9. Borofsky, M.S., Gill, I.S., Hemal, A.K., Marien, T.P., Jayaratna, I., Krane, L.S., et al.: Near-infrared fluorescence imaging to facilitate super-selective arterial clamping during zeroischaemia robotic partial nephrectomy. BJU Int. **111**, 604–610 (2013)
10. Byrn, J.C., Schluender, S., Divino, C.M., Conrad, J., Gurland, B., Shlasko, E., et al.: Three-dimensional imaging improves surgical performance for both novice and experienced operators using the da Vinci robot system. Am. J. Surg. **193**(4), 519–522 (2007)
11. Chandra, V., Nehra, D., Parent, R., Woo, R., Reyes, R., Hernandez-Boussard, T., et al.: A comparison of laparoscopic and robotic assisted suturing performance by experts and novices. Surgery **147**(6), 830–839 (2010)
12. Corker, H.P., Singh, P., Sodergren, M.H., Balaji, S., Kwasnicki, R.M., Darzi, A.W., et al.: A randomized controlled study to establish the effect of articulating instruments on performance in single-incision laparoscopic surgery. J. Surg. Educ. **72**(1), 1–7 (2015)
13. Daskalaki, D., Aguilera, F., Patton, K., Giulianotti, P.C.: Fluorescence in robotic surgery. J. Surg. Oncol. **112**(3), 250–256 (2015)
14. Daskalaki, D., Fernandes, E., Wang, X., Bianco, F.M., Elli, E.F., Ayloo, S., et al.: Indocyanine green (ICG) fluorescent cholangiography during robotic cholecystectomy: results of 184 consecutive cases in a single institution. Surg. Innov. **21**, 615–621 (2014)
15. Gómez-Gómez, E., Carrasco-Valiente, J., Valero-Rosa, J., Campos-Hernández, J.P., Anglada-Curado, F.J., Carazo-Carazo, J.L., et al.: Impact of 3D vision on mental workload and laparoscopic performance in inexperienced subjects. Actas Urol. Esp. **39**(4), 229–235 (2015)
16. Islam, A.: Early surgeon impressions and technical difficulty associated with laparoendoscopic single-site surgery: a Society of American Gastrointestinal and Endoscopic Surgeons learning center study. Surg. Endosc. **25**(8), 2597–2603 (2011)
17. Jafari, M.D., Lee, K.H., Halabi, W.J., Mills, S.D., Carmichael, J.C., Stamos, M.J., et al.: The use of indocyanine green fluorescence to assess anastomotic perfusion during robotic assisted laparoscopic rectal surgery. Surg. Endosc. **27**, 3003–3008 (2013)
18. Klein, M.I., Warm, J.S., Riley, M.A., Matthews, G., Doarn, C., Donovan, J.F., Gaitonde, K.: Mental workload and stress perceived by novice operators in the laparoscopic and robotic minimally invasive surgical interfaces. J. Endourol. **26**(8), 1089–1094 (2012)
19. Lee, G.I., Lee, M.R., Clanton, T., Sutton, E., Park, A.E., Marohn, M.R.: Comparative assessment of physical and cognitive ergonomics associated with robotic and traditional laparoscopic surgeries. Surg. Endosc. **28**(2), 456–465 (2014)
20. Leite, M., Carvalho, A.F., Costa, P., Pereira, R., Moreira, A., Rodrigues, N., et al.: Assessment of laparoscopic skills performance: 2D versus 3D vision and classic instrument versus new hand-held robotic device for laparoscopy. Surg. Innov. **23**(1), 52–61 (2016)
21. Leong, F., Garbin, N., Di Natali, C., Mohammadi, A., Thiruchelvam, D., Oetomo, D., et al.: Magnetic surgical instruments for robotic abdominal surgery. IEEE Rev. Biomed. Eng. (2016) [Epub ahead of print]
22. Letouzey, V., Huberlant, S., Faillie, J.L., Prudhomme, M., Mares, P., de Tayrac, R.: Evaluation of a laparoscopic training program with or without robotic assistance. Eur. J. Obstet. Gynecol. Reprod. Biol. **181**, 321–327 (2014)
23. Manny, T.B., Hemal, A.K.: Fluorescence-enhanced robotic radical cystectomy using unconjugated indocyanine green for pelvic lymphangiography, tumor marking, and mesenteric angiography: the initial clinical experience. Urology **83**, 824–829 (2014)

24. Manny, T.B., Pompeo, A.S., Hemal, A.K.: Robotic partial adrenalectomy using indocyanine green dye with near-infrared imaging: the initial clinical experience. Urology **82**, 738–742 (2013)
25. Martinec, D.: The trade-off between flexibility and maneuverability: task performance with articulating laparoscopic instruments. Surg. Endosc. **23**(12), 2697–2701 (2009)
26. McVey, R., Goldenberg, M., Bernardini, M., Yasufuku, K., Quereshy, F., Finelli, A., et al.: Baseline laparoscopic skill may predict baseline robotic skill and early robotic surgery learning curve. J. Endourol. (2016) [Epub ahead of print]
27. Moore, L.J., Wilson, M.R., Waine, E., McGrath, J.S., Masters, R.S., Vine, S.J.: Robotically assisted laparoscopy benefits surgical performance under stress. J. Robot Surg. **9**(4), 277–284 (2015)
28. Mottrie, A., De Naeyer, G., Schatteman, P., Carpentier, P., Sangalli, M., Ficarra, V.: Impact of the learning curve on perioperative outcomes in patients who underwent robotic partial nephrectomy for parenchymal renal tumours. Eur. Urol. **58**, 127–132 (2010)
29. Nagendran, M., Gurusamy, K.S., Aggarwal, R., Loizidou, M., Davidson, B.R.: Virtual reality training for surgical trainees in laparoscopic surgery. Cochrane Database Syst. Rev. **8**, CD006575 (2013)
30. Payne, T.N., Dauterive, F.R.: A comparison of total laparoscopic hysterectomy to robotically assisted hysterectomy: surgical outcomes in a community practice. J. Minim. Invasive Gynecol. **15**(3), 286–291 (2008)
31. Peitgen, K., Walz, M.V., Holtmann, G., Eigler, F.W.: A prospective randomized experimental evaluation of three-dimensional imaging in laparoscopy. Gastrointest. Endosc. **44**, 262–267 (1996)
32. Rossi, E.C., Ivanova, A., Boggess, J.F.: Robotically assisted fluorescence-guided lymph node mapping with ICG for gynecologic malignancies: a feasibility study. Gynecol. Oncol. **124**, 78–82 (2012)
33. Schols, R.M., Bouvy, N.D., van Dam, R.M., Stassen, L.P.: Advanced intraoperative imaging methods for laparoscopic anatomy navigation: an overview. Surg. Endosc. **27**(6), 1851–1859 (2013)
34. Schols, R.M., Connell, N.J., Stassen, L.P.: Near-infrared fluorescence imaging for real-time intraoperative anatomical guidance in minimally invasive surgery: a systematic review of the literature. World J. Surg. **39**(5), 1069–1079 (2015)
35. Stefanidis, D., Wang, F., Korndorffer Jr., J.R., Dunne, J.B., Scott, D.J.: Robotic assistance improves intracorporeal suturing performance and safety in the operating room while decreasing operator workload. Surg. Endosc. **24**(2), 377–382 (2010)
36. Szeto, G.P., Cheng, S.W., Poon, J.T., Ting, A.C., Tsang, R.C., Ho, P.: Surgeons' static posture and movement repetitions in open and laparoscopic surgery. J. Surg. Res. **172**, e19–e31 (2012)
37. Tanagho, Y.S., Andriole, G.L., Paradis, A.G., Madison, K.M., Sandhu, G.S., Varela, J.E., et al.: 2D versus 3D visualization: impact on laparoscopic proficiency using the fundamentals of laparoscopic surgery skill set. J. Laparoendosc. Adv. Surg. Tech. A **22**(9), 865–870 (2012)
38. Tang, F.J., Qi, L., Jiang, H.C., Tong, S.Y. and Li, Y.: Comparison of the clinical effectiveness of 3D and 2D imaging systems for laparoscopic radical cystectomy with pelvic lymph node dissection. J. Int. Med. Res. (2016) [Epub ahead of print]
39. Tobis, S., Knopf, J.K., Silvers, C., Messing, E., Yao, J., Rashid, H., et al.: Robot-assisted and laparoscopic partial nephrectomy with near infrared fluorescence imaging. J. Endourol. Soc. **26**, 797–802 (2012)
40. Wenzl, R., Lehner, R., Vry, U., Pateisky, N., Sevelda, P., Husslein, P.: Three-dimensional video endoscopy: clinical use in gynecological laparoscopy. Lancet **344**, 1621–1622 (1994)

Bio-Kinematic Design of Individualized Lift-Assist Devices

S.M.F. Reimer, K. Abdul-Sater and T.C. Lueth

Abstract Rising from a chair is a fundamental movement in daily life and a prerequisite for independent functional ability. Yet, it remains one of the most biomechanically demanding activities as it requires high levels of neuromuscular coordination, muscle strength and postural control (Ellis et al. J Biomed Eng 6:113–120 (1984), [3]). While standing up is considered a natural ubiquitous skill it becomes increasingly difficult with age. To prolong the independence of elderly we present a novel computational design procedure for lift-assist devices that are individualized to the user while complying with the limited space within the chair. Given marker-based sit-to-stand motion data task positions are defined to carry out a finite position synthesis of a four-bar linkage that provides user-specific guidance of a seat. The four-bar linkage combined with the lower limb of a user generates a biologically inspired six-bar linkage. Thus, accomplishing a bio-kinematic design of linkages where this contribution provides an exemplary design session.

Keywords Bio-kinematics · Four-bar linkage · Six-bar linkage · Individualized · Lift-assist device · Sit-to-stand · Elderly

1 Introduction

Approximately 10% of the world's population is over 60 years old. By 2050 this proportion will have more than doubled. The greatest rate of increase will be among people aged 85 and older [8]. This group is subject to greater physical and cognitive impairments compared to younger people due to natural age-related changes of the body composition and functional capacity. This has a profound impact on the independence of elderly who risk functional dependence and reliance on friends, family or caregivers and in the worst case risk institutionalization. Both cognitive and physical diminishing abilities address the body including aspects such as awareness, perception, haptics, reaction, balance and basic motor skills. Assistive technologies

S.M.F. Reimer (✉) · K. Abdul-Sater · T.C. Lueth
Technical University of Munich, Munich, Germany
e-mail: samuel.reimer@tum.de

M. Husty and M. Hofbaur (eds.), *New Trends in Medical and Service Robots*,
Mechanisms and Machine Science 48, DOI 10.1007/978-3-319-59972-4_5

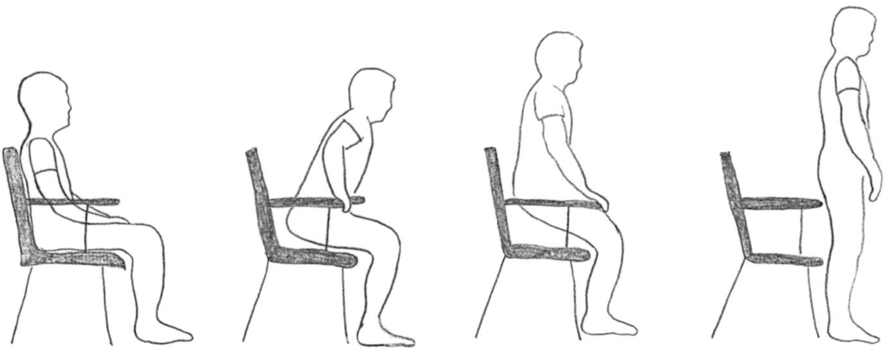

Fig. 1 Qualitative view of the sagittal sit-to-stand movement split into four phases; sitting, hip flexion, chair rise and balance coordination

for the mobility-impaired include the wheelchair, lift aids and other devices, all of which have been around for centuries. However, the individual typically requires assistance to use these devices; whether to push the wheelchair, to lift themselves from the bed to a chair or for guiding the individual through cluttered areas. With fewer caregivers and more elderly expected in the near future, there is a need for improving these devices to provide elderly with independent assistance.

Rising from a chair (visualized in Fig. 1) is one of the most frequent activities of daily living and often described as sit-to-stand (STS) movement. As a precursor to gait, the capacity to rise from a chair may determine physical functional independence. Indeed, chair rise is thought to be the one of the most biomechanically demanding functional tasks [1].

Although mechanical lift-assist devices (LADs) have been recommended for use by elderly, rehabilitation specialists have voiced two major concerns in prescribing these devices. First, it has been suggested that LADs provide a horizontal destabilizing force to the user, thereby predisposing them to falls [9]. Second, it has been hypothesized that LADs may cause accelerated muscle weakness in users due to the decreased muscle activity levels required to rise from a chair. However, to date, no literature was found which substantiated or refuted either concern with LADs.

One way to facilitate the stand-up process is by raising seat height and/or providing chair arm rests for assistance. Both approaches have been found to reduce net moments and joint loading forces acting around the knee in healthy subjects during rising [9]. It is suggested that reductions in joint moments and loading forces are associated with reduced damage to the joint structures [5].

Another possible solution is a passive mechanical LAD which imparts a lifting force only when the user actively initiates STS movement (Fig. 2). The kinematic concept of the LAD is based on a four-bar linkage which consists of two links ((4) and (5)) attached to a coupler (1) which forms the seating surface. Each link is made of two rotary hinges, also known as a 2R chain. These 2R chains guide the motion of the coupler from *sit* configuration (Fig. 2a) to *stand* configuration (Fig. 2b). Due

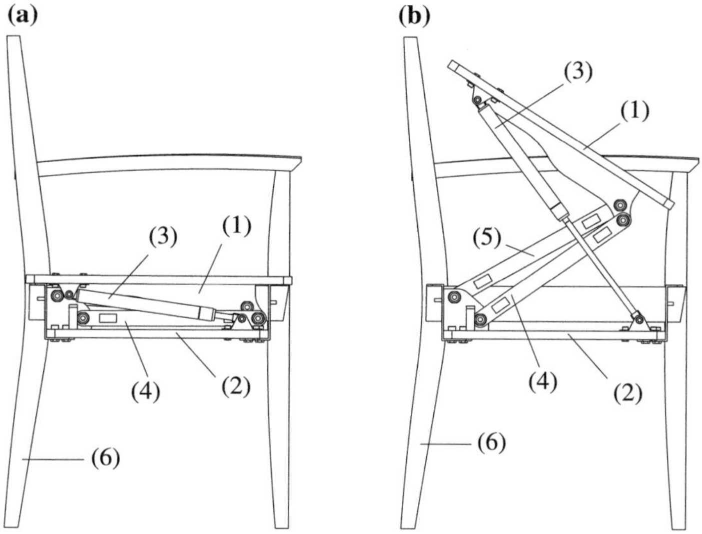

Fig. 2 Conceptual design of a modular lift-assist device (LAD) integrated into a chair (*6*) in *sit* (**a**) and *stand* (**b**) configuration. The LAD consists of a four-bar linkage ((*1*), (*2*), (*4*) and (*5*)) actuated by a gas spring (*3*)

to the fact that the linkage has only one degree of freedom (DOF) it is actuated by a gas spring (3). A gas spring is a robust and simple mechanical solution, compared to the actuation with an electric motor. In addition, it is advantageous in activities of daily living as it reduces complexity, weight and is not dependent on an external energy supply.

Due to the compact design of the four-bar linkage we have been able to construct a LAD as a modular add-on to the original design of the chair. The original seat cushion has been removed from the chair and connected to the coupler of the four-bar linkage (1). The kinematic structure is placed onto a rigid suspension (2) which is easily inserted on to the chair frame (6). Comparable designs have been presented by [2] who have integrated similar kinematic structures into wheelchairs that showed promising support during STS movements.

In this contribution we advance the field of lift-assist devices by introducing an individualization process. Inspired by the four-bar linkage design in Fig. 2 and on previous works by [2] biomechanical parameters and STS movement behavior of the user are captured to synthesize a four-bar linkage that fits to the user.

Four-bar linkages and their analysis are well understood [6] and can be synthesized effortlessly given specific task positions of the coupler. Therefore defining task positions that match those of the STS motion behavior of the user we hypothesize to design a user-specific LAD that causes minimal displacement between seat and contact area of the user's lower limb.

In this contribution we first analyze different kinematic models of the lower limb and which best reflects natural STS movement. This is followed by a dimensional finite position synthesis upon which the computational design procedure of the LAD is based on. Finally we present a preliminary experiment of the computational bio-kinematic design approach based on STS motion data from a volunteer.

2 Bio-Kinematic Representation of Lower Limb and Lift-Assist Device

STS movement has been analyzed extensively [4, 9]. It shows that the motion can be generally split into four phases within the sagittal plane (see Fig. 1). At the beginning the human body is in a stable sitting position. Next, hip flexion occurs which lifts the feet from the ground slightly decreasing ground reaction force. Phase two ends when the body begins to stand up. The final phase lasts until a stable standing position is reached. The kinematic behavior of the lower limb is frequently modeled as a serial kinematic chain which describes shank, thigh and trunk as rigid links connected by revolute joints that mimic ankle, knee and hip joint. Note, that this clearly defines a particularly simplified view point, which, however will be sufficient for our purposes. Linkages studied in this contribution are build from two elementary joints, the rotary hinge, called a *revolute* joint (denoted by R), and a linear slider, or *prismatic* joint (denoted by P).

In order to individualize the LAD to the user's leg geometry and movement we investigated possible simplified kinematic representations that connect the human leg (blue) with the four-bar structure (black) of the LAD as seen in Fig. 3.

Thus, the thigh is considered to be in continuous contact with the seat, i.e. the coupler of the four-bar linkage (see Fig. 3a). However, in this case one can immediately deduce that the structure cannot move because applying the *Chebychev-Grübler-Kutzbach criterion* yields a DOF of $F = 3(n - 1 - g) + \sum_{i=1}^{g} b_i = 3(5 - 1 - 6) +$

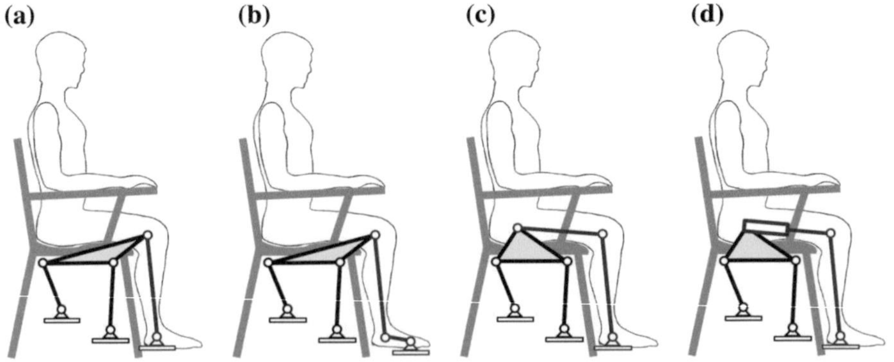

Fig. 3 Kinematic representations of the lower limb (*blue*) and lift-assist device (*black*) as a five-bar (**a**), six-bar (**b**, **c**) and six-bar with prismatic joint (**d**) linkage structure

$6 = 0$, where g and n are the number of revolute joints and links respectively. b_i represents the number of DOF for the ith joint. Hence, to obtain a suitable linkage we must integrate another link and joint either into the LAD or into the human model to achieve 1 DOF.

Increasing the complexity of the LAD is generally unfavorable as this has ramifications on workspace, actuation, weight and cost of the kinematic assembly. However, there exist several scenarios how to implement a suitable joint into the lower limb model. Implementing a joint at the toe as seen in Fig. 3b would imply that there is continuous movement between heel and ground while the user rises from the chair. This is often the case for people whose leg length is shorter than the height of the chair. During STS movement they touch ground first with their toes before their heel is lowered to ground. However, the majority of the STS transition occurs after the person has reached a stable foot position on the ground rendering any further movement of the LAD impossible.

Alternatively, Fig. 3c displays a linkage model with a modeled hip joint. The leg is now modeled as a 3R chain connected to the coupler of the four-bar linkage. The revolute joint situated at the hip is a logical modification as there is generally some rotary movement about the hip when the seat lifts the individual.

Figure 3d replaces the revolute joint at the hip with a prismatic joint. This imitates linear sliding of the hip on the seating surface during STS movement. Hip sliding occurs when the persons pelvis gradually moves forward during seating. Sliding on the seat is generally more uncomfortable and ought to be avoided. Hence, we continue with the 7R linkage configuration as shown in Fig. 3c.

The three different approaches from Fig. 3b–d may all be seen as valid models, if the joint movement in the corresponding R or P joint approximately vanishes during STS motion. This is possible if appropriate kinematic dimensions of the four-bar LAD can be synthesized. Once a four-bar synthesis is completed, kinematic analysis of the six-bar linkage must detect, whether the considered joint motion stays approximately constant.

The system from Fig. 3c is also known as a *Stephenson III* linkage (see Fig. 4). The lower limb model consists of a fixed pivot point at the ankle, $\mathbf{q}_{ankle}$, and two moving pivots each with one DOF representing the knee, $\mathbf{p}_{knee}$, and hip joint, $\mathbf{p}_{hip}$. The hip

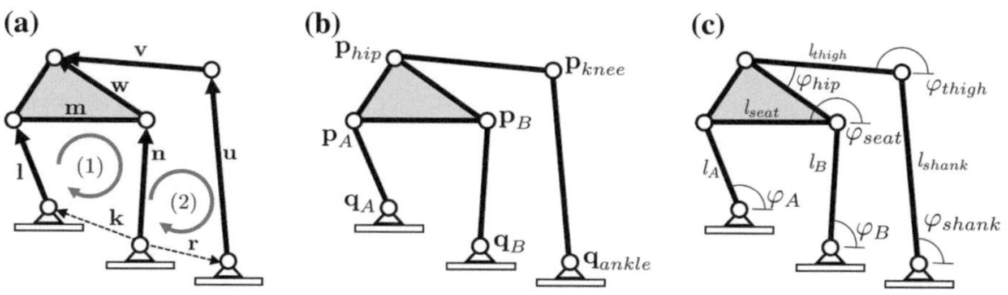

Fig. 4 Nomenclature of links and two closed loops (*1*) and (*2*) (**a**), joints (**b**) and link length and angles of a 7R kinematic interpretation of LAD and lower limb

joint is attached to a coupler of the four-bar linkage which represents the LAD. The LAD consists of two 2R chains, link A which consists of two revolute joints $\mathbf{q}_A$ and $\mathbf{p}_A$ and link B which consists of $\mathbf{q}_B$ and $\mathbf{p}_B$. The length of link A and B is yet to be determined. Once suitable parameters for the two links are found, the movement of the linkage and in particular the movement between lower limb and LAD can be analyzed. In fact, the angle φ_{hip} between the coupler described by $\mathbf{p}_A$, $\mathbf{p}_B$ and $\mathbf{p}_{hip}$ and the thigh described by $\mathbf{p}_{knee}$ and $\mathbf{p}_{hip}$ will be of interest in this approach. Since rotary movement between human leg and seating surface is inevitable, the four-bar link dimensions should satisfy

$$\varphi_{hip} \approx const. \tag{1}$$

within a user-specific range of motion so as to allow a smooth transition of the user from sit-to-stand.

3 Dimensional Finite Position Synthesis

The algebraic synthesis of 2R chains determines the kinematic dimension of the LAD for a given specified set of task positions. Note, that a task position shall represent a location and orientation of the seat and hence also of the user's thigh. The dimensions may be found from the joints in a reference configuration, so that a set of joint coordinates will be determined rather than link length. Hence, task positions must be defined which are based on motion data of the user.

Each 2R chain consists of the unknown fixed pivot $\mathbf{q} = (x_{\mathbf{q}}, y_{\mathbf{q}})^T$ and the unknown moving pivot $\mathbf{p}^i = (x_{\mathbf{p}^i}, y_{\mathbf{p}^i})^T$, where $i = 1, \ldots, n$ defines different, finitely separated configurations of the linkage. Here, vectors will be measured in a fixed coordinate frame W.

In order to describe configuration i of $\mathbf{p}$ in terms of the movement of the thigh we consider another coordinate frame M which is rigidly attached to the thigh which is conveniently located at $\mathbf{p}^i_{knee}$ (see Fig. 5). Thus, the translation of M in the xy-plane of W is measured using the 2×1 translation vector $\mathbf{t}^i_M = \mathbf{p}^i_{knee}$. Orientation of M with respect to W shall be measured using the angle φ^i_{thigh} and shall be described using a proper 2×2 rotation matrix $\mathbf{R}^i_M(\varphi^i_{thigh})$ (see Fig. 5). Parameter $\mathbf{t}^i_M$ and φ^i_{thigh} will be available from a motion tracking system, which captures the stand-up motion of the user. Applying these quantities, the configuration i of $\mathbf{p}$ is obtained using the commonly known *displacement* equation, which can be expressed with respect to a reference configuration

$$\mathbf{p}^i = \underbrace{\mathbf{R}^i_M(\mathbf{R}^1_M)^T}_{\mathbf{R}^{1i}_M(\varphi^{1i}_{thigh})} \cdot \mathbf{p}^1 + \underbrace{\mathbf{t}^i_M - \mathbf{R}^{1i}_M \cdot \mathbf{t}^1_M}_{\mathbf{t}^{1i}_M}, \qquad i = 2, \ldots, n. \tag{2}$$

Note, that Eq. (2) consists of W-frame coordinates only.

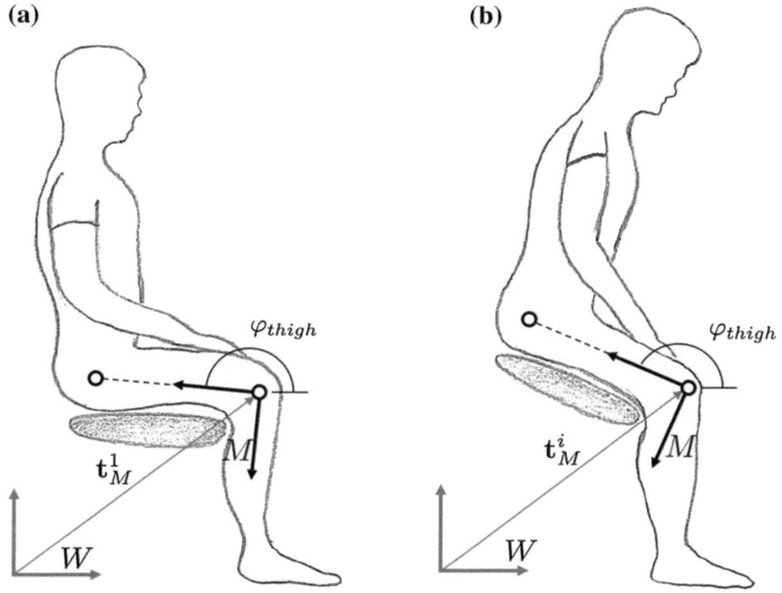

Fig. 5 Task positions of frame *M* in configuration 1 (**a**) and configuration *i* (**b**) with respect to a world coordinate frame *W*

Herein $\varphi_{thigh}^{1i} = \varphi_{thigh}^{i} - \varphi_{thigh}^{1}$ and $\mathbf{t}_M^{1i}$ rotate and translate the seat from configuration 1 to *i* and expresses $\mathbf{p}^i$ through $\mathbf{p}^1$. Equation (2) is the first significant equation in the design procedure since it calculates the pivot points in a reference configuration based on specified movement of the seat. The second equation is represented by the geometric constraint of a 2R chain which is known as the *constant distance constraint*

$$(\mathbf{p}^i - \mathbf{q})^T(\mathbf{p}^i - \mathbf{q}) = l^2, \qquad i = 1, \ldots, n. \tag{3}$$

Subtracting Eq. (3) for $i = 1$ from Eq. (3) for $i = 2, \ldots, n$ eliminates the parameter l. Next, substituting $\mathbf{p}^i = \mathbf{R}_M^{1i} \cdot \mathbf{p}^1 + \mathbf{t}_M^{1i}$ and rearranging yields

$$(\mathbf{p}^1)^T \cdot (\mathbf{E} - \mathbf{R}_M^{1i})^T \cdot \mathbf{q} + (\mathbf{t}_M^{1i})^T \cdot \mathbf{R}_M^{1i} \cdot \mathbf{p}^1 - (\mathbf{t}_M^{1i})^T \cdot \mathbf{q} + \frac{1}{2}(\mathbf{t}_M^{1i})^T \cdot \mathbf{t}_M^{1i} = 0 \tag{4}$$

for $i = 2, \ldots, n$ and where $\mathbf{E}$ is the 2×2 identity matrix. By solving this set of equations we can calculate the coordinates of each link's pivot points in reference configuration 1 of the linkage. Equation (4) is known as the algebraic *design* equation of planar 2R chains, where motion quantities $\mathbf{R}_M^{1i}$ and $\mathbf{t}_M^{1i}$ are given and $\mathbf{q} = (x_\mathbf{q}, y_\mathbf{q})^T$ and $\mathbf{p}^1 = (x_{\mathbf{p}^1}, y_{\mathbf{p}^1})^T$, are four unknown *W*-frame coordinates. Hence, the maximum number of task positions of the thigh is $n = 5$, since then there are four equations in four unknowns.

4 Individualized Computational Bio-Kinematic Design Procedure

Based on the dimensional finite position synthesis we explain further algebraic and computational steps necessary to individualize a four-bar LAD to the user.

Figure 4 illustrates the set of given and undefined parameters. On the one hand there is the 3R chain, $\mathbf{q}_{ankle}$, $\mathbf{p}_{knee}$ and $\mathbf{p}_{thigh}$ defined by the individual. On the other hand there are two unknown 2R chains $\mathbf{q}_A$, $\mathbf{p}_A$ and $\mathbf{q}_B$, $\mathbf{p}_B$ that must be solved for. Additionally there are certain prerequisites that the LAD must ensure. It must guarantee a natural STS transition of the seat such that Eq. (1) is maintained. Secondly the four-bar linkage must fit into the limited space provided by the chair.

4.1 Definition of the Workspace and the Number of Task Positions

The aforementioned algebraic synthesis is able to determine the coordinates of $\mathbf{q}_A$, $\mathbf{q}_B$ $\mathbf{p}_A^1$ and $\mathbf{p}_B^1$. However, it does not necessarily comply with the prerequisite that all coordinates in configuration 1, i.e. the *sit* configuration of the LAD, lie within the dimensions of the chair. From Fig. 3 it is apparent that the workspace for $\mathbf{p}^1$ and $\mathbf{q}$ must lie underneath the seat and between the chair legs. While $\mathbf{q}$ can be located anywhere within this space $\mathbf{p}^1$ is further limited by the fact that it acts as the rotary joint of the seat and therefore $\mathbf{p}^1$ should ideally be attached as close to the seat as possible.

Earlier it was described that a maximum number of $n = 5$ task positions can be defined in order to ensure a continuous user-specific STS movement. When specifying the maximum number of task positions the four-bar linkage will be more likely to follow the movement of the user. In turn, however, we receive four *design* equations in four unknowns. Therefore, none of the parameters of $\mathbf{p}^1$ and $\mathbf{q}$ can be specified such that they are within the workspace of the chair.

Decreasing the number of task positions to $n = 4$ results in three *design* equations. Hence, one of the four unknown parameters can be confined within the workspace of the chair. $\mathbf{p}^1$ is more limited than $\mathbf{q}$. Therefore $x_{\mathbf{p}^1}$ or $y_{\mathbf{p}^1}$ may be preallocated within a particularly narrow space while the three remaining parameters are obtained from solving the three design equations, see [6]. However, this still means that we cannot ensure, whether $\mathbf{p}^1$ lies within the given space. For these reasons we consider $n = 3$, which yields two *design* equations. Thus, we are unrestricted to specify $\mathbf{p}^1$ in regard of the desired space and may solve for $\mathbf{q}$ linearly (see [6]).

4.2 Analysis of STS Motion and Definition of Task Positions

STS movement of the individual can be recorded using marker-based motion capturing cameras which emit infrared light to detect reflective passive markers attached to the human. Markers are positioned at the hip, knee and ankle joint of the lower limb and a reference marker placed onto the chair. This allows for capturing discrete three-dimensional motion data of $\mathbf{p}^i_{hip}$, $\mathbf{p}^i_{knee}$ and $\mathbf{q}_{ankle}$.

Task positions of the seat are derived from captured motion data. Given vector $\mathbf{p}^i_{hip}$ and $\mathbf{p}^i_{knee}$, we can determine the translation $\mathbf{t}^i_M$ and orientation $\mathbf{R}^i_M(\varphi^i_{thigh})$ where $\mathbf{t}^i_M = \mathbf{p}^i_{knee}$ and φ^i_{thigh} is measured from the x-axis of W to the vector from $\mathbf{p}^i_{knee}$ to $\mathbf{p}^i_{hip}$.

The third task position defines the *end* configuration of the supported movement, which could, for example, be assessed by a doctor or physiotherapist depending on the support that the individual requires. The second task position is in between the first' and last'. Repetitions of the STS movement produces a range of possible $\mathbf{p}^i_{hip}$ and $\mathbf{p}^i_{knee}$ values, and therefore a set of different $\mathbf{t}^i_M$ value for $i = 2$ and 3. Note, that the first position is not considered to vary here. Each set defines an upper and lower boundary of possible values for $\mathbf{t}^i_M$ defined by x^i_{min}, x^i_{max} and y^i_{min}, y^i_{max}. Discrete values in this range can be inserted into $\mathbf{t}^i_M$ and $\mathbf{R}^i_M(\varphi^i_{thigh})$ for $i = 2$ and 3. The result is a set of task positions that will yield a set of four-bars each of which may be analyzed with regard to Eq. (1).

4.3 *Exhaustive Search and Kinematic Analysis*

Given the mentioned range of values for $\mathbf{t}^i_M$, $\mathbf{p}^1_A$, $\mathbf{p}^1_B$ and $\mathbf{R}^i_M(\varphi^i_{thigh})$, where $i = 2, 3$, an exhaustive search can be conducted to find real solutions for $\mathbf{q}_A$ and $\mathbf{q}_B$ that are within the boundaries of the chair frame. This yields eight variables for each 2R chain configuration.

An exhaustive search, also known as a *brute-force method* is a well known problem-solving technique of systematically enumerating all possible parameter configurations and may find a solution. With respect to the amount of open parameters it is important to reduce the range of values for each parameter as much as possible to avoid a *combinatorial explosion*.

Should a solution be found it is worth increasing the depth of search within a smaller radius of the open parameters to find a set of solutions for the four-bar linkage configuration.

Once a set of linkage configurations is found a kinematic analysis of the earlier mentioned *Stephenson III* linkage is applied to validate Eq. (1). The solution that satisfies Eq. (1) best is chosen. Retrace from Fig. 4 that φ_{hip} may be calculated easily from a given φ_{thigh} and φ_{seat}.

A linkage analysis determines each of the joints angles for a given input angle. For the linkage φ_{thigh} is the input rotation and φ_A, φ_B, φ_{seat} and φ_{shank} are the unknown output rotations. In order to solve the relationship between input and output angles we introduce a fixed world frame W and split the six-bar linkage into two separate vector loops. The first loop consists of the 4R chain, $\mathbf{q}_A$, $\mathbf{p}_A$, $\mathbf{p}_B$ and $\mathbf{q}_B$, while the second loop is expressed by the 5R chain, $\mathbf{q}_B$, $\mathbf{p}_B$, $\mathbf{p}_{hip}$, $\mathbf{p}_{knee}$ and $\mathbf{q}_{ankle}$ as seen in Fig. 4a.

From each loop two *constraint* equations can be obtained that are

$$\mathbf{f}(\vec{\phi}) = \begin{bmatrix} f_1(\vec{\phi}) \\ f_2(\vec{\phi}) \\ f_3(\vec{\phi}) \\ f_4(\vec{\phi}) \end{bmatrix} = \begin{bmatrix} \mathbf{k} + \mathbf{l} - \mathbf{m} - \mathbf{n} \\ \mathbf{n} + \mathbf{w} - \mathbf{v} - \mathbf{u} - \mathbf{r} \end{bmatrix} = \vec{\mathbf{0}} \tag{5}$$

where $\mathbf{f}$ contains the functions $f_i(\vec{\phi})$ and $\vec{\phi}$ contains the independent variables φ_A, φ_B, φ_{seat} and φ_{shank}. Expending Eq. (5) produces four non-linear equations which can be solved numerically by applying the *Newton-Raphson* method. This requires the evaluation of a matrix, known as the *Jacobian* of the system, which is defined as

$$\mathbf{J} = \begin{bmatrix} \frac{\partial f_1}{\partial \varphi_A} & \frac{\partial f_1}{\partial \varphi_B} & \frac{\partial f_1}{\partial \varphi_{seat}} & \frac{\partial f_1}{\partial \varphi_{shank}} \\ \frac{\partial f_2}{\partial \varphi_A} & \frac{\partial f_2}{\partial \varphi_B} & \frac{\partial f_2}{\partial \varphi_{seat}} & \frac{\partial f_2}{\partial \varphi_{shank}} \\ \frac{\partial f_3}{\partial \varphi_A} & \frac{\partial f_3}{\partial \varphi_B} & \frac{\partial f_3}{\partial \varphi_{seat}} & \frac{\partial f_3}{\partial \varphi_{shank}} \\ \frac{\partial f_4}{\partial \varphi_A} & \frac{\partial f_4}{\partial \varphi_B} & \frac{\partial f_4}{\partial \varphi_{seat}} & \frac{\partial f_4}{\partial \varphi_{shank}} \end{bmatrix}. \tag{6}$$

If $\vec{\phi} = \vec{\phi}^1$ represents the first guess for the solution successive approximations to the solution are obtained from

$$\vec{\phi}^{m+1} = \vec{\phi}^m - \mathbf{J}^{-1} \cdot \mathbf{f}(\vec{\phi}^m). \tag{7}$$

Retrace, that $\vec{\phi}^1$ is easily calculated from the synthesis results.

5 Individualized Lift-Assist Device

Here, we present a preliminary investigation of the aforementioned computational bio-kinematic design procedure with a volunteer. For this experiment we used a digital single-lens reflex camera to capture motion data rather than installing a sophisticated motion tracking system. White markers were positioned onto the hip, knee and ankle joints according to *Helen Hayes* marker placement [7] as seen in Fig. 6.

To avoid excessive movement of the fabric relative to the lower limb we asked the volunteer to wear close-fitting trunks. While sitting the volunteer had his back rest against the backrest of the chair and the arms hold on to the armrests. During STS movement the volunteer was asked to lift himself from the chair using his legs and arms.

The camera was fixed onto a tripod with its imaging plane parallel to the sagittal plane of the volunteer's STS movement and six images were captured representing different task positions of the lower leg during STS movement. Since each captured

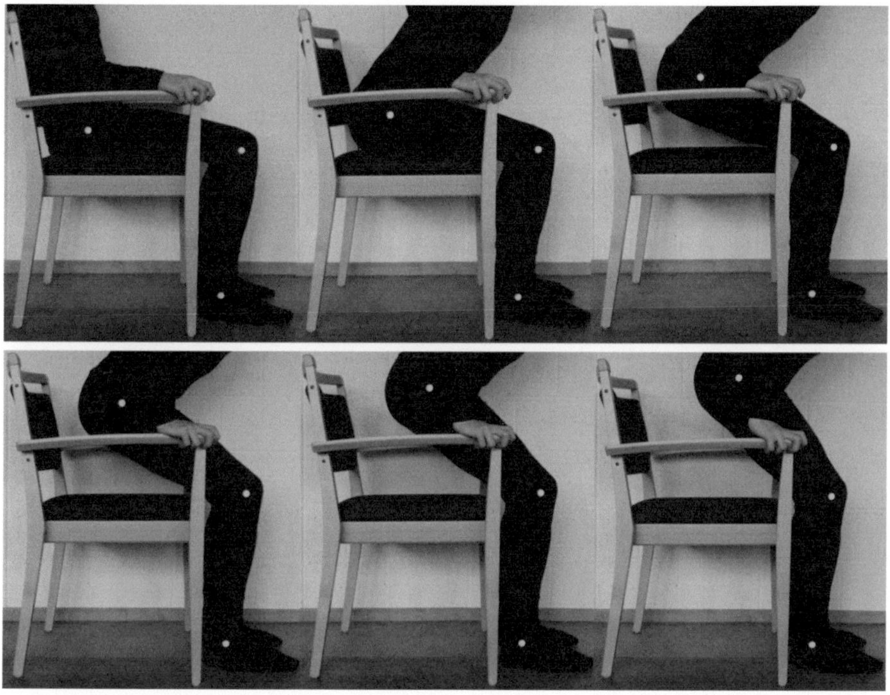

Fig. 6 Sit-to-stand movement of a test person

image has the same format we were able to extract a range of hip, knee and ankle joint positions across multiple STS movements. Joint positions are captured as *pixel* coordinates in reference to a picture coordinate system fixed to the lower left edge of the image. Similarly we defined corner points of the workspace below the chair from the images. The mean values of joint positions are displayed in Table 1.

Table 1 Mean lower limb coordinates of task positions defined in Fig. 6

Task position, i	x_{hip}	y_{hip}	x_{knee}	y_{knee}	x_{ankle}	y_{ankle}
1	1055	716	1467	663	1371	295
2	1086	758	1475	660	1373	298
3	1105	794	1482	659	1371	299
4	1127	838	1487	657	1369	301
5	1147	882	1484	658	1372	298
6	1166	915	481	660	1370	299

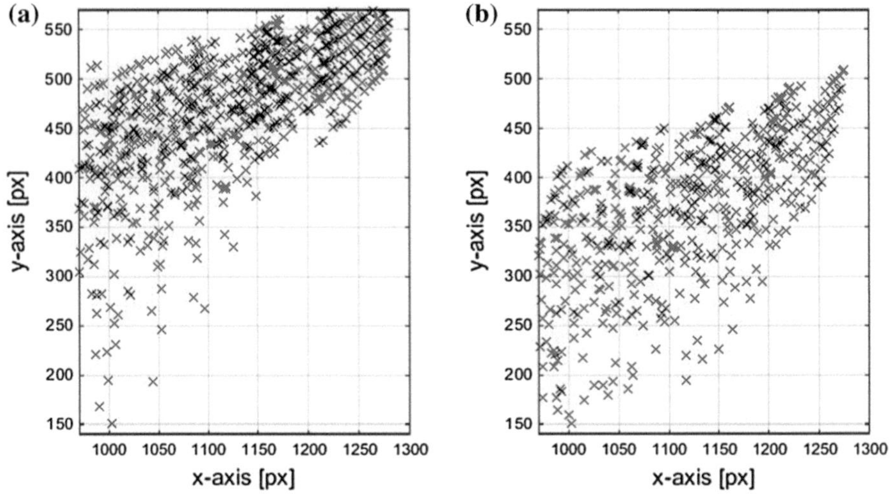

Fig. 7 Results of an exhaustive search for positions of $\mathbf{q}_A$ (**a**) and $\mathbf{q}_B$ (**b**) within the rectangular workspace of the chair

Table 2 Joint positions in *pixel* of the *Stephenson III* linkage

Coordinates	$\mathbf{q}_A$	$\mathbf{p}_A^1$	$\mathbf{q}_B$	$\mathbf{p}_B^1$	$\mathbf{p}_{hip}^1$	$\mathbf{p}_{knee}^1$	$\mathbf{q}_{ankle}$
x	1016	1168	1068	1201	1055	1467	1371
y	422	589	357	549	816	663	298

From Table 1 $\mathbf{t}_M^i$ and $\mathbf{R}_M^i(\varphi_{thigh}^i)$ are easily established. Using a dimensional finite position synthesis with $n = 3$ task positions we selected task position 1, 3 and 5 from Table 1. These values were inserted into an exhaustive search algorithm implemented in MATLAB to find a set of values for $\mathbf{q}_A$ and $\mathbf{q}_B$. Figure 7a and b display the exhaustive search results for $\mathbf{q}_A$ and $\mathbf{q}_B$ respectively. Each task position is varied within a range of values deduced from the images. In addition, values for $\mathbf{p}_A^1$ and $\mathbf{p}_B^1$ are varied within a range close to the seat. The range in the x and y-axis represents the available space within the chair.

From the exhaustive search two random points were chosen for $\mathbf{q}_A$ and $\mathbf{q}_B$. Combined with the joint positions of the hip, knee and ankle joint we receive the following *Stephenson III* configuration shown in Table 2. Finally we were able to analyze the 7R linkage structure using the mentioned *Newton-Raphson* method. The results are seen in Table 2 and Fig. 8. Using φ_{thigh} as the input angle produced a $\Delta\varphi_{hip}$ range of 3.2° between 172–155° of φ_{thigh}, which corresponds to the first 15% of STS movement.

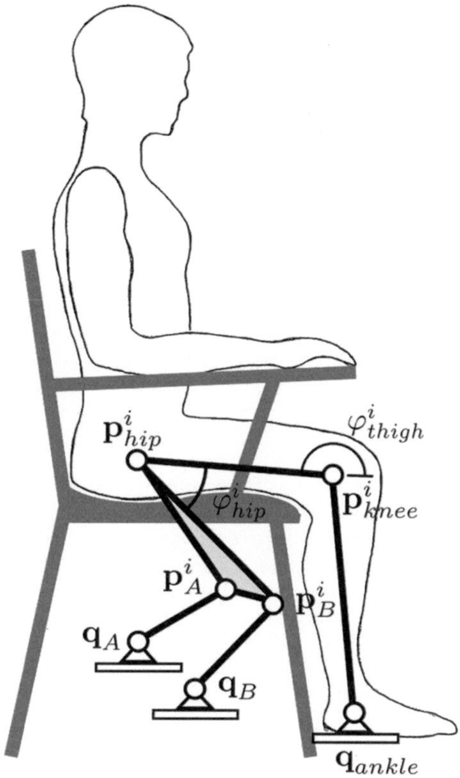

Fig. 8 Individualized four-bar linkage attached to the lower limb model based on the results shown in Table 2

6 Discussion

In this contribution we explained the outline of necessary design steps to synthesize a bio-kinematic LAD. Herein, we analyze a kinematic six-bar linkage that combines both mechanical elements with biological elements of the user to improve support of the STS movement. A four-bar linkage is individualized to the biomechanical parameters of the user and the amount of support the user needs. In the future, a physiotherapist or doctor could determine the extent of lift support and therefore define the task positions of the four-bar linkage and the power that actuates the structure. The swiftly growing rapid prototyping industry could be utilized in an effort to automate the manufacturing process. A kinetostatic analysis is required to analyze the power required to lift the user from the chair and to calculate the forces acting on the joints.

The experiment showed a high density of fixed pivot points within the workspace of the chair that satisfies Eq. (1) within the given range of task positions. However, more experiments are necessary to validate if Eq. (1) satisfies with our hypothesis. A possible design alternative consists of the original kinematic structure presented in Fig. 3d. Here, φ_{hip} is fixed and a prismatic joint is attached to the seat.

We must also emphasize limits to the conceptual design procedure. Given multiple constraints such as workspace and user-specificity there exist a great number of individual parameters that increase the computational cost of an exhaustive search exponentially. In addition, the exhaustive search does not guarantee a solution. Scenarios in which no solutions are found have not been taken into consideration yet as this could require potential changes to the general kinematic structure. Additionally, human parameters such as the ankle, knee an hip joints are modeled as mechanical rotation joints with one DOF. While this simplifies the model it might falsify the actual movement of the lower limb.

Based on kinematic theory this design procedure shows that individualization procedures are possible. This is particularly interesting with regard to the rapidly growing field of wearable devices such as exoskeleton robots. An ergonomic human-machine interface that allows the full range of motion of the human limbs is crucial to the wearability of external devices.

Acknowledgements The authors would like to express their sincere gratitude to the *Alfried Krupp von Bohlen und Halbach-Stiftung* for their generous financial support of this project. In addition, we are extremely grateful to Dr. Stefan Arend, Michael Pfitzer and the staff of the nursing home, *Kuratorium Wohnen im Alter, Luise-Kiesselbach-Haus*, whose insight and feedback has been invaluable to our research. Last but least, we give special thanks to our colleagues Jonas Joachimmeyer, Joachim Kreutzer and Christina Hein for all of their unprecedented support.

References

1. Alexander, N.B., Gross, M.M., Medell, J.L., Hofmeyer, M.R.: Effects of functional ability and training on chair-rise biomechanics in older adults. J. Gerontol. Ser. A: Biol. Sci. Med. Sci. **56**(9), M538–M547 (2001)
2. D'Angelo, L.T., Abdul-Sater, K., Pfluegl, F., Lueth, T.C.: Wheelchair models with integrated transfer support mechanisms and passive actuation. J. Med. Dev. **9**(1), 011,012-1-13 (2015)
3. Ellis, M.I., Seedhom, B.B., Wright, V.: Forces in the knee joint whilst rising from a seated position. J. Biomed. Eng. **6**(2), 113–120 (1984)
4. Kralj, A., Jaeger, R., Munih, M.: Analysis of standing up and sitting down in humans: definitions and normative data presentation. J. Biomech. **23**(11), 1123–1138 (1990)
5. Mak, M.K., Levin, O., Mizrahi, J., Hui-Chan, C.W.: Joint torques during sit-to-stand in healthy subjects and people with Parkinsons disease. Clin. Biomech. **18**(3), 197–206 (2003)
6. McCarthy, J., Michael, J., Soh, G.S.: Geometric Design of Linkages, 2nd edn. Springer, New York (2011)
7. Nair, S.P., Gibbs, S., Arnold, G., Abboud, R., Wang, W.: A method to calculate the centre of the ankle joint: a comparison with the Vicon Plug-in-Gait model. Clin. Biomech. (Bristol, Avon) **25**(6), 582–587 (2010)
8. Pollack, M.E.: Intelligent technology for an aging population: the use of AI to assist elders with cognitive impairment (2005)
9. Wretenberg, P., Lindberg, F., Arborelius, U.P.: Effect of armrests and different ways of using them on hip and knee load during rising. Clin. Biomech. (Bristol, Avon) **8**(2), 95–101 (1993)

Organising Bodyformation of Modular Autonomous Robots Using Virtual Embryogenesis

M. Daushan, R. Thenius, K. Crailsheim and Th. Schmickl

Abstract In this paper the ability of Virtual Embryogenesis system (VE) to initiate and facilitate the build process of a multi-robot organism is presented. According to a single genome, which is spread in the whole organism, substances (morphogenes) are diffused to all neighbouring robots within the organism and new modules are recruited to advance the building process. Different shapes can be built by this system using different, pre-evolved genomes. This ability to build a robotic modular organism is very stable and is not influenced by the environment the controlling genome has evolved in. The presented method is suggested to control modular robots in future applications in dynamic environments, e.g., in interaction with humans.

Keywords Selfassembling robots · Mechatronic design · Autonomous robots · Virtual Embryogenesis

1 Introduction

The method to build autonomous artificial organisms using mobile robotic units (Fig. 1), which have to organise themselves also autonomously (preferentially in a decentral selforganised manner) has been intensely investigated in recent years [5, 14, 19, 29]. A group of individual robots, be it as a swarm of autonomous mobile robotic units, or as a linked robotic organism, is more than the pure sum of its parts. The possibility to dock robots together to a multifunctional organism unlocks a new series of options to solve technical problems [13].

Besides others, one possible task for such groups of autonomous robots is to operate as assistance devices for humans. Autonomous modular robots have the advantage to be able to generate a big variety of "body-shapes", and based on this, perform a even bigger variety of tasks. With this task in mind, one can see the advantages of both configuration modes—swarm and organism. For some tasks, e.g., Cleaning, searching objects, using the mechanics of a swarm, thus increasing the

M. Daushan · R. Thenius (✉) · K. Crailsheim · Th. Schmickl
Karl-Franzens-Universität Graz, Universitätsplatz 2, 8010 Graz, Austria
e-mail: ronald.thenius@uni-graz.at

M. Husty and M. Hofbaur (eds.), *New Trends in Medical and Service Robots*,
Mechanisms and Machine Science 48, DOI 10.1007/978-3-319-59972-4_6

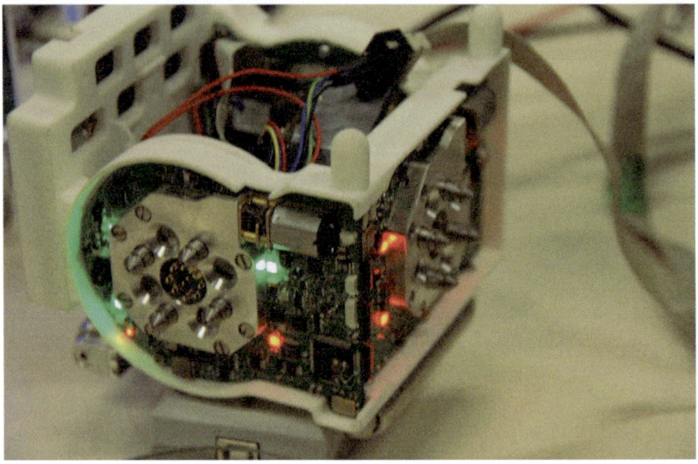

Fig. 1 Mobile autonomous robotic module, developed in the project SYMBRION (please see [29])

searchable space by the number of individuals searching. On the other hand some tasks may require a solid robotic organism, e.g., as a chair or table. The design of such an organism should be closely reflecting the situation this organism is applied to. Several strategies have been investigated to deal with these emerging difficulties [5, 15, 21, 22].

Our approach to this problem is a process of Virtual Embryogenesis (VE) (e.g., [35]) which results in the shape of a multi-robot organism using evolutionary computation. Evolution has been solving these very problems for a long time and provides us with a wealth of inspiring examples for the design and shaping of organisms.

The long tradition of modelling embryogenesis processes in both Biology and Computer Science goes back to Turing [36], one of the grounding fathers of modern Computer Science, who also created one of the first models in this field. Our methodology is constructed to mimic the most basic processes found in real-life embryogenesis and is based on the approach of Evolutionary Developmental Biology (EvoDevo) [1, 2, 17, 38]. The model is implemented as a two-dimensional multi agent simulation in which each cell represents an agent that acts upon its respective individual status and also reacts to the input from surrounding agents. Each cell chooses one or several actions per time step from a catalogue of activities, based on the inputs from the other agents. Encoded in these activities is a genome provided for each individual embryo consisting of several cells. Our VE is natively designed to allow individual cells to connect to each other thus forming an Artificial Neuronal Network (ANN) [31, 35]. This aspect is disregarded in this work, because our focus lies on he morphological aspects of the system. Substances emitted by each cell, the morphogens, trigger the forming of the embryo through genome based behaviours in cells and thus allow specialization of cells which may lead to the development of different tissues within the developing embryo. These behaviours consist of: proliferation (duplication), change of sensitivity to a certain morphogen and the emittance of morphogens. Morphogens spread throughout our virtual embryo via a simplified diffusion process [3, 8, 40, 41]. The resulting gradients in the morphogen act inter alia as positional cues for the cells. A primary gradient [6, 26], emitted by the first cell, which lies in the center of the virtual grid, is provided in each simulation to support this. This behaviour can have three different effects: lateral, vertical and omnidirectional proliferation. Duplication is limited to zero or once each timestep for each cell. The direction chosen from the three possibilities is the direction holding the minimal number of cells. This is done to emphasize the weight of the surrounding cells to the currently duplicating cell. However, if the border of the simulation environment is reached, duplication is prevented in this direction. In contrast to the experiments presented in [4] the environment used in this work is set to a grid of 20 times 20 spatial units, each able to host one agent. This limits the possible outcome of the VE-process to small-scale robotic organisms, which is desirable in our case of building robotic organisms, due to the usual limitation of only a few available robots. To shape a genome for a task as described above, it is necessary to evolve it in an artificial evolutionary system. This brings a known problem into play: controllers developed by artificial evolution in a simulator are separated from application in the "real world" by a so called "reality gap" (e.g., [16]): Every creature, artificial or natural, is always optimised for survival in the physical or virtual environment it evolved. Smallest changes in the physical laws of the environment (e.g., differences in sensor noise between simulation and real world, non-linearity in friction or control of actuators), often lead to a vast loss of efficiency or a complete functional breakdown. In this work we want to show how the VE-process deals with this reality gap.

2 Materials and Methods

2.1 Implementation

The first implementation of the VE paradigm was done in NetLogo [39] to provide a solid base for rapid prototyping and immediate visualization of results [35].

To enable fast computation and to consider certain hardware requirements of the robots a C++ implementation has been developed including all core features of the original NetLogo version. Earlier results of this implementation process were reported in [4]. A short overview over the results of these first experiments is given here, for more details please see [4]. Following an object oriented approach [23] the program consists of a set of classes working scheduled from each other on their given tasks. To represent cells within the virtual two-dimensional world, class 'CellController' has been created. This class was designed to represent a cell within the VE simulation but also to be able to correspond to a robot within a multi-robot organism. To distinguish between these two different situations, the class includes a boolean variable that indicates whether it is executed in robot-mode. We do not use the inheritance concept of C++ [28] as one of our aims is to show that the exact same system, meaning the exact same class that runs on recent computer hardware, is also able to be executed on robotic hardware.

A more detailed description of the VE paradigm is given in [33, 35]. For further details about the features and the fields of usage for VE please see [10, 24, 30, 32].

2.2 Cellular Behaviour

We simulate the embryo as a multi-agent model, in which a single cell is represented by an agent. The space in our model is discrete (see Fig. 3), organised in so called "patches". Each patch can be occupied by only one cell. Cells interact with each other via virtual physics (e.g., limitation of space) and via virtual chemistry. Morphogenes are emitted by cells and diffuse throughout the embryo [3]. The concentration $c_{m,x,y,t}$ of a morphogene m at the position x, y at time step t is calculated according to

$$c_{m,x,y,t} = min(c_{max,m}, cn_{m,x,y,t-1} - d_m), \tag{1}$$

whereby $c_{max,m}$ is the maximum concentration of a morphogene m, $cn_{m,x,y,t}$ is the maximum concentration of the morphogene m in the cell at the position x, y and in all neighbouring cells ("Von Neumann" neighbourhood), at the time step t. The amount of the decrease of the morphogene concentration when diffusing from one cell to another is d_m. When a cell at position x, y emits a morphogene, its value for $c_{m,x,y,t}$ is set according to

$$c_{m,x,y,t} = c_{max,m}. \tag{2}$$

Please note, that no conservation of mass is implemented in our model. This simplification of real physical diffusion processes is necessary to achieve the required computational speed. The results of this abstract diffusion model suffices for our needs to achieve the desired embryogenesis.

2.3 Simulated Genetics

In our model, a cell measures the concentrations of morphogenes every time step and reacts in a preprogrammed way. The concentration of a morphogene needed to trigger a reaction as well as the triggered type of reaction is specified in the genome of the cell. The genome N is a set of n genes G (see Eq. 3). Each gene is a tuple of numeric values (see Eq. 4). These values determine which cell-reaction r is triggered, if a defined morphogene s is present with a concentration higher than c_{min} and lower than c_{max} at the position of the cell in the embryo. All cells share the same genome, which does not change during the embryogenetic process.

$$N = \{G_1, \dots, G_n\} \tag{3}$$

$$G_n = (s, c_{min}, c_{max}, r) \tag{4}$$

The reactions r of cells can be as follows: emission of a morphogene, cell duplication, changes in responsiveness.

Our "genes" are triggered by morphogenes, which is comparable to the mechanisms of gene expression and protein synthesis found in nature. Especially the concepts of second-messenger mechanisms [7] and transcription-coregulator mechanisms found in biological cells [18] were used in a very simplified way for our concept of virtual embryology.

Morphogenes can not only influence the growth of the embryo by inducing cell duplication, but they can also change internal status variables of cells. These values can code for the receptivity for another morphogene or for properties that are necessary for the function of the resulting Bodyshape (e.g., if a cell hase to move its hinge or not).

2.4 Simulated Physics

In case of cell duplication the new cell is placed on one free patch close by. For the given model effects like cell cohesion or pushing of cells were not implemented. This step of reduction of model complexity (compared to the model presented in [35]) was necessary to allow a reduction of the solution space to allow to run the given model on real world robotic hardware.

2.5 Evolution Controller

To find a genome resulting in an embryo that matches an assumed ideal shape, evolutionary computation is applied. Two additional classes are added to the program—class 'Generation' and class 'Evolution'. 'Generation' is in charge of the calculation and administration of all individuals belonging to one generation. As output several created genomes are handed over to 'Evolution' that collects all genomes and also picks a start-genome for the upcoming generation. The very first start-genome may be read in or created randomly.

A template schema, currently consisting of 460 cells, is used for internal representation of the maximum fitness within the evolution process. Fitness points are assigned to each individual according to the number of cells lying within or outside the borders of this template schema. For *ingoal* cells which lie within the template pattern one point is awarded whereas for outliers *outgoal* two points are subtracted. The fitness for each embryo is then calculated using

$$fitness = (ingoal - 2 * outgoal)/maxFitness \tag{5}$$

whereby *maxFitness* holds the maximal achievable fitness value. The resulting individual fitness is a value between 0 and 1 with 1 representing a perfect mapping of the template pattern by the embryo. A value of 0 is awarded if the fitness would be negative or more than 90% of the grid is beset with cells which corresponds to uncontrolled growth (cancer). For more information please see [4].

2.6 Robotic Hardware

We use robotic hardware from the SYMBRION [29] and REPLICATOR [19] EU projects, in particular the robots designed by the Karlsruhe Institute for Technology. These are cubical robots with docking elements, proximity, light and docking sensors on four sides and are described extensively in [11, 12]. Due to their cubical form and their ability to dock to other robots in each direction in 2D, they perfectly correspond to our 2D VE where each cell may have a maximum of four neighbours. On the bottom of the machines are two actuators to provide mobility [12]. The main controller for the robot is a *Blackfin* (ADSP-BF537E from ANALOG DEVICES) board that includes a fixed point digital signal processor and runs an uCLinux [37] operating system. All relevant sensor and actuator information is handled by a high level API (Application Programming Interface) that can be accessed via a C++ interface. From a electronic point of view these robots are identical with the robots mentioned in [4], but differ in their way of locomotion. The tested robots have a caterpillar-drive (see top image in Fig. 4) what allows them to move faster then the robots using a screw-drive, mentioned in [4]. For more details about the mentioned robotic platform please see [19, 29].

3 Experiments and Results

For our applications, VE on multi-robot organisms and evolutionary computation using the C++ version of VE, first results could be obtained.

3.1 Virtual Embryogenesis

The implementation of VE in C++ is able to produce forms similar to a provided template schema using evolutionary computation. These results can be compared with those obtained by using the NetLogo program as the two versions use the same most basic ruleset (see Sect. 1, [35]). Due to the higher complexity in the choice of start genome for each generation and individual reproduction process in the NetLogo implementation, differences in the results build up over time. One of the resulting forms and it's corresponding ideal template schema are shown in Fig. 2.

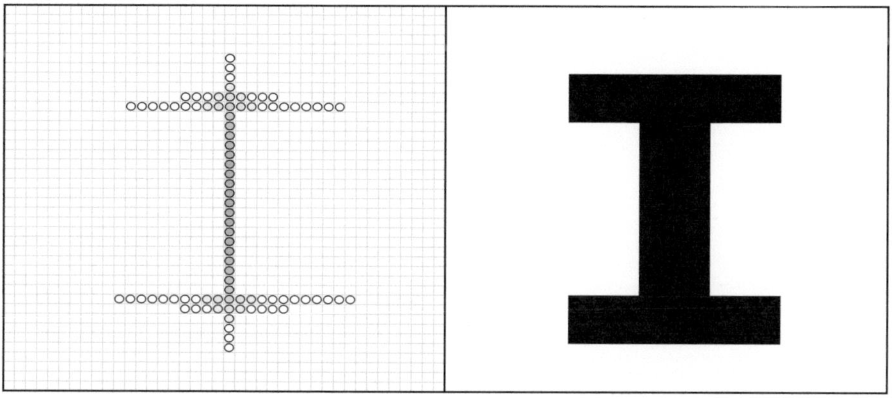

Fig. 2 Plot of a resulting embryo showing the gradient of morphogen 0 in *green* (*left* figure). This shape was produced by assigning fitness points according to the similarity to the template schema depicted in the figure on the *right* side. For each *ingoal* cell one point is awarded whereas two points are subtracted for each cell that overshoots the template pattern (*outgoal*). Resulting negative fitness values for the embryo are set to be zero. Figures from [4]

Fig. 3 Shape of a "snake-like" VE organism, evolved in a simulation environment. *Circles* indicate the position of cells, the *grid* indicates the possible position of cells

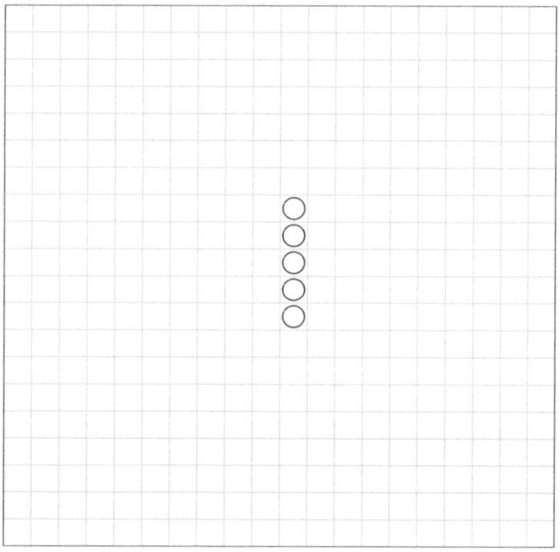

3.2 Test of VE on Swarm of Real-World Robots to Control Body Formation Based on Artificial Evolution

To test the abilities of the VE to organise the process of building a robotic organism consisting of different autonomous robotic units as described in Sect. 2.6.

Three experiments were performed:

1. **Test of VE under conditions of low calculation power**. We tested for the ability of the robots to generate a body-shape with a given genome, using only the limited on-board hardware capacities of the robots' *Blackfin* processor. This first

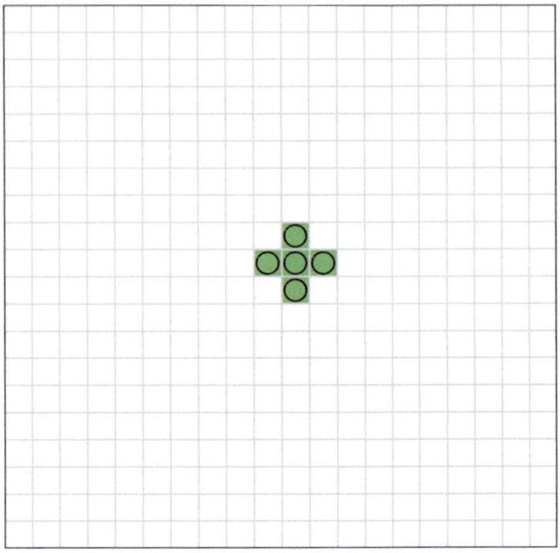

Fig. 4 Shape of a "cross-like" VE organism, evolved in a simulation environment. *Circles* indicate the position of cells, the *grid* indicates the possible position of cells

experiment aimed for a test for the feasibility of the usage of the VE in the given robotic hardware.

2. **Test of VE to cross the reality gap**. In this experiment we investigated if a simple body-shape, which was evolved in a simulation on a standard PC, can be build by the VE process on-board a autonomous robot.
3. **Test of VE to build complex shapes with real-world robotic hardware**. We tested if the VE is also able to built more complex body-shapes. Again the body-shape was evolve on a standard PC in a simulation environment, and then tested on real-world robots.

3.2.1 Test of VE Under Conditions of Low Calculation Power

It showed, that due to the low computational requirements of the VE paradigm, the algorithm is highly suitable for the processors used in the robots of [19, 29]. The process of developing a body-shape on-board a robot using the VE-simulator on the main processor (for hardware details please see Sect. 2.6) needed less than 200 ms. This shows, that the VE works well in an "on-board" situation, and is suitable even for on-board evolutionary developments of body shapes.

3.2.2 Test of VE to Cross the Reality Gap

A simple body-shape for the robotic organism was evolved on a PC (see Fig. 3). The genome was transferred to a robotic unit. Figure 5 shows the resulting building process: The genome of the VE controls the building process by turning on and of visible docking signals on the appropriate side of the autonomous robotic module. As soon as the new module has docked, the genome is transferred to the new module,

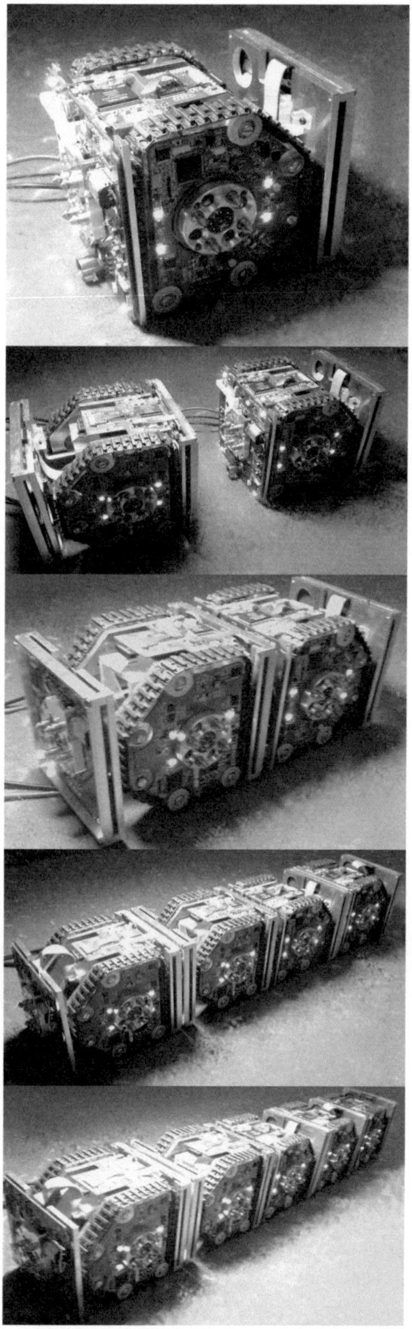

Fig. 5 Growth of a "snake-like" robotic organism, consisting of mobile autonomous robotic units. The growth process is controlled by the VE-algorithm. The genome steering this process was developed in a simple simulation. The outcome of the growth process controlled by the genome with this simulation is depicted in Fig. 3. It shows, that the body shapes of both organisms, in simulation and in real-world, are identical

the information about the current status of the morphogen levels is transferred. In the next step the VE process calculates the new levels of the morphogen in every module of the robotic organism. Please note, that this calculation is done autonomously in every robotic unit (as described in [4]). The resulting new "pattern" of docking signals leads to new robots that dock to the robotic organism: the organism grows. This circle of docking, transferring morphogens and recruiting new modules to join the organism continues until all docking signals are turned off by the genome.

3.2.3 Test of VE to Build Complex Shapes

In this experiment a more complex body-shape was evolved on a PC (see Fig. 4). As described in experiment 2 (see Sect. 3.2.2), the genome was transferred to a autonomous robotic unit, and the growth process of the robotic organism was observed. It showed, that the VE process had no problem to create a robotic organism according to the shape of the virtual embryo evolved in the simulation.

4 Discussion and Outlook

In the work at hand we show that the VE paradigm is suitable for evolving body shapes for a real-world modular robotic organism in an artificial environment. The problem of the "reality gap", mentioned in Sect. 1 is circumvented by the fact that all processes steering the growth of the robotic organism (flow of morphogens between modules (or cells), parsing of the genome) operate on a virtual level, be it in the simulation or on the real-world robotic module. This allows to evolve genomes that produce identical body shapes, in simulation as well as in reality (as depicted in Figs. 3, 4, 5, and 6).

Our bio-inspired VE process shown in this work performs well in both design and construction of multi-robot organisms. Previous investigations in swarm robotics use global information to a large extent [21, 22]. This information consists of the exact positional data of every robot at all time steps. A lot of work that has been don in the field of bio-inspired works on shape development processes depends on the existence of a global positioning system, that often encodes positional information in the genome [9, 20, 25, 42]. Contrasting that, our approach of self-organisation has no necessary requirement of a single robot to be aware of its position at each time step. Positional cues in our organisms are available using morphogen gradients [6, 26] that are based on pure neighbour to neighbour communication. During construction of the organism each robot is equally suited to extend the organism by docking to it. These features of VE provide a high resilience to faults for building virtual and robotic organisms.

As a next step we plan to implement a complete evolutionary algorithm on-board a single robotic unit, and allow it to evolve a body shape for a robotic organism to be built autonomously. We also plan to use the abilities of the VE to control

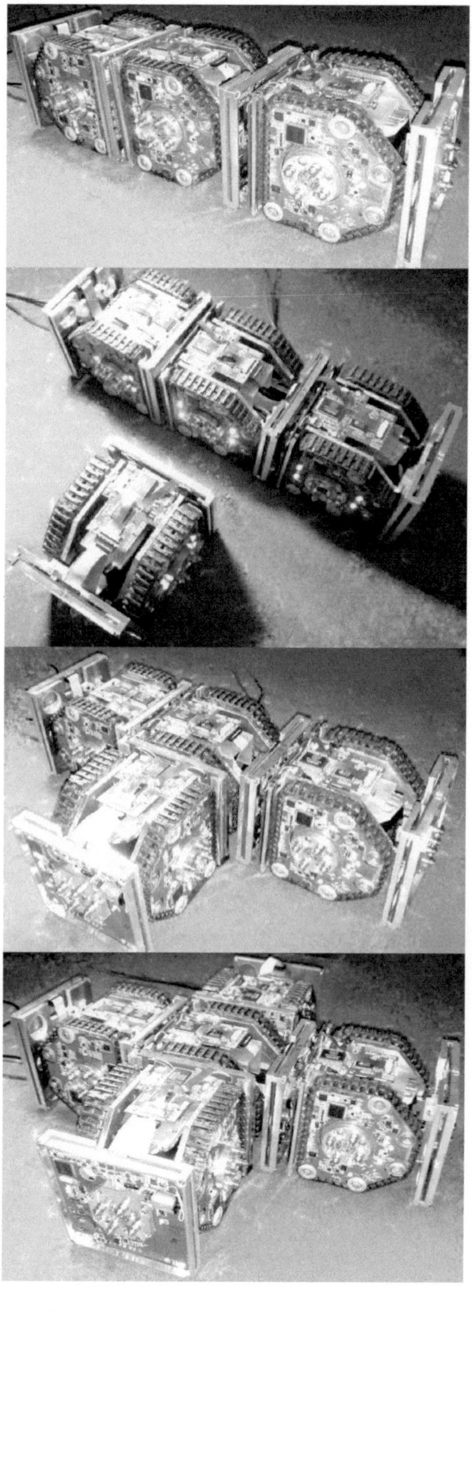

Fig. 6 Growth of a "cross-like" robotic organism, consisting of mobile autonomous robotic units. The outcome of the growth process controlled by the same genome with the simulation is depicted in Fig. 4

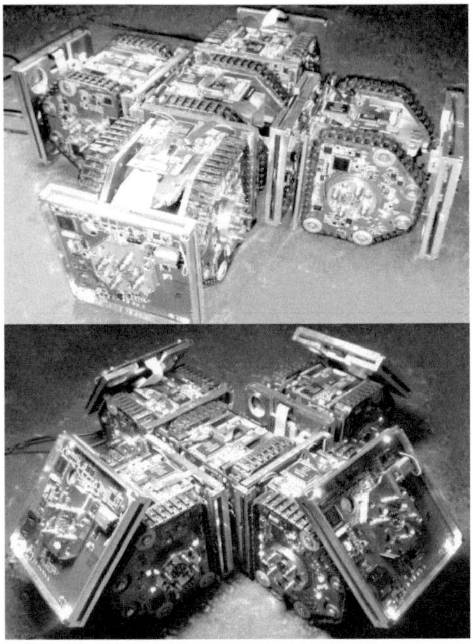

Fig. 7 First experiments with the VE system controlling the movement of the robotic organisms after building. Hinges of individual robotic units can be activated according to a given morphogen concentration

individual agents (as mentioned in [4]) to steer an organism. First investigations and experiments (depicted in Fig. 7) show, that movement of the robotic organism can also be controlled by the same genome, that is able to steers individual agents as well as control the building of the bodyshape [27]. To what degree this described method is able to control all three states of a swarm of modular robots (which are "swarm of autonomous robotic units", "immobile robotic organism while building" and "mobile autonomous robotic organism") is under investigation at the moment. Further plans contain investigations, into the extent a VE system can be used to not only shape robotic organisms, but also the internal controller of an agent (e.g., an ANN as described in [35]. We also plan to test the regenerative abilities of VE (described in [34]) on robotic hardware.

Acknowledgements This work was supported by: EU-ICT project REPLICATOR, no. 216240; EU H2020 FET-Proactive project 'subCULTron', no. 640967.

References

1. Carroll, S.B.: Endless forms: the evolution of gene regulation and morphological diversity. Cell **101**(6), 577–580 (2000)
2. Carroll, S.B.: Endless Forms Most Beautiful: The New Science of Evo Devo. W. W. Norton (2006)

3. Crick, F.: Diffusion in embryogenesis. Nature **225**(5231), 420–422 (1970). doi:10.1038/225420a0
4. Dauschan, M., Thenius, R., Schmickl, T., Crailsheim, K.: Using virtual embryogenesis multi-robot organisms. In: International Conference on Adaptive and Intelligent Systems, ICAIS'11, Klagenfurt, AT, 06–08 Sept 2011. Proceedings, pp. 238–247 (2011)
5. Dorigo, M., Tuci, E., Groß, R., Trianni, V., Labella, T.H., Nouyan, S., Ampatzis, C., Deneubourg, J.L., Baldassarre, G., Nolfi, S., Mondada, F., Floreano, D., Gambardella, L.M.: The SWARM-BOTS project. In: Proceeding of Swarm Robotics, SAB 2004 International Workshop, Santa Monica, pp. 31–44. Springer (2005). http://www.springerlink.com/content/e4klufrqeqe6nvc2
6. Ephrussi, A., Johnston, D.S.: Seeing is believing—the bicoid morphogen gradient matures. Cell **116**(2), 143–152 (2004). doi:10.1016/S0092-8674(04)00037-6
7. Gomperts, B.D., Kramer, I.M., Tatham, P.E.R.: Signal Transduction. Academic Press (2002)
8. Gurdon, J.B., Bourillot, P.Y.: Morphogen gradient interpretation. Nature **413**(6858), 797–803 (2001). doi:10.1038/35101500
9. Jin, Y., Schramm, L., Sendhoff, B.: A gene regulatory model for the development of primitive nervous systems. In: Proceedings of the 15th International Conference on Advances in Neuro-Information Processing—Volume Part I, ICONIP'08, pp. 48–55. Springer, Berlin (2009)
10. Kernbach, S., Hamann, H., Stradner, J., Thenius, R., Schmickl, T., Crailsheim, K., van Rossum, A., Sebag, M., Bredeche, N., Yao, Y., Baele, G., de Peer, Y.V., Timmis, J., Mohktar, M., Tyrrell, A., Eiben, A., McKibbin, S., Liu, W., Winfield, A.F.: On adaptive self-organization in artificial robot organisms. In: The First International Conference on Adaptive and Self-adaptive Systems and Applications (ADAPTIVE'09). IEEE Press (2009)
11. Kernbach, S., Schmickl, T., Hamann, H., Stradner, J., Schwarzer, C., Schlachter, F., Winfield, A.F., Matthias, R.: Adaptive action selection mechanisms for evolutionary multimodular robotics. In: Fellermann, H., Dörr, M., Hanczyc, M.M., Laursen, L.L., Maurer, S., Merkle, D., Monnard, P.A., Støy, K., Rasmussen, S. (eds.) Artificial Life XII (ALife XII), pp. 781–788. MIT Press (2010)
12. Kernbach, S., Scholz, O., Harada, K., Popesku, S., Liedke, J., Raja, H., Liu, W., Caparrelli, F., Jemai, J., Havlik, J., Meister, E., Levi, P.: Multi-robot organisms: state of the art. In: ICRA10, workshop on "Modular Robots: State of the Art", Anchorage (2010)
13. Kornienko, S., Kornienko, O., Nagarathinam, A., Levi, P.: From real robot swarm to evolutionary multi-robot organism. In: Srinivasan, D., Wang, L. (eds.) 2007 IEEE Congress on Evolutionary Computation, pp. 1483–1490. IEEE (2007). http://ieeexplore.ieee.org/lpdocs/epic03/wrapper.htm?arnumber=4424647
14. Levi, P., Kernbach, S. (eds.): Symbiotic Multi-Robot Organisms: Reliability, Adaptability, Evolution. Springer (2010)
15. Mondada, F., Floreano, D., Gambardella, L.M.: The SWARM-BOTS project. Lect. Notes Comput. Sci. **3342**, 31–44 (2005)
16. Moran, I.F., Moreno, A., Merelo, J., Chacon, P. (eds.): Noise and the Reality Gap: The Use of Simulation in Evolutionary Robotics. Springer (1995)
17. Müller, G.B.: Evo-devo: extending the evolutionary synthesis. Nat. Rev. Genet. **8**, 943–949 (2007)
18. Näär, A.M., Lemon, B., Tjian, R.: Transcriptional coactivator complexes. Annu. Rev. Biochem. **70**, 475–501 (2001)
19. REPLICATOR: Project website (2012). http://www.replicators.eu
20. Roggen, D., Federici, D., Floreano, D.: Evolutionary morphogenesis for multi-cellular systems. Genet. Program. Evolvable Mach. **8**, 61–96 (2007). doi:10.1007/s10710-006-9019-1
21. Rubenstein, M., Shen, W.M.: Scalable self-assembly and self-repair in a collective of robots. In: Proceedings of the IEEE/RSJ International Conference on Intelligent Robots and Systems (IROS), St. Louis, Missouri, USA (2009)
22. Rubenstein, M., Shen, W.M.: Automatic scalable size selection for the shape of a distributed robotic collective. In: iros-10, pp. 508–513 (2010)

23. Rumbaugh, J., Blaha, M., Premerlani, W., Eddy, F., Lorenson, W.: Object-Oriented Modeling and Design, 1st edn. Prentice Hall, Inc. (1991)
24. Schmickl, T., Thenius, R., Stradner, J., Hamann, H., Crailsheim, K.: Robotic organisms: artificial homeostatic hormone system and virtual embryogenesis as examples for adaptive reaction-diffusion controllers. In: Kernbach, S., Fitch R. (eds.) IROS 2011 Workshop–Reconfigurable Modular Robotics: Challenges of Mechatronic and Bio-Chemo-Hybrid Systems (2011)
25. Schramm, L., Jin, Y., Sendhoff, B.: Evolutionary synthesis and analysis of a gene regulatory network for dynamically stable growth and regeneration. BioSystems (2010). Submitted
26. Shvartsman, S.Y., Coppey, M., Berezhkovskii, A.M.: Dynamics of maternal morphogen gradients in drosophila. Curr. Opin. Genet. Dev. **18**(4), 342–347 (2008)
27. Stradner, J., Thenius, R., Zahadat, P., Hamann, H., Crailsheim, K., Schmickl, T.: Algorithmic requirements for swarm intelligence in differently coupled collective systems. Chaos, Solitons Fractals (2013). Accepted for publication
28. Stroustrup, B.: The C++ Programming Language, 3rd edn. Addison-Wesley Longman Publishing Co., Inc., Boston, MA, USA (2000)
29. SYMBRION: Project website (2012). http://www.symbrion.eu
30. Thenius, R., Bodi, M., Schmickl, T., Crailsheim, K.: Evolving virtual embryogenesis to structure complex controllers. PerAdaMagazine (2009). doi:10.2417/2201009.003291
31. Thenius, R., Bodi, M., Schmickl, T., Crailsheim, K.: Growth of structured artificial neural networks by virtual embryogenesis. In: Kampis, G., Karsai, I., Szathmáry, E. (eds.) ECAL (2), Lecture Notes in Computer Science, vol. 5778, pp. 118–125. Springer (2009)
32. Thenius, R., Bodi, M., Schmickl, T., Crailsheim, K.: Evolving artificial neural networks and artificial embryology. In: Levi, P., Kernbach, S. (eds.) Symbiotic Multi-Robot Organisms: Reliability, Adaptability, Evolution, pp. 266–268. Springer (2010). doi:10.1007/978-3-642-14547-6
33. Thenius, R., Bodi, M., Schmickl, T., Crailsheim, K.: Using virtual embryogenesis for structuring controllers. In: Hart, E., McEwan, C., Timmis, J., Hone, A. (eds.) 9th International Conference on Artificial Immune Systems, ICARIS 2010, Edinburgh, UK, 26–29 July 2010. Proceedings, Lecture Notes in Computer Science, vol. 6209, pp. 312–313. Springer (2010). doi:10.1007/978-3-642-14547-6_27
34. Thenius, R., Dauschan, M., Schmickl, T., Crailsheim, K.: Regenerative abilities in modular robots using virtual embryogenesis. In: International Conference on Adaptive and Intelligent Systems, ICAIS'11, Klagenfurt, AT, 06–08 Sept 2011. Proceedings, pp. 227–237 (2011)
35. Thenius, R., Schmickl, T., Crailsheim, K.: Novel concept of modelling embryology for structuring an artificial neural network. In: Troch, I., Breitenecker, F. (eds.) Proceedings of the MATHMOD, pp. 1821–1831 (2009)
36. Turing, A.M.: The chemical basis of morphogenesis. Philos. Trans. R. Soc. Lond. Ser. B, Biol. Sci. **B237**(641), 37–72 (1952)
37. Ungerer, G., Dionne, J., Durant, M.: uClinux: Embedded Linux/Microcontroller Project (2008). http://www.uclinux.org
38. Weatherbee, S.D., Carroll, S.B.: Selector genes and limb identity in arthropods and vertebrates. Cell **97**(3), 283–286 (1999)
39. Wilensky, U.: Netlogo. Center for Connected Learning and Computer-Based Modeling, Northwestern University. Evanston, IL (1999). http://ccl.northwestern.edu/netlogo/
40. Wolpert, L.: Positional information and the spatial pattern of cellular differentiation. J. Theor. Biol. **25**(1), 1–47 (1969)
41. Wolpert, L.: One hundred years of positional information. Trends Genet. **12**(9), 359–364 (1996). http://view.ncbi.nlm.nih.gov/pubmed/8855666
42. Wolpert, L.: Principles of Development. Oxford University Press (1998)

Sensor and Control Concept for a Wearable Robot for Manual Load Handling Assistance

P. Stelzer, B. Otten, W. Kraus and A. Pott

Abstract Current wearable robots mostly focus on applications in military, rehabilitation and load lifting in the health sector, while they are hardly used in industry and manufacturing. In this paper, a sensor and control concept for a wearable robot for assistance in manual handling of loads in industry is presented. Special requirements such as low costs, direct contact between the human and the load and easy set-up are addressed. A wall-mounted test stand of an actuated elbow joint was built up to evaluate the proposed sensors and control algorithms. By using a torque sensor in the elbow joint as reference it is shown that low cost force sensors in the forearm can be used to measure the human-robot interaction. A torque-based and a velocity-based impedance control approach are compared which allow the user to move freely while not handling any loads and which also allow to incorporate a human command signal for regulation of force support. The former is shown to be superior to the position-based approach. Further, the influence of the human impedance characteristics onto stability of the controllers is discussed.

Keywords Wearable robots · Exoskeletons · Impedance control · Resistive sensors · Manual load handling

1 Introduction

Manual handling of loads (MHL) is a common task for workers in industry, especially in the sector of logistics and transport. According to the European Agency for Safety and Health at Work, MHL is one of the major causes for musculoskeletal

P. Stelzer (✉) · W. Kraus · A. Pott
Fraunhofer Institute for Manufacturing Engineering and Automation (IPA), Stuttgart, Germany
e-mail: patrick.stelzer@ipa.fraunhofer.de

B. Otten
Helmut Schmidt University, Hamburg, Germany
e-mail: ben.otten@hsu-hh.de

M. Husty and M. Hofbaur (eds.), *New Trends in Medical and Service Robots*, Mechanisms and Machine Science 48, DOI 10.1007/978-3-319-59972-4_7

disorders (MSD), which are the most serious health problem affecting European workers, more than 50% reported to suffer from MSD [1].

Current assistance systems focus on avoiding MHL, examples are cranes, rope balancers or fork lifts. However, most MHL tasks are characterized by an immense diversity of load weights, sizes, shapes and environmental conditions at the workplace and therefore require the flexibility and cognition of human workers. To combine the physical strength of the robot with human's flexibility and cognitive capabilities, assistance systems can be attached directly to the worker. Such systems, referred to as exoskeletons or wearable robots, could then reduce work related injuries and increase productivity by reducing the strain on the musculoskeletal system and maintaining the workers performance constant over a full working day. However, industrial applications have special requirements regarding the sensor and control concept. For acceptance of the system by the worker an easy set up is required, that is a complicated or time-consuming sensor placement is not acceptable. The control of the system must be possible in an intuitive way such that the worker is not impeded in his handling task, which in general requires both hands. The used sensors must be reliable, cost-effective and lightweight.

In the last decades numerous research on wearable robots was done, however, mostly for applications in rehabilitation, military and load lifting in the health sector, e.g., [2–4]. For example, the *muscle suit* from Tokyo University [5] is an upper limb exoskeleton for load lifting in the health sector with pneumatic actuators for the elbow, shoulder and hip joint. The system produces a static support force and no detection of user intention is done. Other exoskeletons detect the user intention by using sensors based on electromyography (EMG) or force [6–9]. However, EMG based sensors are known to be unreliable and strongly user-dependent, see e.g., [10], and they have to be attached to the human skin which makes them not suitable for the given application. Force sensors, on the other hand, are more reliable and easy to integrate, however, mostly multiaxial force cells are used which are costly, relatively big and heavy. Recently, the company Innophys announced to produce an upper limb exoskeleton based on the *muscle suit* which can be controlled by the user via an air tube in the mouth, which is not feasible for long operation times.

Regarding control, current exoskeletons mostly use impedance control which is suitable for use in contact tasks [11]. Commonly two implementations of impedance control exist, originally presented as force-based impedance control and position-based impedance control [12], in the following both approaches will be referred to as impedance and admittance control, respectively. Their differences will be discussed below.

In this paper, a control and sensor concept for an exoskeleton for assistance of workers in MHL tasks in industry is presented. The exoskeleton is not supposed to fully compensate load weights or to augment the human wearer's force capabilities, but to reduce the necessary force input by the user and hence maintain performance and health. In contrast to existing systems our concept is based on cost-effective and lightweight force sensors in the front cuff of the forearm brace which

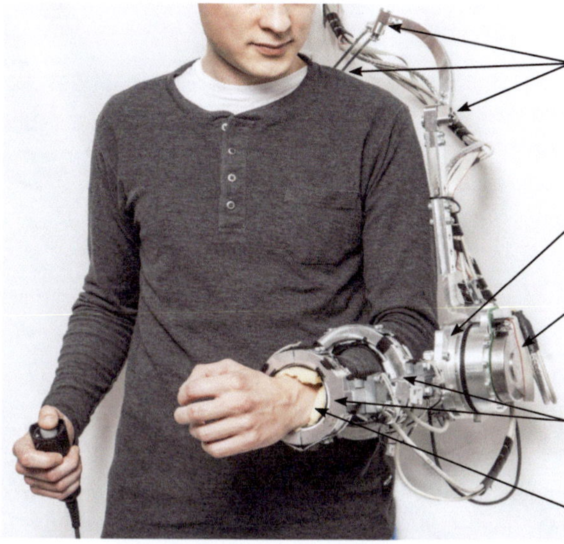

Fig. 1 Wall-mounted test stand of the left arm kinematics with actuated elbow joint, 3-dof shoulder kinematics and forearm brace

can generate a passive movement of the elbow joint according to the worker's intention. An impedance controller is shown to perform better than an admittance controller and stability issues of the control concept are discussed. The control concept allows to incorporate a human control signal for active force support. For this purpose we propose an intelligent sensor glove (see [13, 14]), which is outside the scope of this paper. Hence, the worker does not need to grip a handle or a remote control. For evaluation of the concept a wall-mounted test stand with an actuated elbow joint and a three degree of freedom (dof) shoulder kinematics was built up, see Fig. 1. The actuator is placed directly on the elbow joint to ensure good control performance. The exoskeleton arm is attached to the user via an arm brace at the forearm, consisting of a front and a back cuff. The front cuff comprises a revolute joint allowing pronation and supination of the forearm. Note that this arm exoskeleton is not meant to be wearable, it is used to evaluate the control and sensor concept under constant and repeatable conditions. A body-worn version will be constructed based on the findings of this paper. In Fig. 2 the schematic structure of the system is shown.

The paper is organized as follows: In Sect. 2 the sensor concept for detection of the user intention is presented and verified in measurements, Sect. 3 presents the proposed control algorithms. In Sect. 4 the experimental set-up is described and the proposed controllers are evaluated. Section 5 summarizes the results and gives an outlook.

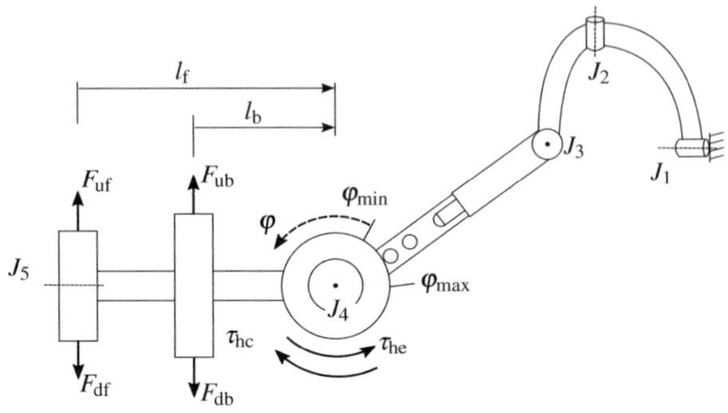

Fig. 2 Schematic structure of the wall-mounted test stand

2 Sensor Concept

In MHL tasks the user needs to grip a a load using his hands, i.e. direct contact between the user and the load is necessary such that the load directly acts on the human hand, not on the exoskeleton construction. In this case force-based sensors at the human-exoskeleton attachment point(s) can only be used to produce a passive movement rather than generate active force support. For this reason, the exoskeleton is supposed to be operated in two different modes. In case the wearer wants to move freely, i.e. if no physical support is required, the exoskeleton must passively follow the wearer's movements and provide full flexibility. This operation mode is referred to as an idle-mode. The second mode, referred to as force-support mode, is given if the user is manually handling loads and needs physical support, i.e. the system must provide force support. In both operating modes the intention of the user needs to be detected. In case of the idle-mode the relevant interaction forces and torques between the user and the exoskeleton can be determined and then transferred to an appropriate movement of the actuated joints. For this purpose, the actuated joints can be equipped with an one-axis torque sensor each. However, to reduce cost and weight, thin-like force sensors in the cuffs of the forearm brace are proposed to replace the torque sensor in the elbow joint. In theory four force sensors, two in each cuff, are necessary to calculate the human-exoskeleton interaction torque τ_{he} around J_4 as

$$\tau_{he} = (F_{df} - F_{uf})\, l_f + (F_{db} - F_{ub})\, l_b, \tag{1}$$

with measured forces in the arm cuffs $F_{df}, F_{uf}, F_{db}, F_{ub}$ and positions of the arm cuffs $l_f = 260$ mm and $l_b = 114$ mm, according to Fig. 2. We propose to use the two sensors in the front cuff only which dominate the measurement as $l_f > l_b$, i.e. reducing the necessary number of sensors by half and reducing the weight of the forearm brace, as the back cuff can be designed much more compact if it does not carry any sensors.

To evaluate this concept the elbow joint was fixed in three different angular positions, an upper, a middle and a lower position. A proband then exerted forces onto the arm brace by pushing its arm up and down. The interaction torque was measured

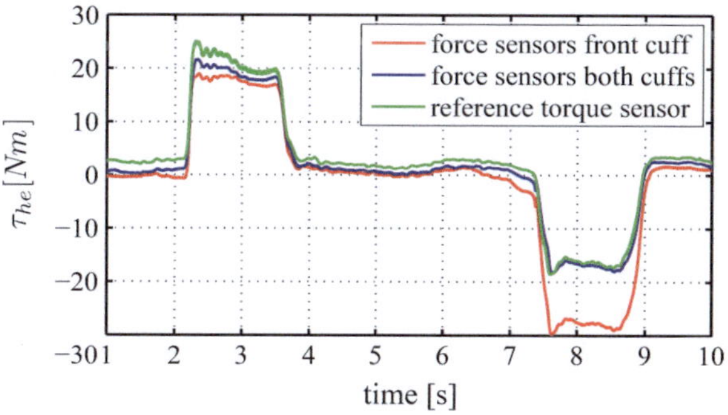

Fig. 3 Human-robot interaction torque for an upward and downward force exertion of the proband

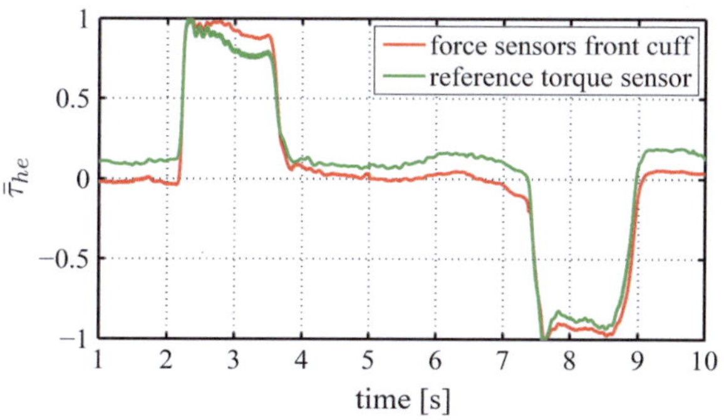

Fig. 4 Normalized human-robot interaction torques measured by the sensors in the front arm cuff and by the torque sensor

using the torque sensor, all four force sensors in both cuffs and only two force sensors in the front cuff. Exemplary for an upward and downward force exertion of the proband the different resulting human-robot interaction torques are depicted in Fig. 3, while the arm brace was fixed in an upper position. In the depicted case, good detection of the human-robot interaction torque using the sensors in both arm cuffs can be observed. However, if we only demand a good qualitative detection of the current desired motion of the human arm rather than the measurement of the precise value of the corresponding interaction torque, using the two sensors in the front cuff is sufficient. This can be seen if we normalize the signals with respect to their maximum absolute value, that is

$$\bar{\tau}_{\mathrm{he}}(t) = \frac{\tau_{\mathrm{he}}(t)}{\max_t(|\tau_{\mathrm{he}}(t)|)}, \tag{2}$$

where $\bar{\tau}_{\mathrm{he}}(t)$ denotes the normalized signal. The normalized signals of the front ring sensors and the torque sensor are depicted in Fig. 4 and show good correlation. Note that the signals of the upward and downward motion were normalized separately.

In the second mode, that is if active force support is required, an additional command signal by the user is necessary, as mentioned above. For this purpose, we propose a sensor glove which provides an intuitive user interface.

3 Control Concept

Two high-level control concepts based on the presented sensor concept are proposed, based on impedance and on admittance control, respectively. Both concepts are (in the linear case) equivalent, however, differences arise in practical implementation. While in admittance control kinematic values are calculated for given forces, in impedance control the inverse calculation is done. The relation between the kinematic and kinetic values is typically given by a second order system, that is both approaches simulate a virtual system in each joint with dynamic behavior

$$J_v \ddot{\varphi}_d + D_v \dot{\varphi}_d + C_v \varphi_d = \tau_{he} - \tau_{hc} =: \tau_h. \tag{3}$$

The angle φ_d denotes the desired elbow joint position, as indicated in Fig. 2. The impedance parameters J_v, D_v and C_v are the desired moment of inertia, damping and stiffness, respectively, for the virtual system, τ_{he} denotes the human-robot interaction torque around the joint and τ_{hc} represents the torque commanded by the user, e.g., by using a sensor glove. The resulting net torque τ_h denotes the total desired torque commanded by the user.

3.1 *Admittance Control Approach*

Based on (3) the proposed admittance control approach calculates a set-point angular velocity for the actuated joints for a measured interaction torque. The angular velocity value is then passed to the low-level motor controller, which carries out velocity control. Velocity control is used as it shows better performance in human-robot cooperation [15], in contrast to position control. Figure 5a depicts the control structure of the admittance control approach. The admittance transfer function can be calculated from (3) as

$$Y(s) = \frac{\mathscr{L}(\dot{\varphi}_d)}{\mathscr{L}(\tau_h)} = \frac{s}{J_v s^2 + D_v s + C_v}, \tag{4}$$

with s denoting the Laplace variable and $\mathscr{L}(\cdot)$ the Laplace transformation. As no static force is desired, stiffness is set to zero, that is $C_v = 0$. It is desirable to set the dynamic parameters for inertia and damping as small as possible in order to achieve high dynamic movements, however, there exist limits in terms of measurement noise and stability. The latter is discussed below. Regarding noise reduction observe that for $C_v = 0$, (4) becomes a first order low-pass filter with cutoff frequency $\omega_c = \frac{D_v}{J_v}$ and static gain $\frac{1}{D_v}$, that is both damping and inertia must be chosen large enough to suppress noise.

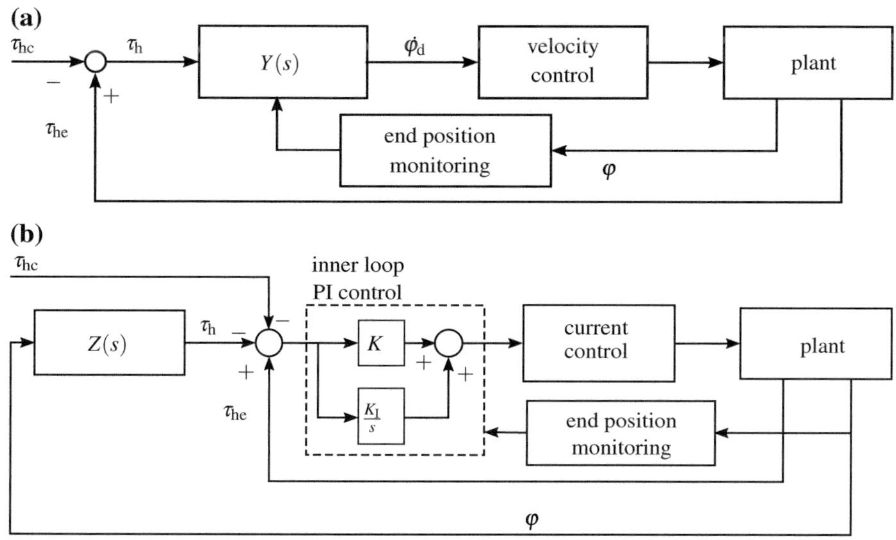

Fig. 5 Structure of **a** the admittance control approach and **b** of the control approach based on impedance control with inner torque control loop

Collision of the robot arm with the end positions is prevented by increasing the damping parameter according to

$$D_v = \begin{cases} D_{v_n} & \text{for} \quad \varphi_{\min} + \gamma < \varphi < \varphi_{\max} - \gamma \\ D_{v_{\max}} \left(1 + \frac{(\varphi_{\min} - \varphi)}{\gamma}\right)^5 + D_{v_n} & \text{for} \quad \varphi \leq \varphi_{\min} + \gamma \\ D_{v_{\max}} \left(1 - \frac{(\varphi_{\max} - \varphi)}{\gamma}\right)^5 + D_{v_n} & \text{for} \quad \varphi \geq \varphi_{\max} - \gamma \end{cases} \tag{5}$$

with elbow angular position φ_d, tuning parameters γ specifying the end zone in which damping increases, D_{v_n} the nominal and $D_{v_{\max}}$ the maximum damping value. Note that damping is only increased if the user's desired movement, indicated by the sign of the interaction torque, is towards the end position.

3.2 *Impedance Control Approach*

In contrast to the admittance control approach presented above, the impedance controller calculates a set-point motor torque, which is fed into the low-level torque controller of the motor controller. Figure 5b depicts the structure of the controller. From (3), the impedance transfer function follows as

$$Z(s) = \frac{\mathscr{L}(\tau_h)}{\mathscr{L}(\varphi)} = J_v s^2 + D_v s + C_v. \tag{6}$$

To achieve high dynamics the impedance parameters are set to zero such that (6) reduces to $\tau_h = 0$, that is the impedance controller degenerates to the special case of a zero torque controller. Even so, it is referred to as impedance controller in the following. To compensate for friction and inertia of the actuator the measured torque is fed back into an inner-loop proportional-integral controller. Note that despite setting the impedance parameters to zero, the system does, of course, not simulate a dynamic behavior corresponding to zero inertia and zero damping. Consider the simplified dynamics of the geared motor joint, that is

$$J\ddot{\varphi} + B\dot{\varphi} + H(\eta) = \tau_h + \tau_m, \tag{7}$$

with inertia J and viscous damping factor B. According to the LuGre model [16], functional H accounts for other friction components, such as hysteresis and the Stribeck effect, and is described by another differential equation with internal state η. Variable τ_m denotes the motor output torque, τ_{hc} is set to zero. Assuming a proportional controller with gain K, it holds $\tau_m = K\tau_h$, hence

$$\frac{J}{1+K}\ddot{\varphi} + \frac{B}{1+K}\dot{\varphi} + \frac{H(\eta)}{1+K} = \tau_h. \tag{8}$$

The inertia and damping felt by the user is hence reduced by the factor $1 + K$.

Collision with the end positions could be prevented by increasing the damping parameter D_v, analogous to the admittance approach. Then, however, online differentiation of the position signal is required, as follows from (6). Alternatively, adjusting the inner-loop PI controller by reducing the proportional gain and setting the integral gain to zero is proposed such that the motor dynamics are scaled according to (8) and the user experiences higher resistance in terms of damping and inertia. For the minimal end position, K is adjusted according to a polynomial function of order four with constraints $K(\varphi_{min} + \frac{\gamma}{2} < \varphi < \varphi_{min} + \gamma) = 0$, $K(\varphi = \varphi_{min}) = -125$ and $K(\varphi = \varphi_{min} - \gamma) = -500$. Similarly, the gain is adjusted when approaching the maximal end position. Anti-windup is used to account for the limitation of the motor current, but not depicted in Fig. 5b.

3.3 On the Stability of the Control Approaches

Various researchers discussed stability of impedance-based controllers in human-robot contact tasks, [17] gives a good overview. In [18] stability of a position based-impedance control was compared to a force-based impedance control in terms of the influence of stiffness and damping, the influence of inertia was outside of the scope. Similarly, in [19] stability of an impedance controller in human-robot

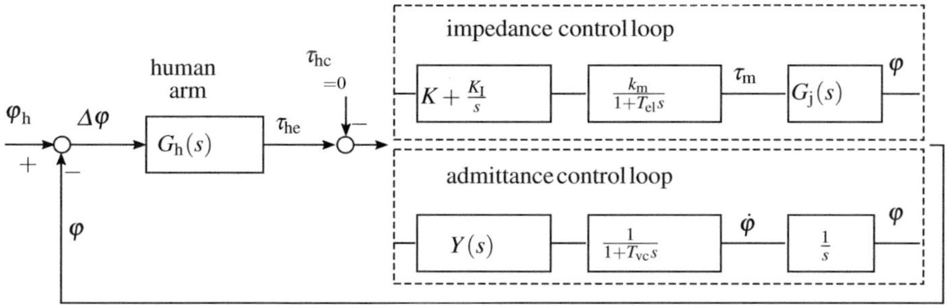

Fig. 6 Linear model of the closed loops of the impedance and admittance controllers

cooperation was investigated. However, influence of inertia and the case with an inner loop controller, as we use in this paper, were not covered.

Stability of the presented impedance-based controllers strongly depends on the human user, who himself is stabilizing the control loop by means of his own impedance characteristics. To achieve stability of the presented admittance and impedance controllers tuning of the impedance parameters and the inner loop proportional gain, respectively, is necessary. To show the influence of these parameters and the human impedance on stability of the given approaches, we derive a linear dynamic model of the control chain. Figure 6 depicts the closed loop of the plant and both the admittance and impedance controller. The human skin muscle model of the arm is modeled as a second-order spring-mass-damper system, similar to the approach in [19], that is

$$G_h(s) = \frac{\mathscr{L}(\tau_{he})}{\mathscr{L}(\Delta\varphi)} = ({l_b}^2 + {l_f}^2)\left(M_h s^2 + D_h s + C_h\right), \tag{9}$$

with human impedance parameters set to $M_h = 0.015\,\text{kg}$, $D_h = 25\,\text{Nsm}^{-1}$ and $C_h = 625\,\text{Nm}^{-1}$, according to [20], and deviation between angular position of the human and the exoskeleton arm $\Delta\varphi = \varphi_h - \varphi$. Note that the impedance parameters need to be scaled by ${l_b}^2 + {l_f}^2$ as they hold for linear deviations Δx_f and Δx_b and forces F_f and F_b acting on the front and back arm cuff, respectively, that is

$$M_h \Delta\ddot{x}_{b,f} + D_h \Delta\dot{x}_{b,f} + C_h \Delta x_{b,f} = F_{b,f}, \tag{10}$$

with $\Delta x_{b,f} = l_{b,f}\sin(\Delta\varphi) \approx l_{b,f}\Delta\varphi$, for small $\Delta\varphi$.

The current and velocity control loops are modeled as first order lags, with time constants determined in measurements as $T_{el} = 0.001$ s and $T_{vc} = 0.01$ s, respectively. The torque constant of the motor is $k_m = 7.05\,\text{NmA}^{-1}$, taking into account the gear ratio. For the dynamics of the joint, viscous damping is assumed, that is

$$G_j(s) = \frac{\mathscr{L}(\varphi)}{\mathscr{L}(\tau_m)} = \frac{1}{J_m s^2 + D_m s}, \tag{11}$$

with viscous damping coefficient $D_\mathrm{m} = 4.5\,\mathrm{Nm\,s\,rad^{-1}}$ and the inertia of the motor and forearm construction calculated as $J_\mathrm{m} = 3\,\mathrm{kgm^2}$ under consideration of the gear ratio.

From Fig. 6 the open loop transfer function of the impedance control loop then calculates as

$$
\begin{aligned}
G_{0\mathrm{I}}(s) &= \frac{\mathcal{L}(\varphi)}{\mathcal{L}(\Delta\varphi)} \\
&= \frac{({l_\mathrm{b}}^2 + {l_\mathrm{f}}^2)k_\mathrm{m}(KM_\mathrm{h}s^3 + (KD_\mathrm{h} + K_\mathrm{I}M_\mathrm{h})s^2 + (KC_\mathrm{h} + K_\mathrm{I}D_\mathrm{h})s + K_\mathrm{I}C_\mathrm{h})}{(J_\mathrm{m}T_\mathrm{el} + D_\mathrm{m}T_\mathrm{el}T_\mathrm{h})s^4 + (D_\mathrm{m}T_\mathrm{el} + J_\mathrm{m})s^3 + D_\mathrm{m}s^2}.
\end{aligned}
\tag{12}
$$

For the given parameter values (12) has two stable poles and two poles in the origin of the complex plane. Stability strongly depends firstly on the human stiffness M_h and secondly on the proportional gain K and the virtual inertia J_v for the impedance and admittance approach, respectively.

Figure 7a gives the Nyquist plots of (12) for varying proportional gains and given human stiffness. Obviously, decreasing the gain leads to instability, in the given case

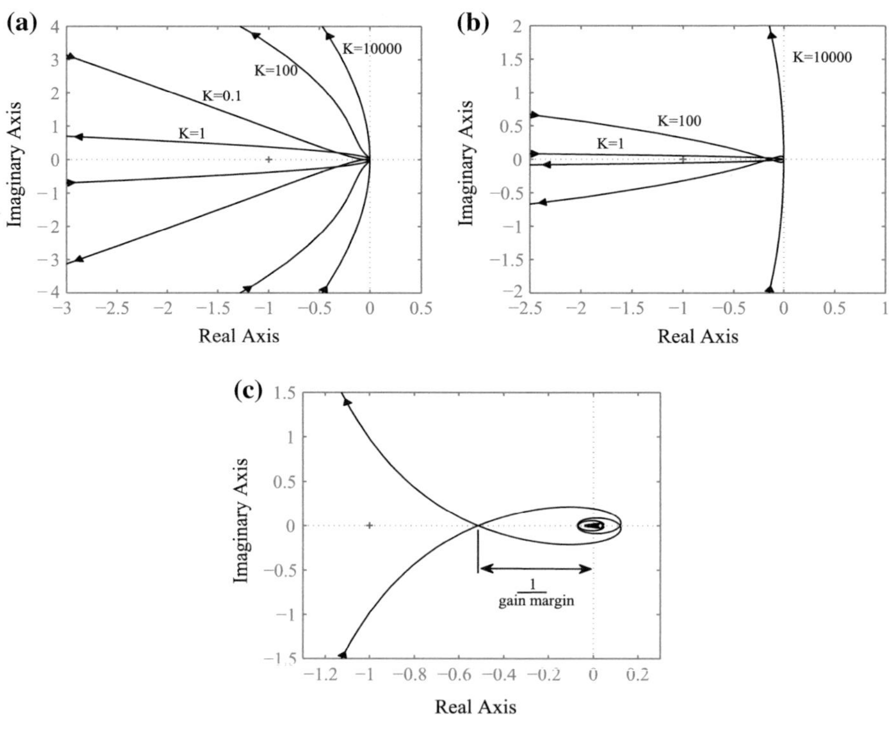

Fig. 7 Nyquist plots of the impedance control open loop for various proportional gains K and fixed human stiffness **a** $C_\mathrm{h} = 625\ \mathrm{Nm^{-1}}$ and **b** $C_\mathrm{h} = 62,500\ \mathrm{Nm^{-1}}$ and **c** in presence of an output time delay of 1 ms

this occurs at $K = 0.1$ (observe the arrows indicating the direction of increase of frequency), according to the Nyquist criterion. Note that due to a double integrator in the open loop the locus needs to be closed at infinity to check for stability. Similarly, in Fig. 7b the Nyquist plots are given for the same gains but a higher human stiffness. In this case, $K = 100$ already leads to instability of the closed loop. Increasing K stabilizes the loop in case of a stiff environment, however, there exist upper bounds. Firstly, oscillations increase due to measurement noise, and secondly, the control loop becomes instable in presence of time delays, e.g., due to communication delays. In Fig. 7c the Nyquist plot of (12) is given, for $K = 250$ and $C_\mathrm{h} = 625\,\mathrm{Nm}^{-1}$. An output time delay of 1 ms is incorporated, representing possible communication delays. The depicted case is stable, however, increasing K by the factor of approx. 2 will give an instable closed loop.

Similar results for stability analysis of the admittance controller are obtained, but not plotted here. Decreasing J_v leads to higher dynamics and a stable loop in presence of stiff environments with the same constraints applying in terms of time delays.

4 Evaluation

The proposed controllers in combination with the two force sensors in the front arm cuff were tested on the test stand depicted in Fig. 1. The elbow joint is actuated by a brushless DC motor (Maxon EC 90 flat) in conjunction with a Harmonic Drive gear (type HFUC-20-100-2A) with a reduction ratio of 100 : 1. The nominal output torque of the drive section is 44 Nm at a nominal angular velocity of 26 rpm. The used motor controller (Maxon EPOS 70/10) can be configured for position, velocity or current control. An incremental rotary encoder is used for motor low level control and for end position monitoring. In the front cuff of the arm brace two resistive force sensors (Tekscan FlexiForce A201) are used to detect the human-robot interaction torque, according to Sect. 2. The used sensors have been shown to be suitable for control applications [21]. A one-axis torque sensor in the elbow joint is used as reference signal, it is based on strain gauges and able to detect torques up to 30 Nm. Its signal is compensated for the weight of the forearm construction. The controllers are realized in MATLAB/SIMULINK in conjunction with a rapid prototyping system (dSPACE DS1103), providing serial, digital and analogue interfaces. The real-time application is running on 10 kHz, however, an update of the joint's angular position is provided by the serial communication interface every 4 ms only, that is at 250 Hz. The user activates the device using a dead-man switch in the right hand. The human command torque τ_hc is set to zero, that is no sensor glove is used. The parameters of the admittance controller were chosen as $J_\mathrm{v} = 0.1\,\mathrm{kgm}^2$ and $D_\mathrm{v} = 0.1\,\mathrm{Nms}$, the proportional gain of the impedance controller was set to $K = 10000$, the integral gain to $K_\mathrm{I} = 1$. These parameters revealed good dynamic behavior while maintaining stability and noise suppression of the force signal.

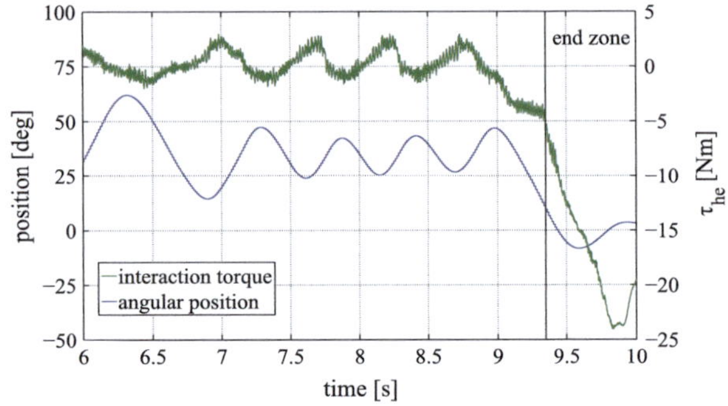

Fig. 8 Interaction torque and measured angular position of the arm for an oscillating movement

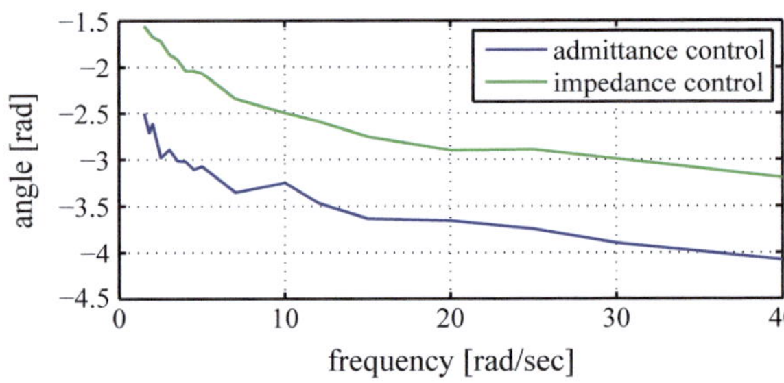

Fig. 9 Measured phase plot of the admittance and impedance control loops for interaction torque as input signal and position response

Both the admittance and impedance control approach showed good results in terms of realizing a movement of the elbow joint according to the user's intention. In Fig. 8 the motor position and the interaction torque for an oscillating movement using impedance control are given. At the end of the plotted section the proband moves towards the minimal end position and enters the end zone at approx. 9.4 s, as indicated by the vertical line. The proportional gain is then reduced according to (8) and the user needs to exert a significant higher torque, which gives an intuitive feedback that the end position is reached. The arm stops slightly after the defined end position, which is acceptable, as φ_{min} is defined before the hardware end position. Hence, it is not even necessary to switch to velocity control mode to stop the motor at the end position. Compared to the impedance controller, the admittance controller was felt by various probands to be less dynamic than the impedance control approach. For objective comparison of both approaches, sinusoidal input force signals were simulated while no user was wearing the exoskeleton arm. The phase delays of the corresponding measured position were determined for various frequencies of the force signals, see Fig. 9. Significant higher phase delays using the admittance controller can be observed compared to the impedance controller, which correlates with the subjective feeling reported by the probands.

5 Discussion and Conclusion

In this paper, a concept for an exoskeleton for assistance in MHL tasks in industry was presented. In contrast to existing systems, the presented approach focuses on the special requirements in industry and MHL tasks regarding cost, weight and an intuitive control interface. No bio-signals but light and economic force sensor were proposed for the forearm to allow easy and fast set-up of the system. It was shown that two sensors in the front cuff of the arm brace only can be used to control the elbow joint, while still providing a revolute joint for pronation and supination of the forearm. In measurements they were shown to provide good detection of the human-robot interaction torque, a torque sensor in the elbow joint was used as reference signal. An impedance and admittance control approach based on the force sensor concept were compared, which allow free movement of the user while wearing the robot and not handling any load. Force support mode is incorporated by using an external user command signal, e.g., by means of a sensor glove. This approach allows the user to handle loads directly using his hands without need to handle a grip. For both approaches a linear model of the closed control chain was derived to identify the influence of the control parameters, human impedance characteristics and possible time delays onto stability. Calculations revealed that even for a significant higher stiffness than the standard human stiffness value, stability can be achieved by appropriate tuning of the controllers.

A test stand with an actuated elbow joint was built up to evaluate the proposed concept. Both control approaches revealed good performance, while the impedance approach showed to be superior. Probands reported it to behave more dynamically, which was confirmed in measurements.

Future work targets at building up a lightweight arm construction based on the presented control and sensor concept, comprising of two actuated joints and a torque sensor in the shoulder joint.

Acknowledgements This work was supported as a Fraunhofer Master Project.

References

1. Schneider, E., Irastorza, X.: Osh in figures: work-related musculoskeletal disorders in the eu—facts and figures. https://osha.europa.eu/en/publications/reports/TERO09009ENC (2010)
2. Hayashi, T., Kawamoto, H., Sankai, Y.: Control method of robot suit HAL working as operator's muscle using biological and dynamical information. In: IEEE/RSJ International Conference on Intelligent Robots and Systems, pp. 3063–3068 (2005)
3. Kazerooni, H., Steger, R.: The berkeley lower extremity exoskeleton. J. Dyn. Syst. Meas. Control **128**(1), 14 (2006)
4. Perry, J.C., Rosen, J., Burns, S.: Upper-limb powered exoskeleton design. IEEE/ASME Trans. Mechatron. **12**(4), 408–417 (2007)
5. Muramatsu, Y., Umehara, H., Kobayashi, H.: Improvement and quantitative performance estimation of the back support muscle suit. In: Annual International Conference of the IEEE Engineering in Medicine and Biology Society, pp. 2844–2849 (2013)

6. Gunasekara, J., Gopura, R., Jayawardane, T., Lalitharathne, S.: Control methodologies for upper limb exoskeleton robots. In: IEEE/SICE International Symposium on System Integration, pp. 19–24 (2012)
7. Khan, A.M., Yun, D.W., Ali, M.A., Han, J., Shin, K., Han, C.: Adaptive impedance control for upper limb assist exoskeleton. In: IEEE International Conference on Robotics and Automation (ICRA), pp. 4359–4366 (2015)
8. Nagarajan, U., Aguirre-Ollinger, G., Goswami, A.: Integral admittance shaping for exoskeleton control. In: IEEE International Conference on Robotics and Automation (ICRA), pp. 5641–5648 (2015)
9. Singh, R.M., Chatterji, S., Kumar, A.: A review on surface EMG based control schemes of exoskeleton robot in stroke rehabilitation. In: International Conference on Machine Intelligence and Research Advancement (ICMIRA), pp. 310–315 (2013)
10. Kiguchi, K., Hayashi, Y.: An EMG-based control for an upper-limb power-assist exoskeleton robot. IEEE Trans. Syst. Man Cybernet. Part B (Cybernetics), 1064–1071 (2012)
11. Vukobratović, M.: How to control robots interacting with dynamic environment. J. Intel. Robot. Syst. **19**(2), 119–152 (1997)
12. Hogan, N.: Impedance control: an approach to manipulation. In: 1984 American Control Conference, pp. 304–313 (1984)
13. Stelzer, P., Kraus, W., Pott, A.: Sensor glove for an intuitive human-machine interface for exoskeletons as manual load handling assistance. In: International Symposium on Robotics 2016 (2016). Forthcoming
14. Otten, B., Stelzer, P., Weidner, R., Argubi-Wollesen, A., Wulfsberg, J.: A novel concept for wearable, modular and soft support systems used in industrial environments. In: Hawaii International Conference on System Sciences 2016 (2016)
15. Duchaine, V., Gosselin, C.M.: General model of human-robot cooperation using a novel velocity based variable impedance control. In: 2nd Joint EuroHaptics Conference and Symposium on Haptic Interfaces for Virtual Environment and Teleoperator Systems (WHC), pp. 446–451 (2007)
16. Canudas de Wit, C., Olsson, H., Astrom, K.J., Lischinsky, P.: A new model for control of systems with friction. IEEE Trans. Autom. Control **40**(3), 419–425 (1995)
17. Pons, J.L.: Wearable robots: biomechatronic exoskeletons. Hoboken, N.J. (ed.), Wiley (2008)
18. Lawrence, D.A.: Impedance control stability properties in common implementations. In: IEEE International Conference on Robotics and Automation, pp. 1185–1190 (1988)
19. Tsumugiwa, T., Yokogawa, R., Yoshida, K.: Stability analysis for impedance control of robot for human-robot cooperative task system. In: IEEE/RSJ International Conference on Intelligent Robots and Systems (IROS), pp. 3883–3888 (2004)
20. Minyong, P., Mouri, K., Kitagawa, H., Miyoshi, T., Terashima, K.: Hybrid impedance and force control for massage system by using humanoid multi-fingered robot hand. In: IEEE International Conference on Systems, Man and Cybernetics, pp. 3021–3026 (2007)
21. Lebosse, C., Renaud, P., Bayle, B., Mathelin, M.D.: Modeling and evaluation of low-cost force sensors. IEEE Trans. Robot. **27**(4), 815–822 (2011)

Unilateral Teleoperation Design for a Robotic Endoscopic Pituitary Surgery System

M.İ.C. Dede, O.W. Maaroof, G. Ateş, M. Berker, İ. Işıkay and Ş. Hanalioğlu

Abstract The aim of this study is to develop a teleoperation system which will be used to support the endoscopic pituitary surgery procedures. The proposed system aims to enable the surgeon to operate with three different operation tools (one of them is the endoscope) simultaneously. By this way, it is expected that the productivity of the surgical operation will be improved and the duration of the operation will be shortened. In the proposed system, a main control unit that can be attached to any of the surgical tools that are used in the operation (other than the endoscope) will be developed to capture the motion of the surgeon's hand motion as demanded by the surgeon, to process the captured motion and to send it to the robot that handles the endoscope. In this way, the endoscope will be directed simultaneously by the surgeon throughout the operation while he/she is using the other surgical tools with his/her two hands. In this paper, the study to determine the type and processing of information that is sent from the surgeon's side to the endoscope robot is presented.

Keywords Endoscopic pituitary surgery · Robotic surgery · Pituitary surgery · Minimally invasive surgery · Teleoperation

M.İ.C. Dede (✉) · O.W. Maaroof · G. Ateş
Izmır Institute of Technology, İzmir, Turkey
e-mail: candede@iyte.edu.tr

O.W. Maaroof
e-mail: omarmaaroof@iyte.edu.tr

G. Ateş
e-mail: gizemates@iyte.edu.tr

M. Berker · İ. Işıkay · Ş. Hanalioğlu
Hacettepe University, Ankara, Turkey
e-mail: mberker@hacettepe.edu.tr

İ. Işıkay
e-mail: ilkayisikay@gmail.com

Ş. Hanalioğlu
e-mail: sahinhanalioglu@gmail.com

M. Husty and M. Hofbaur (eds.), *New Trends in Medical and Service Robots*,
Mechanisms and Machine Science 48, DOI 10.1007/978-3-319-59972-4_8

1 Introduction

In last 20 years, many groups have been working on controlling motion of medical imaging systems such as laparoscope, endoscope by robotic systems. In order to reduce the amount of people in surgeries and reduce the duration, controlling the robotic system by the surgeon is preferred. One of the most important points is how the control demands will be sent to the robot. Since the surgeon sends the control demands to the robot, these demands should be acquired in an intuitive way so that the surgeon's concentration will not be deviated from the primary focus, the surgery itself. Being a technological device, these robotic systems bring some technical problems alongside similar to other technical devices that are already in use in all operating rooms. Among these, the most significant one is the safety. For safety, some redundant safety mechanisms are utilized in different levels. Another constraint is the need of technical training for the surgeon to use these systems. Additionally, even if robots have reached higher precision levels during operation, they are still slower than the human. Furthermore, robots should occupy as little place as possible in the operation room and whenever it is required they should move or restrain the motion of the optical system. All these topics should be considered in designing a surgical robot independent from the operation type.

Robots are generally categorized into two as the active or the passive robots. Active surgical robot systems are capable of recognizing the changes in the environment and organize their duties accordingly. As an example, ROBODOC [1] is an active robot which is used in femur operations. In passive surgical robot systems (also called the master-slave robot systems), the surgeon provided the motion inputs to the slave system via the master system. The control of the slave system is achieved by using these inputs in its control algorithm during surgery. In addition to these, in some semi-active systems such as NeuroMate [2], the surgeon provides the directions. In another type of robotic surgery, the robot and the surgeon handle and direct the surgical tool together. Mako Surgical Corp. product [3] that is used in arthroscopic knee surgeries is a good example of these type of robots.

One of the important advantages of passive systems is the capability of scaling the motion demands which are received from the master system to increasing the sensitivity of the slave system. The tremor problem in surgeon's hand while holding the endoscope for long hours can be resolved by using the master-slave systems and filtering out the tremors within the master systems. Another advantage is that slave system can have six or more degrees-of-freedom (DoF) and the surgeon can enter inputs not only by his/her hands but also fingers and elbow for the slave system. Therefore, flexibility of the system increases [4].

In the literature, there are neurosurgical systems in which these passive systems are used. One of them is developed by Mitsuishi et al. [5] and his group for microscopic neurosurgery. Although this system provides the necessary precision levels, it can be used only by surgeons who are trained to use this systems. Furthermore, the surgery completion duration is reported to be increased. Another commercial system is named NeuroArm and it is the one of the most comprehensive passive robots until now, which is reported to be used in many surgeries [6]. It is able to perform stereotactic and microsurgery with real time MRI. Additionally, this system provides haptic feedback to the surgeon. However, among all the surgical systems, probably the most well-known one is the da Vinci® surgical system. Although its main use is in laparoscopic procedures, it is adapted for also transnasal endoscopic surgeries [7]. However, due to the large size of the system and complicated structure, it is not suitable for neurosurgical applications.

Pituitary tumor is a frequently observed tumor type, which causes important health problems from visual loss through hormonal imbalances [8]. In the management of this tumor, endoscopic endonasal pituitary surgery is a modern treatment method that is cost-efficient and more preferable than open-skull or microscopic transsphenoidal pituitary tumor surgeries [9]. In this surgery, to obtain internal images, an optical system called endoscope is inserted and directed by the surgeon starting from the nostril of the patient, through the naval cavity to the sphenoid sinus, which is right in front of the saddle-shaped hole named Sella Turcica in the skull base where the pituitary gland is located. The tumor is removed by the special surgical tools, which are also inserted through the nostrils [10]. Recent studies showed that endoscopic pituitary surgery leads to at least equal or even more tumor resection rates, better clinical results, higher patient comfort, less hospitalization duration and cost-efficiency in the long run compared to the microscopic surgery [9, 11, 12]. These mentioned reasons make endoscopic pituitary surgery increasingly more preferable among both surgeons and patients. One of the biggest problems in this operation is that the surgeon has to handle and control the endoscope during the whole surgery. This situation causes the surgeon to get tired and not to use the hand holding the endoscope to operate with other tools, which reduce the efficiency and prolongs the duration of the procedure that typically lasts for 2–4 h. Some solutions have been offered to compensate for this problem such as having an assistant to handle the endoscope, using a fixed endoscope holder, endoscopes handled by robots that are controlled via variety of methods. In Fig. 1, it can be observed that surgeon is using his left hand to hold the

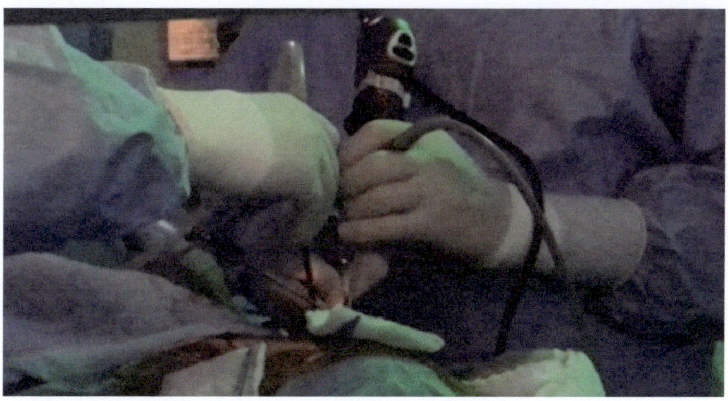

Fig. 1 Cooperation of the surgeon and the assistant throughout the surgery

endoscope and the other hand to operate with a surgical tool while the assistant is helping him to use up to two more surgical tools. This type of procedure is needed very often during this type of surgery.

Due to the limitations of the previously developed systems and including an assistant that is expected to follow the demands of the surgeon precisely, the use of these methods is problematic in clinical applications. The objective of our work is to provide a new robotic surgery system that enables the surgeon to use his/her two hands efficiently at the same time. This system is designated to be a master-slave teleoperation system to handle and control the positioning of the endoscope inside the surgery area. In this paper, among the other novel approaches for the proposed system, the determination of the information to be acquired and to be sent from the master system and the processing type of this information for the slave input is presented. Next section describes the previous work conducted on developing robotic systems to handle and direct optical systems in minimally invasive surgeries. The teleoperation architecture is explained in the third section which is followed by the preliminary experimentation result for the information exchange and control of the robot handling the endoscope. The paper is concluded with the discussions and conclusions based on the presented experimental results.

2 Background on Robotic Endoscopic Surgery

A straightforward and quick solution for holding the endoscope during the surgery for 2–4 h is to devise a stable holder which can be directed by the surgeon manually whenever required. Some of these endoscope holders are designed as passive holder mechanisms with simple mechanical joint locks such as Martin's Arm [13], ASSISTO [14], Endoboy [15], and TISKA [16]. Another type of holders has pneumatically controlled joint locks such as UNITRAC [17] and POINT SETTER [18], which also include mechanical balancing systems. Another passive mechanism presented in [19] is also mechanically balanced which can be positioned and oriented manually. All of these passive endoscope holders and other similar devices still need much effort from the surgeon or assistant whenever a change of view for endoscope is needed. Therefore, the endoscope holders are not the ultimate solution to maximize the efficiency of endoscopic surgeries.

In the survey of Nishikawa [20], positioning systems used in surgical robot systems are classified into three groups based on the level of autonomy: (i) non-autonomous systems, (ii) semi-autonomous systems, and (iii) full-autonomous systems. In another review presented in [21] an analysis on FDA approved robots devoted to endonasal surgery was conducted to expose the advantages and disadvantages of these systems. Taniguchi et al. [22] reported 27 different endoscopic surgical robots developed in between the years 1994–2009. Eight of them were used on humans, others were either experimented on animals or presented as a model. In most of these systems, a commercially available endoscope is directed by a robot arm which is controlled by the surgeon via a control-panel.

One of the oldest examples of the robot controlled imaging systems is developed by Taylor et al. [23]. This system is composed of a four-axis robotic arm and a joystick, which can easily plugged-into laparoscopic instruments in order to control robot holding the camera. Even if joystick sounds a good and easily implementable solution, this system could not be commercialized widely because it degraded the performance of surgeon in using the instruments.

Another important example was developed by Casals et al. [24] for laparoscopic surgeries in which an industrial robot was used. In this system, force sensors are placed on the connections in order to prevent the dangerous situations for the patient. Surgeon controlled the camera by the input commands received from his/her head movements. However, it is difficult for the surgeon to keep his/her head stable throughout the surgery. Hence, this work also could not find use in surgeries. Narwell et al. [25] developed another method which uses a footswitch in order to control the robot handling the endoscope. However, this system also was not widely used since it did not provide a suitable way for the surgeon carry out the surgery without spending extra effort to control the robot. Wei et al. [26] offered another solution for all problematic points of previous works. In this system, a stereo camera acquires the motion of instruments used by surgeon and robot controlling the laparoscope mimics these motions. The surgery robot using this method, Aesop, is employed in over 1000 surgeries. However, this method relies on only stereo camera feedback and because of the resolution and speed limitations, it is not able to detect small and quick movements. Also, it reflects every motion of target instrument which may cause some dangerous situations during the surgery.

Researchers used various methods to acquire control demands from the surgeon to direct the endoscope during the surgery. There are some other examples in which the control demands are acquired by voice commands [27], by head motions [28], and by both joystick and voice commands [29]. In addition, KaLAR system [30] acquires the control demands by voice command and also includes an auto-tracking control. The commercially available VIKY system [31] has a foot pedal and voice recognition system to acquire control demands and it also uses image processing methods to make the robot follow the movements of surgical instruments. In Lapman robotic system [32], a joystick called LapStick® is fixed on a surgical tool as another way to acquire control demands. Emaro [33] is a commercially available air-powered surgical assistive robot that handles and controls the position of the endoscope by acquiring the control demands from the foot buttons and a gyroscope that is located on the forehead of the surgeon. The endoscope robot system FREE [34] is under development and in this system it is proposed to acquire the control demands from the gyroscope attached to the surgeon's foot. Infrared signals send from a headset worn by the surgeon is tracked and used as control demands in the EndoAssist system [35]. In 2010, Rilk et al. [36] fused all the control demand acquiring methods in the previous works (voice, footswitch etc.). In addition to this, in this system, endoscope images are processed and robot is driven to keep the surgical instruments in the middle of the display.

In the works discussed above, various ways are proposed and used to acquire control demands to drive the robot handling the endoscope. In the light of the previous experiences our aim is to develop a teleoperation system architecture in which the surgeon will be able to send control demands in an intuitive way with minimal effort of the surgeon. The next section describes the general teleoperation architecture to be used specifically for the endoscopic pituitary surgery.

3 Teleoperation System Architecture

Generally, in teleoperation systems the master and slave robot systems are in different places but in this work, both robot systems are in the same place. In this teleoperation architecture, master system is a main control unit mounted on a surgical tool that the surgeon uses frequently during surgery, the aspirator. This main control unit is composed of two main parts as the 3-axis gyroscope and the electronic control board acquiring and transferring the sensor signals wirelessly to the slave system. Assuming that the surgeon uses his/her right hand for critical operations such as drilling, the main control unit is attached on and motions are proposed to be acquired from the aspirator tool used by the left hand of the surgeon.

The slave system is a robot arm whose end-effector is the endoscope. Robot arm is used in order to direct the endoscope only inside the surgical area. Different from the examples in literature, this slave robot arm is to be placed into the surgical area by the surgeon and retrieved back from the surgical area again by the surgeon whenever it is necessary. In this way, entering and retrieving processes, which are less critical in operation, can be done in a much faster way. Another advantage of this approach is that the system can be passively backdriven and retrieved from the surgical area in case of an unexpected failure.

The slave system consists of two main mechanisms; a weight-balanced six DoF carrier part, which can be passively backdriven by the surgeon and an active robot, which is driven by the control demands sent from the main control unit.

After the surgeon adjusts the endoscope image settings, the operating procedure of the system during the surgery is as follows:

(1) The surgeon places the endoscope, which is attached to the robot, inside the surgical area. At this stage, brakes are on for all the actuators of the robot, which is positioned in the middle of its workspace. The demonstration of the surgeon placing the endoscope inside the surgical area is presented in Fig. 2.
(2) The main control unit is mounted on the aspirator to be used.
(3) The surgeon activates the data flow between the main control unit and the slave system by pressing the activation button on main control unit whenever there is a need to change the direction of the endoscope. As long as the button pressed, main control unit remains active and it transfers the control demand information to slave robot. While the slave robot is driven to its required position, the compliant control algorithm implemented for the control of the robot prevents the transfer of unnecessary amounts of forces to the patient.

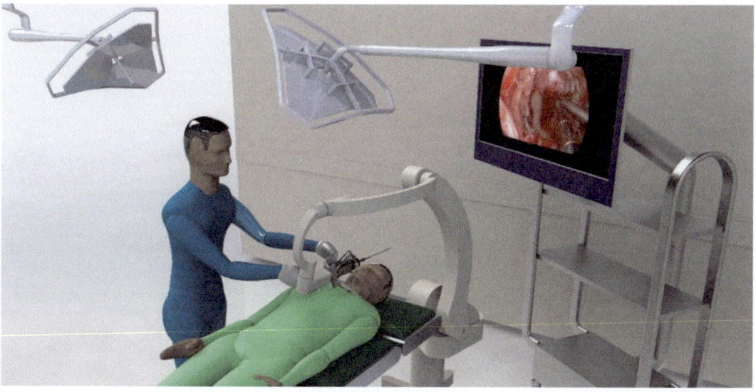

Fig. 2 Endoscope placement procedure

(4) When the endoscope reaches the desired position, the activation button is released and the robot remains in that position.
(5) When the lens of endoscope gets dirty, surgeon retrieves the endoscope from surgical area for cleansing. Then the 5-step procedure is repeated.

Taniguchi et al. [22] state that yaw, pitch and insertion (surge) motions are necessary motions of an endoscope inside the surgical area. It should be noted that in our system, the motions that require larger workspace and more DoF, such as entering the endoscope into the surgical area and retrieving it back from the surgical area, are accomplished by the surgeon manually by backdriving the 6 DoF carrier system. Therefore, the active slave robot system is designed to have 3 DoF motion identified as yaw, pitch and surge. In accordance, control demands from the surgeon should be acquired for these identified motions.

In order to issue control demands for the slave robot, surgeon activates the button placed on the main control unit and the orientation change is measured via the gyroscope in terms of angular velocity in three axes as pitch, roll and yaw. Angular velocities about yaw and pitch axes are used as control demand for slave robot about the same axes however; angular velocity measured about the roll axis is used for issuing control demand for the surge motion of the endoscope along its shaft direction. The representation of the information flow from the gyroscope axes to the 3 DoF robot arm is given in Fig. 3. It should be noted that the presented mechanism of the slave robot is given for general representation of its motion capabilities. Nevertheless, the workspace of the slave is spherical and it is limited due to safety reasons after the analysis for the minimal required workspace.

The next section describes the experimental setup to imitate the teleoperation architecture provided in this section to investigate the use of two different methods of controlling the endoscope robot.

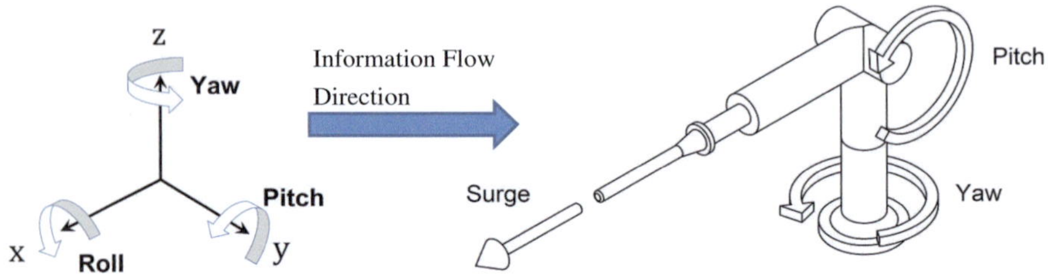

Fig. 3 The representation of information flow from the gyroscope axes to the 3 DoF slave robot arm

4 Experimentation Setup for Testing the Usability of the Teleoperation Architecture

The experimental setup is composed of a replica of a surgical tool with an embedded gyroscope to be used as the master system and a virtual representation of the slave robot. The virtual slave robot is a spherical robot arm and a camera viewpoint is placed at the tip point of this robot arm. The surgeon handling the master system is shown in Fig. 4a. While the surgeon uses the replica of the surgical tool, he can also view the surgical area from the computer screen. This view is generated by the virtual camera placed at the tip of the slave robot. As the robot is moved by the processed control demands, the view of the virtual surgical area changes accordingly. This provides the sense that the surgeon is controlling a real robot that is handling the camera since during a surgery; the surgeon constantly looks at the endoscope image presented on a screen.

During the experimentation, although the surgeon does not see the slave robot, it is shown in Fig. 4b to provide a sense of how the virtual reality system works. The virtual slave robot presented in Fig. 4b is the 3 DoF spherical robot arm and right in front of it, there is a screenshot of the surgical area. As there is a change in the

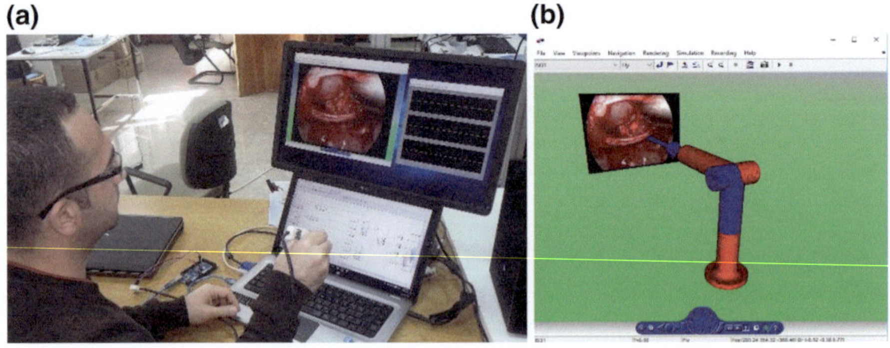

Fig. 4 **a** The surgeon handling master system while observing the endoscope's visual feedback. **b** The virtual representation of the slave robot

orientation and the position of the robot's tip point, the portion of the visualized screenshot changes and this creates the effect of controlling the real endoscope robot.

The replica of the surgical tool, which is produced by using an additive manufacturing system, is shown in Fig. 5. The main control unit on this tool is composed of a gyroscope unit and a push-button.

In the experimental setup, the gyroscope of the inertial measurement unit (IMU) named GY-88 MPU-6050™ by MotionTracking™ Devices is used. This sensor offers four different sensitivity measures. In the scope of this work, resolution is relatively more important than full scale range; therefore, FS_SEL = 0 setting is selected to set the range as ±250°/s and sensitivity as 131 LSB/(°/s). In order to receive and process the measurements obtained from gyroscope, Arduino Mega 2560 board is used. I2C protocol is used for the communication between microprocessor and gyroscope in order to have a noise-free acquisition of the sensor measurements. The processed sensor measurements are forwarded to Matlab via serial port as control demands for the slave robot in real time by using Real Time Windows Target at a sampling frequency of 50 Hz. This rate is enough for visualization of the surgical area. The connection details of the gyroscope and the push-button are shown in Fig. 6. The LED is placed to warn the surgeon the push-button is pressed and the data is being transferred to the slave system.

4.1 Main Control Unit's Algorithm

The flowchart of the main control unit is shown in Fig. 7. It is observed from the figure that the system initiates as soon as it is connected to the power. In the first step, I2C and serial communication protocols should be declared since all the wiring between the gyroscope and the Arduino board should be known by the

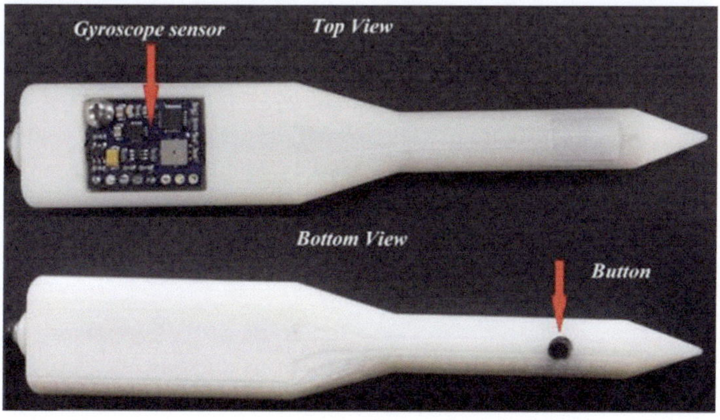

Fig. 5 Replica of a surgical tool and the main control unit's components

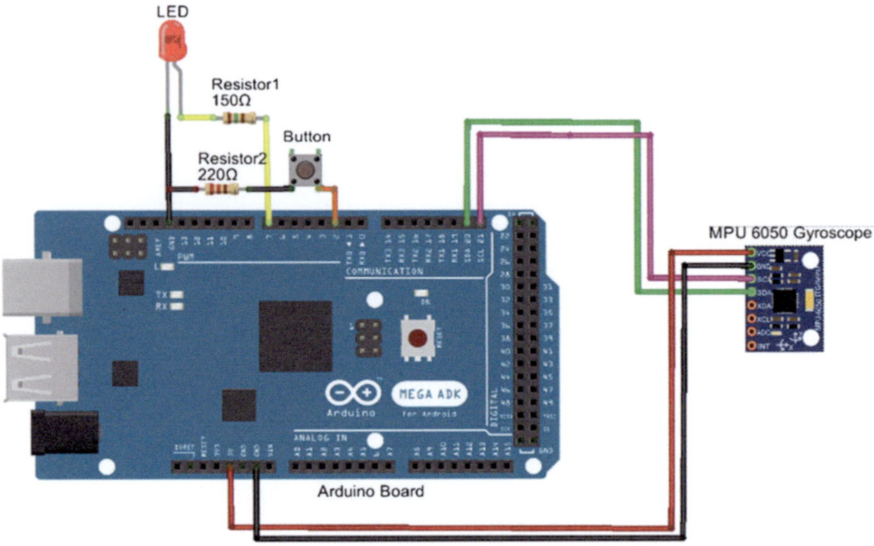

Fig. 6 Wiring of the gyroscope and the push-button to the Arduino board

microprocessor before receiving any signal. Then, the baudrate of serial communication is specified. After these, identification starts and gyroscope measurements are acquired and kept in predefined variables. This process repeats in each 80 ms.

The push-button, which is presented in Figs. 5 and 6, is used to either allow or prevent the data flow from the Arduino board to Matlab. The state of the button is checked continuously and if the button is pressed, data flow is allowed and the speed information is sent to Matlab. Otherwise, only "zero" value is sent through serial port. The reason of sending "zero" value instead of sending "nothing" is that the serial communication would be required to be reconfigured every time the push-button is pressed. Thus, it would degrade the performance of the system.

In the main control unit, there is also an indicator light (LED) to indicate the data flow condition. If the light is on, it means that the system is ready for the data to be sent but currently there is no data being sent. If the light is off, that means there is a loaded data flow over serial link. The situation of this light is dependent on the condition of the push-button. The program is terminated stopping the hardware-in-the-loop simulation built in Matlab Simulink.

4.2 Teleoperation Modes

Although the acquired signal from the gyroscope is angular rate, while processing and converting this signal into control demands to drive the slave robot, two different methodologies can be applied. These methodologies are described as:

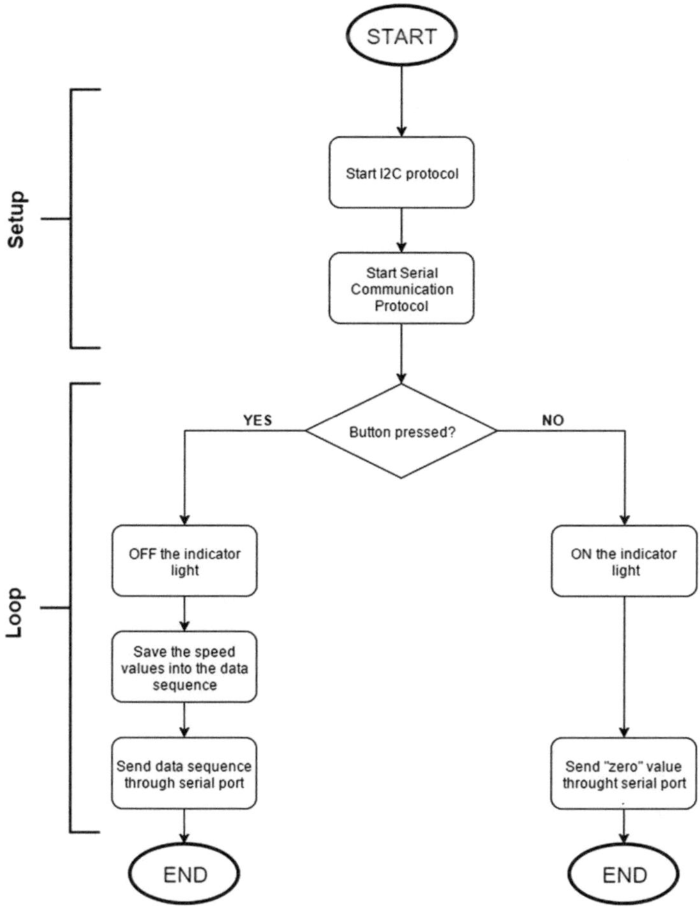

Fig. 7 The flowchart of the program on Arduino board

Displacement-to-displacement method: In this method, the angular rate measured from the gyroscope is processed to find angular displacements in pitch, roll and yaw axes and they are mapped to the control demands for the slave robot in terms of *angular displacements* in pitch and yaw axes and *translational displacement* along the surge axis, respectively. Definition of the axes is provided in Fig. 3. The mathematical relationships to apply this method are given in (1)–(3).

$$S_i = sat\left(K_S \int R_r dt + S_{i-1}\right); \quad i = 0, 1, 2, \ldots \tag{1}$$

$$Y_i = sat\left(K_Y \int Y_r dt + Y_{i-1}\right); \quad i = 0, 1, 2, \ldots \tag{2}$$

$$P_i = sat\left(K_P \int P_r dt + P_{i-1}\right); \quad i = 0, 1, 2, \ldots \tag{3}$$

As it is explained in the flowchart, each time the push-button is pressed, real-time gyroscope measurements are sent to the slave system and also pressing the push-button increases the *i* count by 1 in (1)–(3). In the initial conditions, S_0, Y_0 and P_0 values are set to zero and the S_1, Y_1 and P_1 values are updated as long as the push-button is pressed. After the push-button is released S_1, Y_1 and P_1 values are stored for the next time the push-button will be pressed. S_i, Y_i and P_i are the *i*th displacement demand along surge axis, *i*th angular displacement demands about the yaw and pitch axes, respectively. R_r, Y_r and P_r are the angular rates measured from the gyroscope about roll, pitch and yaw axes. Finally, K_s, K_y and K_p are the gains used scale the workspaces of the main control unit attached surgical tool and the slave robot handling the endoscope. If these gains are selected to be larger, then with a smaller motion of the main control unit attached surgical tool, a larger displacement demand for the slave robot will be issued. Additionally, saturation is used in (1)–(3) in order to limit the workspace of the slave robot (to simulate the real case scenario).

Displacement-to-velocity method: In this method, the measured angular rates are processed to find angular displacements in pitch, roll and yaw axes and they are mapped to the control demands for the slave robot in terms of *angular rates* in pitch and yaw axes and translational velocity along the surge axis, respectively. The mathematical relationships to apply this method are given in (4)–(6).

$$S_i = sat\left[\int \left(K_S \cdot \sigma \int R_r dt\right) dt + S_{i-1}\right]; \quad i = 0, 1, 2, \ldots \tag{4}$$

$$Y_i = sat\left[\int \left(K_Y \cdot \sigma \int Y_r dt\right) dt + Y_{i-1}\right]; \quad i = 0, 1, 2, \ldots \tag{5}$$

$$P_i = sat\left[\int \left(K_P \cdot \sigma \int P_r dt\right) dt + P_{i-1}\right]; \quad i = 0, 1, 2, \ldots \tag{6}$$

The parameters, initial conditions and the applications of the formulas for this method are almost the same with the previous method. The only difference is that in the first integrations, a reset signal is utilized to reset the result of the first integration in (4)–(6) to zero whenever the push-button in the master side is released. Therefore, whenever the push-button is not pressed σ values in (4)–(6) becomes equal to 0 and otherwise it is equal to 1. In this way it is guaranteed that the control demand in terms of velocity sent to the slave system is a zero command and the slave robot will not be operated until the push-button is pressed.

5 Conclusions

This work is dedicated to investigating the most suitable way of control demand acquisition from the surgeon in order to control an endoscope robot during the endoscopic pituitary surgery. Even before constructing the robot to control the endoscope, a simulation of the surgery is developed only to evaluate the ease of sending control demands to the slave robot, which is also called the endoscope robot in this work. Experimental setup is devised as a hardware-in the-loop simulation in which the control signals are acquired from a gyroscope and processed to drive a virtual slave robot with a camera that can replicate the visual information in the related surgery. In this study, there is no haptic feedback and the virtual robot is directed by only motion demands in a kinematics mode simulation environment. Therefore, 80 ms of sampling rate is sufficient to evaluate the teleoperation methods. Two different methods to drive the endoscope robot have been developed and the neurosurgeons from Hacettepe University tested the system with these methods. The first method is very similar to moving the cursor with the mouse on a screen. Although the workspace scaling ratios are increased, it was found to be requiring too much motion during a surgery. It should be recalled that the main controller with the gyroscope is mounted on the suction tube and this tool is inside the surgical area during the control of the endoscope robot. The displacement-to-velocity method is evaluated to be much easier to be operated with minimal effort especially when the workspace scaling ratio is increased. In this method, although the surgeon moves the suction tube in the required direction by a minimal amount and just stops there while pressing the push-button, the slave robot still continues to move the endoscope in the required direction. As a result of these evaluations, the displacement-to-velocity method was found to be the most convenient way of sending control demands to the endoscope robot.

Acknowledgements This work is supported in part by The Scientific and Technological Research Council of Turkey via grant numbers 115E725 and 115E726.

References

1. ROBODOC: "The ROBODOC® Surgical System" ROBODOC®: Professionals. Available via ROBODOC. http://www.robodoc.com/professionals.html
2. Renishaw plc. "neuromate®": neuromate® stereotactic robot. Available via RENISHAW. http://www.renishaw.com/en/neuromate-stereotactic-robot–10712
3. MAKO Surgical Corp.: "MAKOplasty®". MAKOplasty® | MAKO Surgical Corp. Available via Stryker. http://www.makosurgical.com/makoplasty
4. Sekhar, L.N., Tariq, F., Kim, L.J., Pridgeon, J., Hannaford, B.: Commentary: virtual reality and robotics in neurosurgery. Neurosurgery **72**, A1–A6 (2013)
5. Mitsuishi, M., Morita, A., Sugita, N., Sora, S., Mochizuki, R., Tanimoto, K., Baek, Y.M., Takahashi, H., Harada, K.: Master–slave robotic platform and its feasibility study for micro-neurosurgery. Int. J. Med. Robot. Comput. Assist. Surg. **9**, 180–189 (2013)

6. Sutherland, G.R., Latour, I., Greer, A.D.: Integrating an image-guided robot with intraoperative MRI. Eng. Med. Biol. Mag. **27**, 59–65 (2008)
7. Kupferman, M.E., DeMonte, F., Levine, N., Hanna, E.: Feasibility of a robotic surgical approach to reconstruct the skull base. In: Skull Base-An Interdisciplinary Approach, vol. 21, pp. 79–82 (2011)
8. Levy, A.: Pituitary disease: presentation, diagnosis, and management. J. Neurol. Neurosurg. Psychiatry **75**(Suppl 3), iii47–iii52 (2004)
9. Komotar, R.J.: Endoscopic endonasal compared with microscopic transsphenoidal and open transcranial resection of giant pituitary adenomas. Pituitary **15**(2), 150–159 (2012)
10. Laws, E.R., Wong, J.M., Smith, T.R., de Los, Reyes K., Aglio, L.S., Thorne, A.J., Cote, D.J., Esposito, F., Cappabianca, P., Gawande, A.: A checklist for endonasal transsphenoidal anterior skull base surgery. J. Neurosurg. **30**, 1–6 (2015)
11. Almeida, J.P., De Albuquerque, L.A., Dal Fabbro, M., Sampaio, M., Medina, R., Chacon, M., Gondim, J.: Endoscopic skull base surgery: evaluation of current clinical outcomes. J. Neurosurg. Sci. (2015)
12. Berker, M., Işikay, I., Berker, D., Bayraktar, M., Gürlek, A.: Early promising results for the endoscopic surgical treatment of Cushing's disease. Neurosurg. Rev. **37**(1), 105–114 (2014)
13. Marina Medical, Sunrise, FL. Available via marinamedical. http://www.marinamedical.com/product/martins-arm-table-assistant-set
14. GEOMED Medizin-Technik, Tuttlingen, Germany. Available via geomed. http://www.ge-omed.de./index.php?id=60&L=1
15. MIKROLAND Endobloc Company, Rue du Patis, France. Available via mikroland-endobloc. http://www.mikroland-endobloc.fr/gb/_index-gb.html
16. Schurr, M.O., Arezzo, A., Neisius, B., Rininsland, H., Hilzinger, H.U., Dorn, J., Roth, K., Buess, G.F.: Trocar and instrument positioning system TISKA. Surg. Endosc. **13**, 528–531 (1999)
17. Aesculap, Inc., Center Valley, PA. Available via Aesculap. https://www.aesculapusa.com/assets/base/doc/DOC905_Unitrac_Retraction_and_Holding_Brochure.pdf
18. MİTAKA KOHKİ CO., LTD., Japan. Available via karlstorz. https://www.karlstorz.com/cps/rde/xbcr/karlstorz_assets/ASSETS/2149000.pdf
19. Kuo, C.H., Lai, S.J.: Design of a novel statically balanced mechanism for laparoscope holders with decoupled positioning and orientating manipulation. J. Mech. Robot. **8**, 015001-015001-10 (2016)
20. Nishikawa, A.: The surgeon-robot interface for controlling the position of a laparoscope. Jpn. Soc. Comput. Aided Surg. **6**, 69–74 (2004)
21. Trévillot, V., Garrel, R., Dombre, E., Poignet, P., Sobral, R., Crampette, L.: Robotic endoscopic sinus and skull base surgery: review of the literature and future prospects. Eur. Ann. Otorhinolaryngol. Head Neck Dis. **130**, 201–207 (2013)
22. Taniguchi, K., Nishikawa, A., Sekimoto, M., Kobayashi, T., Kazuhara, K., Ichihara, T., Kurashita, N., Takiguchi, S., Doki, Y., Mori, M., Miyazaki, F.: Classification, design and evaluation of endoscope robots. In: Baik, S.H. (ed.) Robot Surgery. InTech, Rijeka (2010)
23. Taylor, R.H., Funda, J., Eldridge, B., Gomory, S., Gruben, K., LaRose, D., Talamini, M., Kavoussi, L., Anderson, J.: A telerobotic assistant for laparoscopic surgery. Eng. Med. Biol. Mag. **14**, 279–288 (1995). IEEE
24. Casals, A., Amat, J., Laporte E.: Automatic guidance of an assistant robot in laparoscopic surgery. In: Proceedings of the IEEE Conference on Robotics and Automation, Minneapolis, Minnesota, vol. 1, pp. 895–900 (1996)
25. Narwell, N.I., Weker, D.R., Wang, Y.: A Force controllable macro-micro manipulator and its application to medical robotics. JPL Computer Motion Inc. Rapor no: N94- 30441 (1994)
26. Wei, G.Q., Arbter, K., Hirzinger, G.: Real-time visual servoing for laparoscopic surgery. Controlling robot motion with color image segmentation. Eng. Med. Biol. Mag. **16**, 40–45 (1997). IEEE
27. Wang, Y., Laby, K.P., Uecker, D.R., Mangaser, A.A., Ghodoussi, M.: Automated Endoscope System For Optimal Positioning. Patent no: US5878193 (1999)

28. Nishikawa, A., Hosoi, T., Koara, K., Daiji, N., Hikita, A., Asano, S., Miyazaki, F., Sekimoto, M., Miyake, Y., Yasui, M., Monden, M.: Real-time visual tracking of the surgeon's face for laparoscopic surgery. In: Niessen, W.J., Viergever, M.A. (eds.) Medical Image Computing and Computer-Assisted Intervention—MICCAI 2001, pp. 9–16 (2001)
29. Buess, G.F., Arezzo, A., Schurr, M.O., Ulmer, F., Fisher, H., Gumb, L., Testa, T., Nobman, C.: A new remote-controlled endoscope positioning system for endoscopic solo surgery. Surg. Endosc. **14**, 395–399 (2000)
30. Lee, Y.J., Kim, J., Ko, S.Y., Lee, W.J., Kwon, D.S.: Design of a compact laparoscopic assistant robot: KaLAR. In: Proceedings of the International Conference on Control Automation and Systems, pp. 2648–2653 (2003)
31. VIKY, EndoControl, Inc., Dover, DE. Available via endocontrol-medical. http://www.endocontrol-medical.com
32. Lapman. Available via medsys. http://www.medsys.be/documents/lapman_leaflet.pdf
33. Emaro: The World's First Pneumatic Endoscope Manipulator Holds Promise for Quality Surgery. Available via Tokyo Institute of Technology. http://www.titech.ac.jp/english/news/pdf/tokyotechpr20150731_emaro_en.pdf
34. Chan, J.Y., Leung, I., Navarro-Alarcon, D., Lin, W., Li, P., Lee, D.L., Liu, Y.H., Tong, M.C.: Foot-controlled robotic-enabled endoscope holder (FREE) for endoscopic sinus surgery: a cadaveric feasibility study. Laryngoscope **126**, 566–569 (2016)
35. Aiono, S., Gilbert, J.M., Soin, B., Finlay, P.A., Gordan, A.: Controlled trial of the introduction of a robotic camera assistant (Endo Assist) for laparoscopic cholecystectomy. Surg. Endosc. Other Interv. Tech. **16**, 1267–1270 (2002)
36. Rilk, M., Kubus, D., Wahl, F.M., Eichhorn, K.W., Wagner, I., Bootz, F.: Demonstration of a prototype for robot assisted Endoscopic Sinus Surgery. In: 2010 IEEE International Conference on Robotics and Automation (ICRA), Anchorage, AK, pp. 1090–1091, May 2010

Kinematic and Dynamic Modeling of a Multifunctional Rehabilitation Robot UHP

A. Mancisidor, A. Zubizarreta, I. Cabanes, P. Bengoa and J.H. Jung

Abstract The design of a suitable controller that handles robot-human interaction is one of the critical tasks in rehabilitation robotics. For this purpose, an accurate model of the robot is required. The Universal Haptic Pantograph (UHP) is a novel upper limb rehabilitation robot that can be configured to perform arm or wrist exercises. This work is focused on the latter, solving the kinematic model by the use of the closure loop equations, while Lagrangian formulation is used to estimate the interaction force. In order to prove the effectiveness of the model, several experimental tests are carried out. Results demonstrate that the mean motion error is less than 1 mm, and the estimated force error less than 10%.

Keywords Rehabilitation robots · Kinematic modeling · Dynamic modeling · Experimental validation

1 Introduction

Cerebrovascular diseases are the third most reason of death and the first cause of physical disability. Every year, more than 15 million strokes are diagnosed, and near 33 million people have disabilities due to the sequels of stroke [3, 13].

Hemiplegia is one of the most common stroke sequels, i.e. complete or partial paralysis of one side of the body. Currently, there is no surgical or pharmacological treatment, but according to various researches, thanks to brain plasticity, patients may recover most of their abilities by performing proper rehabilitation exercises [5, 10]. However, these treatments are time consuming and require constant supervision

A. Mancisidor · A. Zubizarreta (✉) · I. Cabanes · P. Bengoa
Department of Automatics and System Engineering, University of the Basque Country (UPV/EHU), Alameda Urquijo s/n, 48013 Bilbao, Spain
e-mail: asier.zubizarreta@ehu.eus

J.H. Jung
Rehabilitation Area, Health Division, TECNALIA Research and Innovation, Mikeletegi Pasealekua 1-3, 20009 Donostia-San Sebastian, Spain
e-mail: jehyung.jung@tecnalia.com

M. Husty and M. Hofbaur (eds.), *New Trends in Medical and Service Robots*, Mechanisms and Machine Science 48, DOI 10.1007/978-3-319-59972-4_9

of a physiotherapist to prove effective, which increases their economic cost, and lead to the reduction of rehabilitation times.

In recent years, rehabilitation robots have been proposed as a complement to traditional physiotherapy approaches [17]. Robots emulate and replicate the motions and forces produced by a physiotherapist, executing longer, more accurate and higher frequency treatments. In addition, robots can be used as a measurement tool that quantifies forces and/or movements, with the objective of evaluating patients progress and adapting the exercises to their needs. And using a graphical interface, a virtual reality environment can be built, so that the patient is encouraged to continue with the rehabilitation process.

The first rehabilitation robots were designed in the late eighties, and since then, many more have been proposed [1, 6]. Although there have been important advances in the area, there are still unresolved issues that need further studies, such as the design of appropriate, robust and safe control.

In the literature, several approaches are proposed to control the human-robot interaction in rehabilitation robotics: force control [14], computed torque control [9], admittance control [15], impedance control [2, 12] or algorithms using EMG signals [4, 11]. However, the implementation of these controllers requires, in most cases, a proper mathematical model of the robotic device, and the use of expensive force sensors.

In this article, kinematic and dynamic models of the Universal Haptic Pantograph (UHP) [8] are presented. The UHP is an upper limb rehabilitation robot with the ability to change its structure to perform different training exercises. This work is focused on one of the most complex modes, on the so-called Wrist mode, which is used to execute wrist training exercises. The developed models will be used to implement sensorless control approaches, with the goal of estimating the human-robot interaction force and motion during the rehabilitation exercises.

The article is organized as follows: in Sect. 2 the UHP rehabilitation robot is described; in Sect. 3 its kinematic and dynamic models are obtained for the Wrist mode; in Sect. 4, to validate the models, several experimental cases are carried out; finally, the most important ideas and future work are summarized in the conclusions.

2 Universal Haptic Pantograph

The Universal Haptic Pantograph (UHP) robot is designed to execute upper limb training rehabilitation exercises after a stroke [7, 8]. One of the main advantages of the UHP is the possibility to vary its mechanical structure by using lockable/unlockable joints, allowing different types of exercises with the same robot. This way, the UHP can perform rehabilitation of the shoulder, elbow and the wrist by proper configuration of the robot.

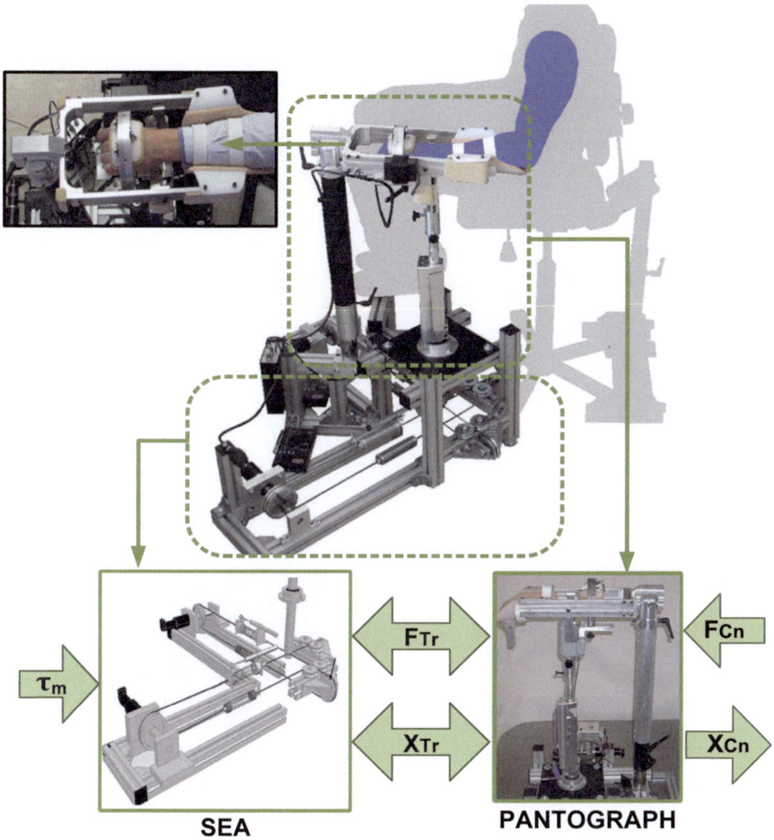

Fig. 1 Universal Haptic Pantograph (UHP)

Among the upper limb rehabilitation robots, the rehabilitation of the wrist is one of the more complex and least developed. The UHP provides a mechanical configuration that allows to perform pronation/supination, radial/unradial and flexion/extension wrist movements.

In order to allow these motions, the UHP is designed as the coupling of two subsystems. The interaction with the patient is carried out by a Pantograph structure (Fig. 1), while its actuation (i.e. the force feedback and sensing) is carried out by two perpendicular SEAs (Series Elastic Actuator). As both subsystems are connected, the torque exerted by the motors ($\tau_{\mathbf{m}}$) and the force exerted by the patient ($\mathbf{F}_{\mathbf{Cn}}$) are transmitted bilaterally between both subsystems in the form of force ($\mathbf{F}_{\mathbf{Tr}}$) and motion ($\mathbf{x}_{\mathbf{Tr}}$).

The drive system is composed by two perpendicular SEAs with two Maxon 40 rotative motors (m_1 and m_2), four elastic springs (S_A, S_B, S_C and S_D) and a series of pulleys. The SEA subsystem is connected to the Pantograph in the transmission point ($\mathbf{P}_{\mathbf{Tr}}$) (Fig. 2).

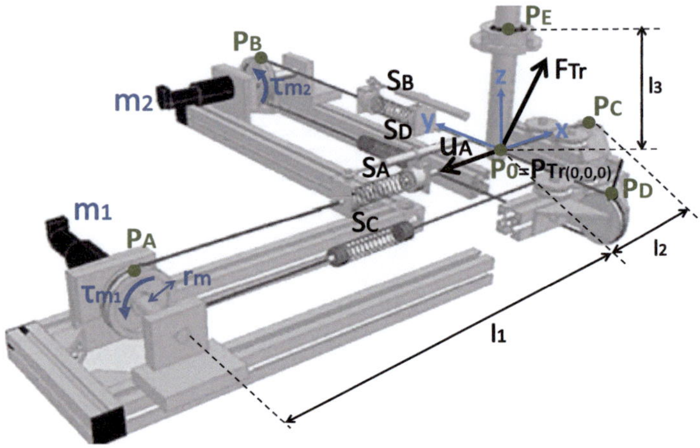

Fig. 2 Series elastic actuator (SEA)

Fig. 3 Pantograph in Wrist mode

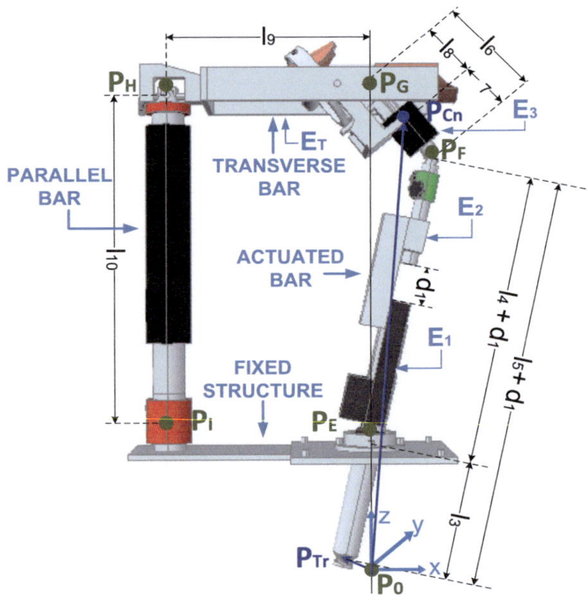

Force and motion transmission is carried out by using cables so that force ($\mathbf{F_{Tr}}$) and motion ($\mathbf{x_{Tr}}$) is transmitted to the Pantograph in two perpendicular directions (x and y). This way, motor m_1 and springs S_A and S_C actuate in the x direction of $\mathbf{P_{Tr}}$ (x_{Tr}), while motor m_2, S_B and S_D actuate in the y axis direction (y_{Tr}).

The Pantograph (Fig. 3) is composed by a fixed structure, three mobile bars (actuated, transverse and parallel), and five joints (spherical joint $\mathbf{P_E}$, lockable universal joint $\mathbf{P_F}$, revolute joint $\mathbf{P_G}$, lockable revolute joint $\mathbf{P_H}$ and lockable universal joint $\mathbf{P_I}$). The actuated bar is composed by three elements ($\mathbf{E_1}$, $\mathbf{E_2}$, $\mathbf{E_3}$), separated by a variable length slider and a $\mathbf{P_F}$ universal joint.

In Wrist mode, joint $\mathbf{P_H}$ is partially locked and joint $\mathbf{P_I}$ is fully locked. Therefore, the parallel bar is always normal to the fixed structure, and the transverse bar ($\mathbf{E_T}$) is locked in parallel to the fixed structure, but allowing rotations along its axis $\overrightarrow{\mathbf{P_H P_G}}$ (i.e., l_{10} is constant). In order to allow actuated bar motion, the slider d_1 is used and the universal joint $\mathbf{P_F}$ is unlocked. Hence, hemispherical motions can be generated in the hand grip, conducting wrist training exercises in all possible directions.

The equilibrium position of the UHP is achieved when the actuated bar is in vertical position (Fig. 3), defining the origin of the base reference frame $\mathbf{P_0}$ ($\mathbf{x_{Tr}} = \overrightarrow{\mathbf{P_0 P_{Tr}}} = [0\ 0\ 0]^T$).

3 Kinematic and Dynamic Modeling

As mentioned previously, a proper mathematical model of the robot is required to implement the robot patient-force interaction controller. Therefore, in this section UHP kinematic and dynamic models are presented. First, in Sect. 3.1 the drive system SEA model is obtained. Then, in Sect. 3.2 the model of the Pantograph in Wrist mode is calculated.

3.1 The Drive System SEA Model

Kinematic Model of the SEA

First, the drive system kinematics is analyzed, which is composed by two perpendicular SEA systems, with one rotary actuator in each, and two sets of springs, being the upper ones sensorized by means of linear potentiometers.

Hence, the main goal of this section is to define the relationship between measurable variables, motor rotation angle ($\mathbf{q_m} = [q_{m_1}\ q_{m_1}]^T$), upper springs variable length (n_{S_A} and n_{S_B}), and output contact motion ($\mathbf{x_{Tr}} = \overrightarrow{\mathbf{P_0 P_{Tr}}}$).

From Fig. 2, considering that the cables are stiff and both SEAs dimensions identical,

$$\begin{aligned} \overrightarrow{\mathbf{P_0 P_{Tr}}} &= \overrightarrow{\mathbf{P_0 P_A}} + \overrightarrow{\mathbf{P_A P_{Tr}}} \\ \overrightarrow{\mathbf{P_0 P_{Tr}}} &= \overrightarrow{\mathbf{P_0 P_B}} + \overrightarrow{\mathbf{P_B P_{Tr}}} \end{aligned} \tag{1}$$

Operating these equations,

$$\overrightarrow{\mathbf{l_A}} = \overrightarrow{\mathbf{P_A P_{Tr}}} = \overrightarrow{\mathbf{P_0 P_{Tr}}} - \overrightarrow{\mathbf{P_0 P_A}} = \begin{bmatrix} x_{Tr} \\ y_{Tr} \\ z_{Tr} \end{bmatrix} + \begin{bmatrix} l_1 \\ 0 \\ 0 \end{bmatrix}$$
$$\overrightarrow{\mathbf{l_B}} = \overrightarrow{\mathbf{P_B P_{Tr}}} = \overrightarrow{\mathbf{P_0 P_{Tr}}} - \overrightarrow{\mathbf{P_0 P_B}} = \begin{bmatrix} x_{Tr} \\ y_{Tr} \\ z_{Tr} \end{bmatrix} - \begin{bmatrix} 0 \\ l_1 \\ 0 \end{bmatrix} \quad (2)$$

where l_1 is the distance from the equilibrium point to the position of the motor, and $\overrightarrow{\mathbf{l_i}}$ is the distance between $\mathbf{P_i}$ and the transmission point $\mathbf{P_{Tr}}$, $i = A, B, C, D$ (Fig. 2).

If each vector module is calculated, the relationship between distances l_A and l_B and $\mathbf{x_{Tr}} = [x_{Tr}\ y_{Tr}\ z_{Tr}]^T$ is obtained,

$$l_A = \left|\overrightarrow{\mathbf{l_A}}\right| = \sqrt{(x_{Tr} + l_1)^2 + y_{Tr}^2 + z_{Tr}^2}$$
$$l_B = \left|\overrightarrow{\mathbf{l_B}}\right| = \sqrt{x_{Tr}^2 + (y_{Tr} - l_1)^2 + z_{Tr}^2} \quad (3)$$

On the other hand, the variable length of springs S_A and S_B (n_{S_A}, n_{S_B}) depends on distances l_A, l_B and the rotation angle of the motors (q_{m_1}, q_{m_2}),

$$n_{S_A} = l_A + q_{m_1} r_m - l_1$$
$$n_{S_B} = l_B + q_{m_2} r_m - l_1 \quad (4)$$

where r_m is the pulley radius.

Therefore, using Eqs. 3 and 4, the relationship between the motion transmission $(\mathbf{x_{Tr}})$ and the measured variables $(q_{m_1}, q_{m_2}, n_{S_A}, n_{S_B})$ can be calculated,

$$n_{S_A} - q_{m_1} r_m = \sqrt{(x_{Tr} + l_1)^2 + y_{Tr}^2 + z_{Tr}^2} - l_1$$
$$n_{S_B} - q_{m_2} r_m = \sqrt{x_{Tr}^2 + (y_{Tr} - l_1)^2 + z_{Tr}^2} - l_1 \quad (5)$$

As $\mathbf{x_{Tr}}$ has three variables (x_{Tr}, y_{Tr} and z_{Tr}), a third equation is required to solve the equation system. For that purpose the motion of the actuated bar is analyzed. The actuated bar presents a spherical joint $\mathbf{P_E}$ with respect to a fixed structure. Hence, the motion of $\mathbf{P_{Tr}}$ $(\mathbf{x_{Tr}})$ is constrained to the surface of a sphere of radius l_3,

$$x_{Tr}^2 + y_{Tr}^2 + (l_3 - z_{Tr})^2 = l_3^2 \quad (6)$$

Equations 5 and 6 define the input-output kinematic model of the SEA. However, in order to fully define the motion of the SEA subsystem, the nonsensorized lower springs deformation n_{S_C} and n_{S_D} must be calculated. For that purpose, a similar procedure as the one applied for the sensorized ones is applied,

$$l_C = \left|\vec{\mathbf{l_C}}\right| = \left|\overrightarrow{\mathbf{P_C P_{Tr}}}\right| = \left|\overrightarrow{\mathbf{P_0 P_{Tr}}} - \overrightarrow{\mathbf{P_0 P_C}}\right| = \sqrt{(x_{Tr} - l_2)^2 + y_{Tr}^2 + z_{Tr}^2}$$
$$l_D = \left|\vec{\mathbf{l_D}}\right| = \left|\overrightarrow{\mathbf{P_D P_{Tr}}}\right| = \left|\overrightarrow{\mathbf{P_0 P_{Tr}}} - \overrightarrow{\mathbf{P_0 P_D}}\right| = \sqrt{x_{Tr}^2 + (y_{Tr} + l_2)^2 + z_{Tr}^2} \tag{7}$$

Hence, the variable length of the lower springs (n_{S_C}, n_{S_D}) in terms of the motors rotation angle (q_{m_1}, q_{m_2}) and the transmission motion ($\mathbf{x_{Tr}}$),

$$n_{S_C} = l_C + q_{m_1} r_m - l_2 = \sqrt{(x_{Tr} - l_2)^2 + y_{Tr}^2 + z_{Tr}^2} + q_{m_1} r_m - l_2$$
$$n_{S_D} = l_D + q_{m_2} r_m - l_2 = \sqrt{x_{Tr}^2 + (y_{Tr} + l_2)^2 + z_{Tr}^2} + q_{m_2} r_m - l_2 \tag{8}$$

Dynamic Model of the SEA

Once defined the kinematic model of the SEA, its dynamic model can be calculated. As the SEA is based on a motor-spring actuation, the exerted force will be obtained based on the spring forces that are transmitted through the cables.

The magnitude of each spring force F_{S_i} depends on its variable length n_{S_i} and its spring constant k_{S_i}, while its direction depends on the transmission motion $\mathbf{x_{Tr}}$,

$$\mathbf{F_{S_i}}(n_{S_i}, \mathbf{x_{Tr}}) = k_{S_i}\, n_{S_i}\, \mathbf{u}_i \tag{9}$$

where $\mathbf{u}_i$ is the unitary direction vector of $\mathbf{P_{Tr}P}_i$, $i = A, B, C, D$, which depends on $\mathbf{x_{Tr}}$, as calculated in Sect. 3.1.

As the transmission point is fixed to the cables, the transmitted force vector $\mathbf{F_{Tr}}$ can be calculated by adding the forces transmitted by all cables attached to this point,

$$\mathbf{F_{Tr}} = \mathbf{F}_{S_A} + \mathbf{F}_{S_B} + \mathbf{F}_{S_C} + \mathbf{F}_{S_D} = \sum_{i=A}^{D} \mathbf{F}_{S_i} \tag{10}$$

On the other hand, the actuation torque exerted by each motor $j = 1, 2$ is calculated by using their inertia coefficient I_{m_j}, the torsional viscous friction coefficient B_{m_j}, and the Coulomb friction torque defined with coefficient F_{c_j} and β_j [16],

$$\tau_{m_j} - \tau_{S_j} = I_{m_j}\, \ddot{q}_{m_j} + B_{m_j}\, \dot{q}_{m_j} + F_{c_j}\, \tanh(\beta_j\, \dot{q}_{m_j}) \tag{11}$$

where $\tau_{S_1} = \tau_{S_{AC}}$ in motor m_1 and $\tau_{S_2} = \tau_{S_{BD}}$ in motor m_2 define the equivalent torques exerted by the springs,

$$\tau_{S_{AC}} = \tau_{S_A} + \tau_{S_C} = \mathbf{F}_{S_A}\, r_m + \mathbf{F}_{S_C}\, r_m$$
$$\tau_{S_{BD}} = \tau_{S_B} + \tau_{S_D} = \mathbf{F}_{S_B}\, r_m + \mathbf{F}_{S_D}\, r_m \tag{12}$$

3.2 Pantograph Model in Wrist Mode

In this section the kinematic and dynamic models of the Pantograph on Wrist mode are analyzed.

Kinematic Model of the Pantograph

First, its kinematic model, that relates the motion the contact point $\mathbf{P_{Cn}}$, whose position is defined by $\mathbf{x_{Cn}} = [x_{Cn}\ y_{Cn}\ z_{Cn}]^T$, and the transmission point $\mathbf{P_{Tr}}$, whose position is defined by vector $\mathbf{x_{Tr}} = [x_{Tr}\ y_{Tr}\ z_{Tr}]^T$, is calculated based on the kinematic loop equation from Fig. 3,

$$\overrightarrow{\mathbf{P_E P_F}} + \overrightarrow{\mathbf{P_F P_G}} + \overrightarrow{\mathbf{P_G P_E}} = \mathbf{0} \tag{13}$$

Solving for $\mathbf{x_{Cn}}$,

$$\begin{bmatrix} x_{Cn} \\ y_{Cn} \\ z_{Cn} \end{bmatrix} = -\frac{(l_4 + d_1)\, l_8}{l_3 l_6} \begin{bmatrix} x_{Tr} \\ y_{Tr} \\ z_{Tr} \end{bmatrix} + \begin{bmatrix} 0 \\ 0 \\ l_3 + l_{10} + \frac{l_8(l_4+d_1-l_{10})}{l_6} \end{bmatrix} \tag{14}$$

As it can be seen in Eq. 14, d_1 must be calculated to solve the equation system. As l_6 is a constant distance,

$$l_6 = \left|\overrightarrow{\mathbf{l_6}}\right| = \sqrt{\left(\frac{l_4 + d_1}{l_3} x_{Tr}\right)^2 + \left(\frac{l_4 + d_1}{l_3} y_{Tr}\right)^2 + \left(\frac{l_4 + d_1}{l_3} z_{Tr} + l_{10} - (l_4 + d_1)\right)^2} \tag{15}$$

Combining this expression with Eq. 6 and operating, d_1 can be obtained in terms of the Cartesian components of $\mathbf{x_{Tr}}$,

$$d_1 = l_{10} - l_4 + \frac{-l_{10} z_{Tr}}{l_3} \pm \sqrt{\left[\frac{l_{10} z_{Tr}}{l_3} - l_{10}\right]^2 - l_{10}^2 + l_6^2} \tag{16}$$

Hence, Eqs. 14 and 16, define the relation between the input ($\mathbf{x_{Tr}}$) and the output motion ($\mathbf{x_{Cn}}$) of the Pantograph is obtained.

The speed problem is completely defined from the calculation of the Jacobian matrices relating the output variables speed ($\dot{\mathbf{x}}_{\mathbf{Cn}}$) with the time derivative of the input variables ($\dot{\mathbf{x}}_{\mathbf{Tr}}$). Therefore, derivating Eqs. 14 and 16 with respect to time the $\mathbf{J_x}$ Jacobian can be calculated,

$$\dot{\mathbf{x}}_{\mathbf{Cn}} = \underbrace{\mathbf{J_x}}_{3x3} \dot{\mathbf{x}}_{\mathbf{Tr}} \tag{17}$$

Dynamic Model of the Pantograph

The dynamic model of the Pantograph is used to determine the relationship between the transmission force ($\mathbf{F_{Tr}}$) and the contact force vectors ($\mathbf{F_{Cn}}$) depending on the transmission motion ($\mathbf{x_{Tr}}$). For that purpose, the Lagrangian formulation is used.

In Wrist mode not all the elements of the robot move, as the fixed base and the parallel bar are locked, so their energy will be zero. In addition, the transverse bar ($\mathbf{E_T}$) can only rotate along its axes (no potential energy) and the actuated bar elements ($\mathbf{E_1}$, $\mathbf{E_2}$, $\mathbf{E_3}$) present both rotation and translation motions due to the slider, the universal joints and the rotation of the transverse bar (Fig. 3).

Hence, kinetic (**K**) and potential (**U**) energies,

$$\mathbf{L} = \mathbf{K}_{E_T} + \mathbf{K}_{E_1} + \mathbf{K}_{E_2} + \mathbf{K}_{E_3} - (\mathbf{U}_{E_1} + \mathbf{U}_{E_2} + \mathbf{U}_{E_3}) \tag{18}$$

where,

$$\mathbf{K}_{E_i} = \frac{1}{2}\, m_{E_i}\, \mathbf{v}^T_{CM_{E_i}}\, \mathbf{v}_{CM_{E_i}} + \frac{1}{2}\, \omega^T_{CM_{E_i}}\, \mathbf{I}_{E_i}\, \omega_{CM_{E_i}} \tag{19}$$

$$\mathbf{U}_{\mathbf{E_i}} = m_{E_i}\, g\, h_{CM_{E_i}} \tag{20}$$

where, m_{E_i} is the mass, $\mathbf{I}_{E_i}$ is the inertia, CM_{E_i} is the mass center and $h_{CM_{E_i}}$, $\mathbf{v}_{CM_{E_i}}$ and $\omega_{CM_{E_i}}$ are the height, linear velocity and angular velocity of the mass center of the element E_i.

Kinetic and potential energies of elements $\mathbf{E_1}$ and $\mathbf{E_2}$ are defined depending on the transmission motion ($\mathbf{x_{Tr}}$) and the ones of $\mathbf{E_3}$ and $\mathbf{E_T}$ can be obtained based on the contact motion ($\mathbf{x_{Cn}}$). The calculation of each term can be easily accomplished, and it is not detailed in this work due to space constraints. So, the Lagrangian function of the Pantograph will depend on these two sets of variables ($\mathrm{L}(\mathbf{x_{Tr}}, \dot{\mathbf{x}}_{\mathbf{Tr}}, \mathbf{x_{Cn}}, \dot{\mathbf{x}}_{\mathbf{Cn}})$).

Therefore, in order to calculate the dynamic model, the Lagrangian formulation is applied to the Lagrangian defined in Eq. 18,

$$\mathbf{D_{Tr}}\ddot{\mathbf{x}}_{\mathbf{Tr}} + \mathbf{C_{Tr}}\dot{\mathbf{x}}_{\mathbf{Tr}} + \mathbf{G_{Tr}} = \frac{d}{dt}\left(\frac{\partial \mathbf{L}}{\partial \dot{\mathbf{x}}_{\mathbf{Tr}}}\right) - \frac{\partial \mathbf{L}}{\partial \mathbf{x_{Tr}}} = \sum \lambda_i \frac{\partial \Gamma(\mathbf{x_{Tr}}, \mathbf{x_{Cn}})}{\partial \mathbf{x_{Tr}}} + \mathbf{F_{Tr}} \tag{21}$$

$$\mathbf{D_{Cn}}\ddot{\mathbf{x}}_{\mathbf{Cn}} + \mathbf{C_{Cn}}\dot{\mathbf{x}}_{\mathbf{Cn}} + \mathbf{G_{Cn}} = \frac{d}{dt}\left(\frac{\partial \mathbf{L}}{\partial \dot{\mathbf{x}}_{\mathbf{Cn}}}\right) - \frac{\partial \mathbf{L}}{\partial \mathbf{x_{Cn}}} = \sum \lambda_i \frac{\partial \Gamma(\mathbf{x_{Tr}}, \mathbf{x_{Cn}})}{\partial \mathbf{x_{Cn}}} + \mathbf{F_{Cn}} \tag{22}$$

where, $\Gamma(\mathbf{x_{Tr}}, \mathbf{x_{Cn}}) = \mathbf{0}$ is the closure equation that relates the input and output variables (Eq. 13), and inertia $\mathbf{D_i}$, Coriolis $\mathbf{C_i}$ and gravity $\mathbf{G_i}$ terms can be easily calculated by grouping acceleration, velocity and gravitational terms.

If the model is to be defined in terms of $\mathbf{x_{Tr}}$, and considering that $\partial \mathbf{x_{Cn}}/\partial \mathbf{x_{Tr}} = \mathbf{J_x}$,

$$\mathbf{F_{Tr}} = \mathbf{D}\ddot{\mathbf{x}}_{\mathbf{Tr}} + \mathbf{C}\dot{\mathbf{x}}_{\mathbf{Tr}} + \mathbf{G} + \mathbf{F_E} \tag{23}$$

where,

$$\mathbf{D} = \mathbf{D_{Tr}} + \mathbf{J_x}^T \mathbf{D_{Cn}}\,\mathbf{J_x}$$

$$\mathbf{C} = \mathbf{C_{Tr}} + \mathbf{J_x}^T \mathbf{C_{Cn}}\,\mathbf{J_x} + \mathbf{J_x}^T \mathbf{D_{Cn}}\,\dot{\mathbf{J}}_\mathbf{x}$$

$$\mathbf{G} = \mathbf{G_{Tr}} + \mathbf{J_x}^T \mathbf{G_{Cn}}$$

$$\mathbf{F_E} = -\mathbf{J_x}^T \mathbf{F_{Cn}}$$

This equation defines the relationship between the transmission force ($\mathbf{F_{Tr}}$), the transmission motion ($\mathbf{x_{Tr}}$) and the contact force ($\mathbf{F_{Cn}}$).

4 Experimental Validation

Several experimental tests have been carried out to demonstrate the effectiveness of the calculated kinematic and dynamic models. For that purpose, the calculated models have been implemented in Matlab, and its results are compared with those obtained from the experimental tests with the UHP prototype.

In order to perform the experimental validation data captured from the UHP robot is used: both motors encoders that measure the motors rotation angle ($\mathbf{q_m}$) and the linear-potentiometers that measure the variable lengths of springs S_A and S_B (n_{S_A}, n_{S_B}). In addition, a force sensor has been integrated to measure contact force ($\mathbf{F_{Cn}}$) and a 3 axis inclinometer has been attached to the Pantograph, so that the x and y inclination angle can be measured, and the x_{Tr} and y_{Tr} variables are estimated easily.

Parameters of the UHP elements have been experimentally identified, while the motor-pulley parameters have been identified using the Grey-box procedure [16]. Real prototype parameters are summarized in Table 1 (The inertia tensors are defined as centroidal, hence, only diagonal components are detailed).

Three tests have been carried out to validate the models. First, the UHP kinematic model in Wrist mode is validated. For this purpose, motors are induced to perform a sinusoidal motion with 5 s period and no contact force is applied. Motor rotation angles ($\mathbf{q_m}$), variable length of the upper springs (n_{S_A}, n_{S_B}) and actuated bar angles are measured and used to estimate the contact motion ($\mathbf{x_{Cn}}$).

In Fig. 4, the real and estimated values of $\mathbf{x_{Cn}}$ x and y componentes are observed. As it can be seen, the mean error is smaller than one millimeter and the maximum error is 6 mm.

The second test is used to validate the dynamic model of the drive system SEA. As forces of the SEA are related to the spring motion, the test is based on the estimation of the spring measurements and forces. For this test, the Pantograph is locked in the equilibrium position ($\mathbf{x_{Tr}} = [0\,0\,0]^T$) and the motors execute a sinusoidal motion with 5 s period. In this case, motors torques ($\tau_\mathbf{m}$) and rotation angles ($\mathbf{q_m}$) and variable length of the upper springs (n_{S_A}, n_{S_B}) are measured, along with the actuated bar orientation using the inclinometer.

Table 1 Parameters of the UHP prototype

Parameter	Value	Parameter	Value
l_1	0.575 m	r_{p_1}	0.047 m
l_2	0.15 m	r_{p_2}	0.0325 m
l_3	0.18 m	I_{m_1}	0.003615 N s^2/rad
l_4	0.46 m	I_{m_2}	0.002742 N s^2/rad
l_5	0.64 m	B_{m_1}	1.02×10^{-7}N s/rad
l_6	0.202 m	B_{m_2}	5.27×10^{-9}N s/rad
l_7	0.12 m	F_{c_1}	0.840395 N m
l_8	0.268 m	F_{c_2}	0.731213 N m
l_9	0.268 m	β_1	4223.98
l_{10}	0.662 m	β_2	4318.25
		k_{S_i}	4000 N/m
m_{E_1}	0.882 kg	I_{E_1}	[13.50.49 13.4] 10^{-3}kg m^2
m_{E_2}	1.25 kg	I_{E_2}	[9.70.599.51] 10^{-3}kg m^2
m_{E_3}	1.23 kg	I_{E_3}	[4.91.963.61] 10^{-3}kg m^2
m_{E_T}	1.55 kg	I_{E_T}	[4013.528] 10^{-3}kg m^2

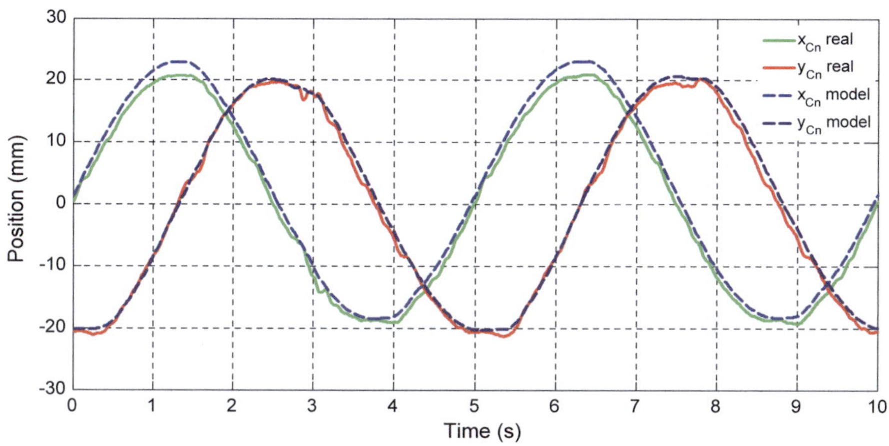

Fig. 4 Kinematic model validation test results

Based on the inclinometer data, the real $\mathbf{x_{Tr}}$ is obtained. Combining it with the measured motor position $\mathbf{q_m}$ and torque $\tau_\mathbf{m}$, the spring force $\mathbf{F_{Si}}$ is estimated, and using the spring constant, the variable length of the springs S_A and S_B (n_{S_A}, n_{S_B}) is calculated.

In Fig. 5, the real and estimated values of n_{S_A} and n_{S_B} are observed. In this case, the mean error is half millimeter and the maximum error is smaller than 3 mm.

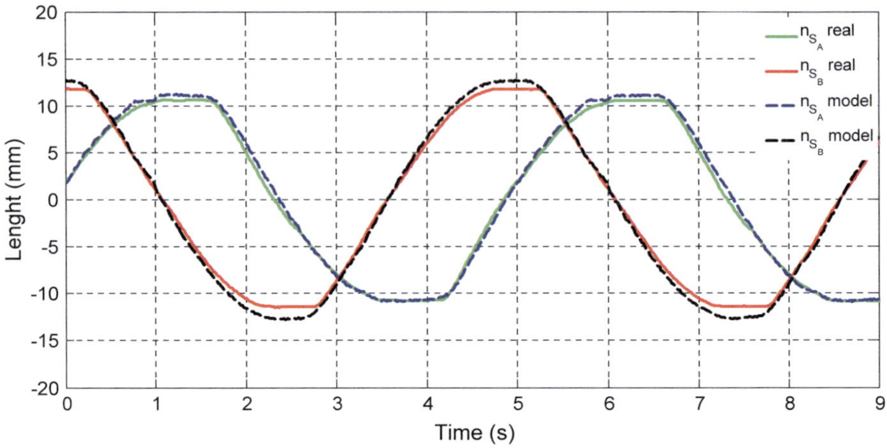

Fig. 5 Drive systems dynamic model validation test results

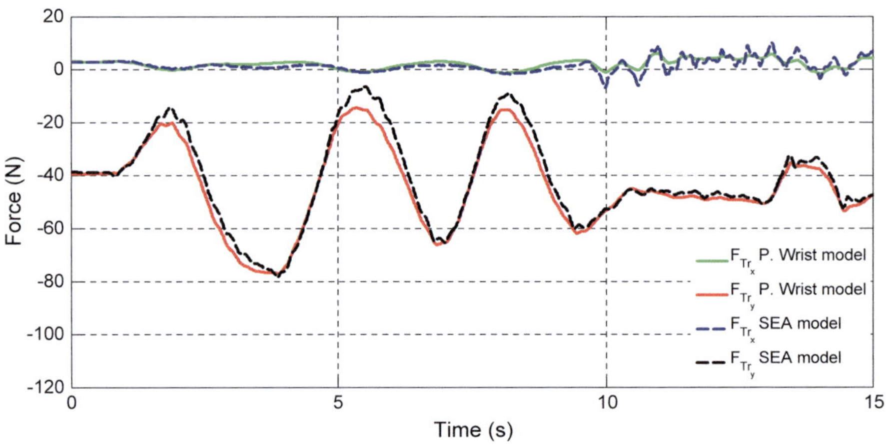

Fig. 6 UHP dynamic model validation test results

In the final test, the dynamic model of the UHP robot in Wrist mode is validated. In order to achieve this, the UHP will execute a trajectory, while the user exerts external force. In this case, motor rotation angles ($\mathbf{q_m}$), variable length of the upper springs (n_{S_A}, n_{S_B}), actuated bar angles and the contact force ($\mathbf{F_{Cn}}$) are measured.

Using these measurements the transmission force ($\mathbf{F_{Tr}}$) is calculated based on the dynamic model of SEA, validated in the previous section. In addition, the transmission force is also estimated by using the contact force measurement and the dynamic model of the Pantograph on the Wrist mode. The latter is considered to be the more accurate.

In Fig. 6, the values of $\mathbf{F_{Tr}}$ obtained with the dynamic model of the SEA and with the dynamic model of the Pantograph are observed. As it can be seen, the mean error is 5 N and the error is always less than the 10%.

5 Conclusions

In this work kinematic and dynamic models of a multifunctional rehabilitation robot UHP (Universal Haptic Pantograph) are presented. The UHP provides various functionality modes that provide different rehabilitation exercises. This work focuses on the Wrist mode.

The UHP robot modeling is divided in two parts: the drive system, which is based on a Serial Elastic Actuator system, and a Pantograph. To solve the kinematic model, the closure equations are used, while Lagrangian formulation is used to calculate the dynamic model of the robot.

To verify the models, a set of experimental tests have been carried out. Results show that the model works properly in all relevant scenarios. The motion mean error in the contact point ($\mathbf{P_{Cn}}$) is one millimeter while the transmission force ($\mathbf{F_{Tr}}$) error is smaller than the 10%.

The calculated kinematic and dynamic model are critical to perform proper control of the robot-patient interaction. The proposed models will be used to estimate the force and motion of this interaction without the direct measurement of the contact force, hence, reducing the economical cost of the robot.

Acknowledgements This work was supported in part by the Basque Country Governments (GV/EJ) under grant PRE-2014-1-152, UPV/EHU's UFI11/28 project, Spanish Ministry of Economy and Competitiveness' MINECO & FEDER inside the DPI-2012-32882 project, Spanish Ministry of Economy and Competitiveness' BES-2013-066142 grant, Euskampus, FIK and Spanish Ministry of Science and Innovation PDI-020100-2009-21 project.

References

1. Babaiasl, M., Mahdioun, S.H., Jaryani, P., Yazdani, M.: A review of technological and clinical aspects of robot-aided rehabilitation of upper-extremity after stroke. Disabil. Rehabil. Assist. Technol. 1–18 (2015). doi:10.3109/17483107.2014.1002539
2. Carignan, C., Tang, J., Roderick, S.: Development of an exoskeleton haptic interface for virtual task training. IEEE/RSJ Int. Conf. Intell. Robots Syst. (IROS) **2009**, 3697–3702 (2009). doi:10.1109/IROS.2009.5354834
3. Corbyn, Z.: A growing global burden. Nat. **510**(7506), S2–S3 (2014). doi:10.1038/510S2a
4. Gopura, R.A.R.C., Kiguchi, K., Li, Y.: SUEFUL-7: a 7DOF upper-limb exoskeleton robot with muscle-model-oriented EMG-based control. IEEE Int. Conf. Intell. Robots Syst. 1126–1131 (2009). doi:10.1109/IROS.2009.5353935
5. Harwin, W.S., Patton, J.L., Edgerton, V.R.: Challenges and opportunities for robot-mediated neurorehabilitation. Proc. IEEE **94**(9), 1717–1726 (2006). doi:10.1109/JPROC.2006.880671

6. Maciejasz, P., Eschweiler, J., Gerlach-Hahn, K., Jansen-Troy, A., Leonhardt, S.: A survey on robotic devices for upper limb rehabilitation. J. Neuroeng. Rehabil. **11**(3), 1–29 (2014). doi:10.1186/1743-0003-11-3
7. Oblak, J., Matjačić, Z.: Design of a series visco-elastic actuator for multi-purpose rehabilitation haptic device. J. Neuroeng. Rehabil. **8:3**(1), 1–13 (2011). DOI 10.1186/1743-0003-8-3
8. Perry, J.C., Oblak, J., Jung, J.H., Cikajlo, I., Veneman, J.F., Goljar, N., Bizoviar, N., Matjai, Z., Keller, T.: Variable structure pantograph mechanism with spring suspension system for comprehensive upper-limb haptic movement training. J. Rehabil. Res. Dev. **48**(4), 317–334 (2011). doi:10.1682/JRRD.2010.03.0043
9. Rahman, M.H., Ouimet, T.K., Saad, M., Kenné, J.P.: Development and control of a wearable robot for rehabilitation of elbow and shoulder joint movements. IEEE Ind. Electron. Soc. 1506–1511 (2010). doi:10.1109/IECON.2010.5675459
10. Sawaki, L.: Use-dependent plasticity of the human motor cortex in health and disease. IEEE Eng. Med. Biol. Mag. **24**(1), 36–39 (2005). doi:10.1109/MEMB.2005.1384098
11. Song, Z., Zhang, S., Gao, B.: Implementation of resistance training using an upper-limb exoskeleton rehabilitation device for elbow joint. J. Med. Biol. Eng. **34**(2), 188–196 (2014). doi:10.5405/jmbe.1337
12. Stienen, A.H.A., Hekman, E.E.G., Ter Braak, H., Aalsma, A.M.M., Van Der Helm, F.C.T., Van Der Kooij, H.: Design of a rotational hydro-elastic actuator for an active upper-extremity rehabilitation exoskeleton. 881– 888 (2008). doi:10.1109/BIOROB.2008.4762873
13. Thrift, A.G., Cadilhac, D.A., Thayabaranathan, T., Howard, G., Howard, V.J., Rothwell, P.M., Donnan, G.A.: Global stroke statistics. Int. J. Stroke **9**, 6–18 (2014). doi:10.1111/ijs.12245
14. Vertechy, R., Frisoli, A., Dettori, A., Solazzi, M., Bergamasco, M.: Development of a new exoskeleton for upper limb rehabilitation. IEEE Int. Conf. Rehabil. Robot. (ICORR) **2009**, 188–193 (2009). doi:10.1109/ICORR.2009.5209502
15. Wen, Y., Rosen, J., Li, X.: PID admittance control for an upper limb exoskeleton. IEEE Am. Control Conf. 1124–1129 (2011). doi:10.1109/ACC.2011.5991147
16. Wernholt, E.: Nonlinear identification of a physically parameterized robot model. SYSID 143–148 (2006). doi:10.3182/20060329-3-AU-2901.00016
17. Zhou, S.H., Fong, J., Crocher, V., Tan, Y., Oetomo, D., Mareels, I.: Learning control in robot-assisted rehabilitation of motor skills a review. J. Control Decis. **7706**, 1–25 (2016). doi:10.1080/23307706.2015.1129295

Minimally Actuated Four-Bar Linkages for Upper Limb Rehabilitation

E. Xydas, A. Mueller and L.S. Louca

Abstract In the previous years the scientific community dealt extensively with designing, developing and testing robot-based rehabilitation systems. Besides the benefits that resulted for disabled people, this twenty-year endeavor has helped us improve our understanding of the neuroplasticity mechanisms in the Central Nervous System (CNS) and how these are triggered through the interaction with the physical world and especially through interaction with robots. In these systems, most of the state-of-the-art arrangements are based on multi-Degree of Freedom (DOF) open kinematic chains. They also employ sophisticated control hardware as well as high-profile actuators and sensors. The state-of-the-art technology that is integrated in these arrangements, increases the cost and at the same time requires the presence of trained employees that are able to maintain and operate such systems. Another option, are mechanisms that are based on four- and six-bar linkages. These are closed kinematic chain designs that can generate a variety of paths, yet they can do so with much less flexibility and adaptation possibilities. Despite the reduced flexibility over their robotic counterparts these mechanisms are attractive due to their reduced cost, simplicity and low external power requirement. This paper elaborates on the synthesis, analysis, simulation and passive control of four-bar linkages that can be used in upper limb rehabilitation and extends previous work by simulating the mechanism-impaired user interaction using a dynamic multibody system model. The emphasis in this work has been on straight-line

E. Xydas (✉) · L.S. Louca
Mechanical and Manufacturing Engineering Department, University of Cyprus, Latsia, Cyprus
e-mail: evagoras.xydas@nu.edu.kz

L.S. Louca
e-mail: lslouca@ucy.ac.cy

E. Xydas
Nazarbayev University, Mechanical Engineering Department, Astana, Kazakhstan

A. Mueller
Johannes Kepler University, Institute of Robotics, Linz, Austria
e-mail: a.mueller@jku.at

M. Husty and M. Hofbaur (eds.), *New Trends in Medical and Service Robots*, Mechanisms and Machine Science 48, DOI 10.1007/978-3-319-59972-4_10

trajectory generation, but this established methodology can be applied for developing mechanisms with higher complexity and more complex trajectories.

Keywords Rehabilitation · Four-bar linkage · Minimum-jerk-trajectory · Reaching · Straight line motion

1 Introduction

Despite the wide use of closed kinematic chain designs in industry, these have not been employed for human-machine interaction [1–6]. Instead, multi-DOF and open kinematic chain designs are used for most of the applications involving human robot interaction and assistive robotics as well as robotic rehabilitation [7–11]. The main function that is considered in this paper is the guidance of the user's hand along paths that resemble the natural ones, with respect to temporal and spatial characteristics [12–14]. Inarguably, the multi-DOF approach provides flexibility and freedom for adaptation but at the same time, it also provides less robustness. Such a design is more susceptible to unstable movement as well as to singularities and vibrations. Also the higher number of actuators and sensors that are needed further increases the cost of these systems.

Furthermore, the computer, software and complex electronics that accompany these systems require routine technical support and maintenance, which raises the cost even more. Such provisions and resources are usually available at medium and large centers in the western world. Nevertheless, the biggest percentage of disabled people worldwide live in developing countries [15]. The neurorehabilitation services in most of these countries are either inexistent or inadequate and overall, the availability of trained professionals is far from sufficient [16]. In the 1970s and the early 1980s, community based rehabilitation was proposed and promoted by the world bodies as an approach that is suitable for developing countries with limited resources in order to provide wider coverage of services. A key element of this approach is the transfer of minimally-adequate rehabilitation skills to family members and other volunteers in the community. Also, one of the aims of the 2014–2021 World Health Organization (WHO) Global disability action plan is "to strengthen and extend rehabilitation, habilitation, assistive technology, assistance and support services, and community-based rehabilitation," [17]. Furthermore, the World Federation for Neurorehabilitation (WFNR) in their 2015 call for action for improving neurorehabilitation in developing countries supports Community Based Rehabilitation (CBR) services as "the most appropriate way forward in developing countries" [18].

The current and previous work by the authors addressed the issue of developing rehabilitation devices that are more cost-effective than the conventional robotic systems [1–4], as well as simpler in use and ergonomics. With the use of the proposed mechanisms generic paths can be generated as a result of structural and topological constraints rather than by coordinated actuation of the multiple DOFs.

The simpler and most widely used mechanism of this kind is the four-bar linkage, a 1-DOF linkage. Despite its simplicity, by changing its geometrical characteristics a specific path can be produced. A vast amount of published work describes various methods for synthesis, analysis and design of four-bar linkages for achieving a wide variety of tasks [19, 20]. This work is focused on the design, inertial parameter optimization and passive control of four-bar linkages for achieving natural temporal characteristics along linear trajectories [12]. The main model that is used as a reference for the speed profile along the whole range of linear movement is the Minimum Jerk Model (MJM). The model establishes that when people perform reaching tasks on a plane (i.e. a table), they naturally track a straight line and that the hand velocity is governed by a smooth curve and depicted by the model. Providing rehabilitation along straight lines can be both desirable and beneficial as it addresses the most basic level of movement that humans can perform with their hands. Furthermore, straight-line motion requirement is an ideal basis for an initial design that can be later modified for curved motion generation, given the versatility of four-bars in this respect. Figure 1 depicts three well known straight line generation mechanisms. The mechanisms (from left to right) are the Watt's, Hoeken's and Chebyshev's and have been analyzed kinematically and dynamically in [3]. The analysis that is carried out in this and previous work mainly employs the Chebyshev's mechanism but it can be applied for most straight-line generating four-bar linkages.

The previous work has shown that by integrating passive elements (springs) on a four-bar linkage natural straight-line hand trajectories can be generated with minimal external power [2, 3]. Further work established a numerical optimization procedure that identifies a set of linear springs that can act as passive control elements [1]. Finally, a parametric investigation showed that the external torque requirement could be further reduced by varying the Center of Gravity (CG) of the mechanism's links [4]. The work in this paper outlines the previous research and further extends it by simulating the interaction of an impaired user with the mechanism. The simulation is performed in Alaska multibody-dynamics software [21].

The current work is presented through the following sections: First a background section presents the main hand movement model that is employed in this work (Minimum Jerk Model) as well as the method by which the impaired user

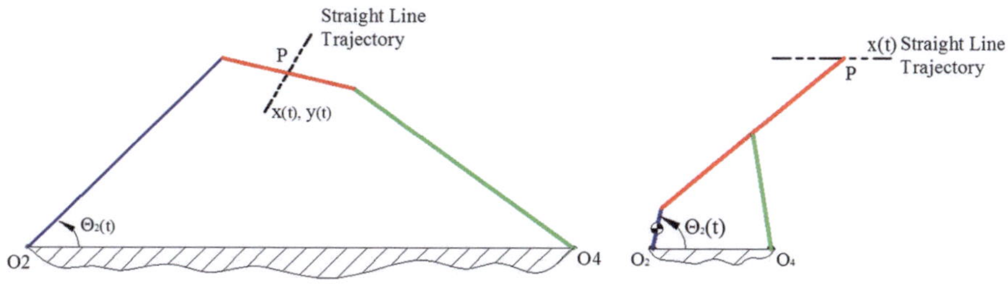

Fig. 1 Straight line generating mechanisms: Watt's, Hoeken's and Chebyshev's

interaction force has been established. Then the main principles that are applied in kinematic and kinetostatic analysis of the four-bar linkage are shown. The main purpose of this analysis is the establishment of the required input torque that can cause the mechanism to move under the velocity profile specified by the MJM. The fourth section elaborates on the identification of springs as passive control elements that can reduce the external torque requirement. Finally the results of the user-mechanism interaction simulation are presented, followed by discussion and conclusions.

2 Background

2.1 Minimum Jerk Model (MJM)

A frequently employed approach for predicting spatio-temporal trajectories of reaching tasks is to minimize a cost function in order to generate a time-space dependent trajectory equation. Among various cost functions, the model that accounts for the largest body of data, while being attractively simple is the MJM [12]. In this case, the trajectory equations are generated by minimizing a jerk-based cost function, jerk being the derivative of acceleration. The result is a fifth order polynomial for each coordinate:

$$x_{MJM}(\tau) = x_i + (x_i - x_f)\left(-10\tau^3 + 15\tau^4 - 6\tau^5\right) \quad (1)$$

$$y_{MJM}(\tau) = y_i + (y_i - y_f)\left(-10\tau^3 + 15\tau^4 - 6\tau^5\right) \quad (2)$$

where, $\tau = t/t_f$ is the normalized time that takes values ranging from 0 to 1. Also, $\{x_i|y_i\}$ and $\{x_f|y_f\}$, are the coordinates of initial and final positions.

Here, the MJM is applied in its 1-dimensional form along the x direction, where (2) is disregarded and only (1) is employed. As an example Fig. 2 shows the position for a 1-dimensional straight-line motion of 0.1 m length duration of 2 s, as generated by Eq. (1).

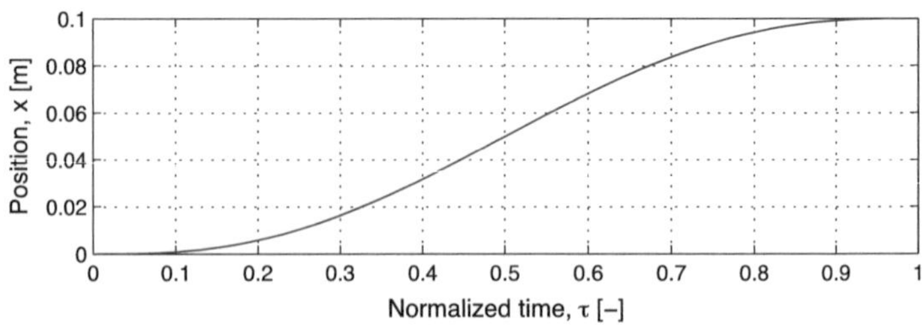

Fig. 2 Position profile for a MJM trajectory

2.2 User Force

Before moving to detailed design and manufacturing it is important to perform simulations that account for the human user as well. When the mechanism moves without any external force, the springs, motor and the controller only account for the effect of the inertial forces in order to generate a MJM motion at the coupler point as in Fig. 1. Given a non-impaired user interacting with the mechanism, ideally, zero interaction force will be generated at the coupler since the user will move in a natural way and will have the same velocity as the coupler point of the mechanism. In practice, this force will be minimal just after a few repetitions, and given a fixed target and a predetermined time requirement. In the case of a user with a neuro-disability, the generated motion will differ from the MJM trajectory; the user will tend to be either faster or slower than the reference movement, opposing in this way the arrangement's design temporal motion. For simulation purposes this force is calculated based on experimental measurements with users with Multiple Sclerosis (MS) as presented in previous work by the authors [22, 23]. In Fig. 3 the comparison of people with MS and an MJM generated trajectory is shown. Note that the MJM trajectory is normalized for 0.5 s while in reality the measurements refer to a variety of durations. The validity of this approach is established statistically in [22] where seven people with Multiple Sclerosis participated in the experiments. It can be seen that until 0.35 s the impaired users' average is slow, while after that he is becoming faster than the reference.

The next step is the transformation of positional difference to interactive force. It is achieved by considering an imaginary spring that connects the user's hand with the mechanism (coupler point 'P') (Fig. 4). The idea of using an imaginary spring for calculating interaction force has been used extensively in the case of force haptic-interface systems [24 cited in 25]. In the specific case and given the lack of experimental data for force, this method is ideal for representing the interaction between the user and the mechanism, where forces are generated based on the different motion potentials. With the imaginary spring, and depending on the lag or lead of the user with respect to the coupler point, a design coupler force is calculated.

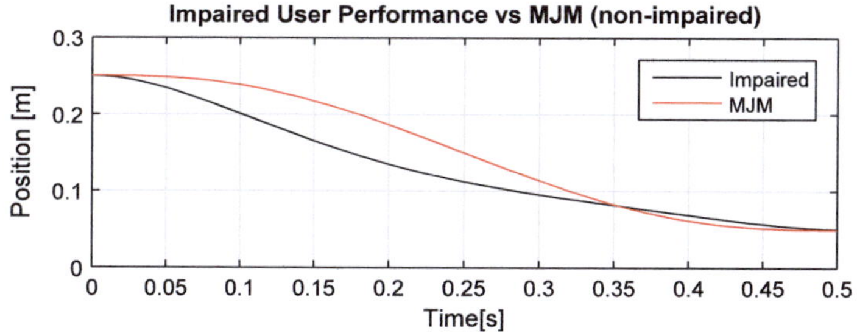

Fig. 3 Position difference between impaired users (MS) and MJM generated trajectory

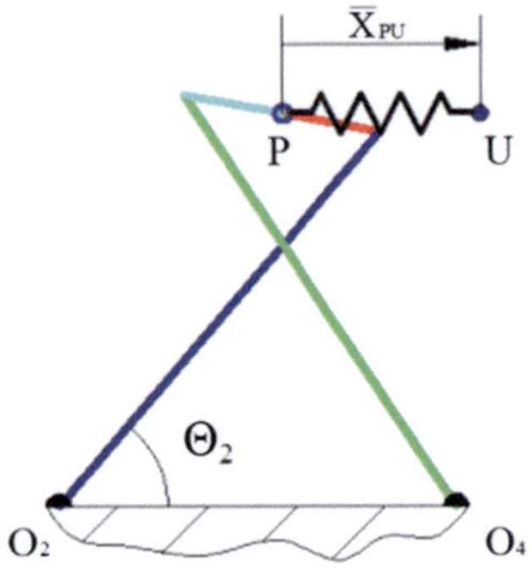

Fig. 4 Liner spring model of user-mechanism interaction

The spring force $\overline{F}_{PU}$ will can be calculated by Eq. (3) where k_{PU} is the spring stiffness.

$$\overline{F}_{PU} = k_{PU} \cdot \overline{X}_{PU} \tag{3}$$

The spring stiffness is calculated using a maximum force value of 15 N and the maximum difference between the user trajectory and the MJM trajectory. This difference is taken from the data that refer to Fig. 2 and is equal to 0.0533 m. The maximum force of 15 N is based on measurements performed by authors in previous work [23] and will also serve as a safety limit in the final design. Given the maximum positional difference and the maximum force, the spring stiffness is equal to:

$$k_{PU} = \frac{|\bar{F}_{PU}(\max)|}{|\bar{X}_{PU}(\max)|} = \frac{15\,\mathrm{N}}{0.0533\,\mathrm{m}} = 281.4\frac{\mathrm{N}}{\mathrm{m}} \tag{4}$$

The force along the rest of the trajectory is calculated using the resulting spring stiffness and Eq. (3). It is shown in Fig. 5.

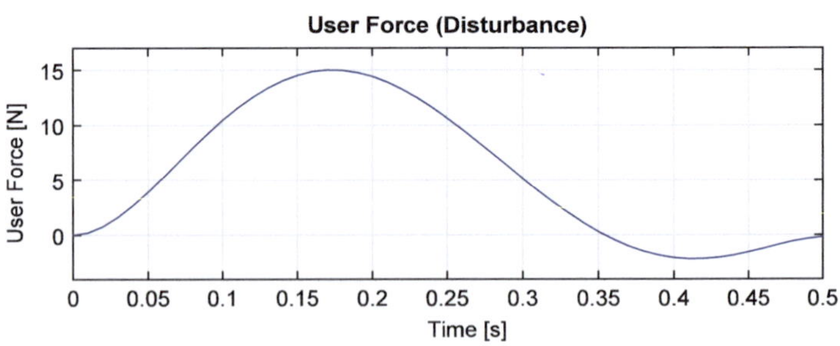

Fig. 5 User-mechanism interaction force

2.3 Straight Line Four-Bar Linkage for Generating a MJM Velocity Profile

Among the straight line four-bar linkages that have been considered in this work, the Chebyshev's mechanism is chosen for the further analysis as it is relatively symmetric and can lead to more meaningful parametric studies. The mechanism is synthesized and designed so that the coupler point can cover a 0.3 m straight-line trajectory. For avoiding extreme torque values at the boundaries, only a length of 0.2 m of the straight-line trajectory is considered. The duration of the motion is set to be 0.5 s. Note that the natural duration of any reaching task towards a target is standard and is given by the Fitts' Law [13]. With respect to Fig. 5, the coupler point P has to move for 0.2 m, under the temporal specification prescribed by the MJM (Fig. 2). More specifically, the position of coupler point 'P' is:

$$x(t) = 0.25 + (0.05 - 0.25)\left(10\left(\frac{t}{0.5}\right)^3 - 15\left(\frac{t}{0.5}\right)^4 + 6\left(\frac{t}{0.5}\right)^5\right) \qquad (5)$$

where the values 0.25 and 0.05 refer to the initial and final positions, x_i and x_f (in meters), and 0.5 is the movement duration in seconds as explained above. A kinematic analysis that considers the required position, velocity and acceleration was carried out. For a complete analysis refer to [1]. The following geometric characteristics were used (Table 1).

Figure 6 shows the simulated geometry of the Chebyshev's mechanism and the generated straight line trajectory. Figure 7 shows the corresponding angular velocities of the three links, i.e. the inverse kinematics solution.

Following the kinematic analysis a kinetostatic analysis is performed for calculating the input torque T_{12} that can generate the required spatio-temporal characteristics when applied to the mechanism.

Further analysis investigated the effect of adding a flywheel at the input link O_2 (Fig. 8). The flywheel increases the input torque requirement, but at the same time it reduces the sensitivity of the mechanism to disturbance (impaired user motion). Essentially the flywheel increases the inertial resistance of the arrangement and consequently the required input torque, while the generated motion remains the same. For countering the increased input torque requirement, stiffer springs are needed and once those are active the external input torque is again minimized, with the difference that a bigger user force will be needed for altering the mechanism's inherent motion. The optimum flywheel size and overall inertial characteristics are

Table 1 Geometric characteristics

Link	Length (m)
1 (ground)	0.3000
2 (input) + flywheel	0.3750
3 (coupler)	0.1500
4 (output)	0.3750

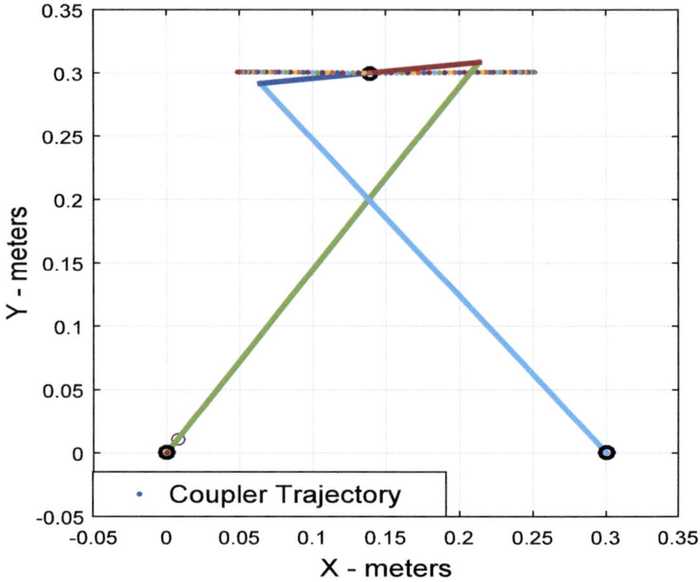

Fig. 6 Straight line generated by the simulated Chebyshev's Mechanisms

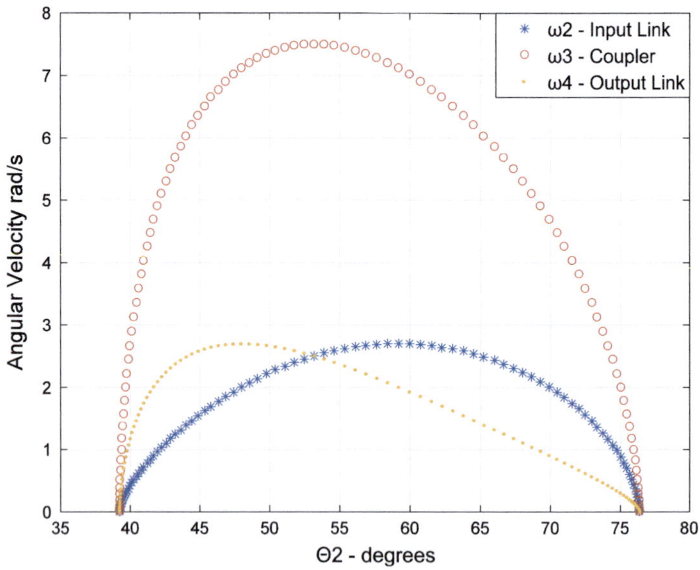

Fig. 7 Angular velocities of the links that respect to MJM movement at point P

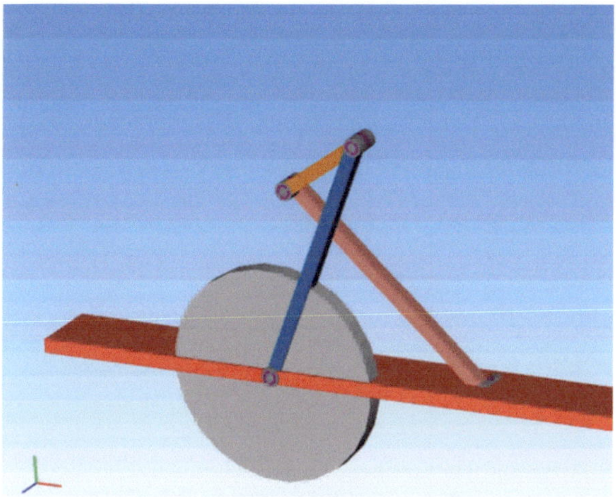

Fig. 8 Alaska simulation model of the Chebyshev mechanism with a flywheel

Table 2 Design parameters

Link	Mass (kg)	Moment of inertia (kg m^2)	Length (m)
1 (ground)	–	–	0.3000
2 (input) + flywheel	5.3831	0.0803	0.3750
3 (coupler)	0.1532	2.8733×10^{-4}	0.1500
4 (output)	0.3831	0.0045	0.3750

part of further investigation by the authors. For the kinetostatic analysis the following parameters were employed (Table 2).

The flywheel itself has a mass of 5 kg and a radius of 0.15 m. For a more detailed kinematic and kinetostatic analysis of the proposed system refer to [2].

The resulting input torque T_{12} is shown in Fig. 9.

3 Design of the Passive Control Elements

3.1 Linear Torsional Springs

After the required input torque for generating a natural motion profile is known (Fig. 9), instead of using external power alone for the generation of that torque, a combination of spring-elements and an external actuator can be used. These springs can be either linear or torsional springs. In the case of torsional springs the immediate approach for establishing the spring characteristics is to approximate the required input torque with a linear function that can be generated with the use of two linear springs. In Fig. 10 a linear approximation of the required input torque is

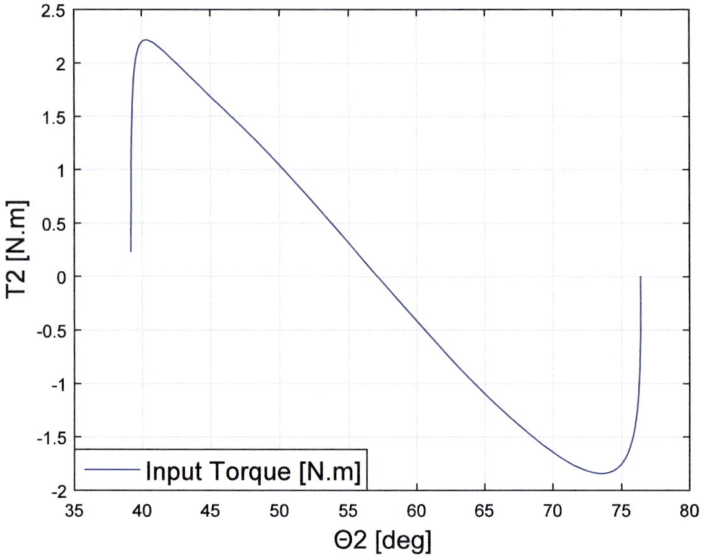

Fig. 9 Required input torque T_{12} for generating a MJM motion at the coupler point P

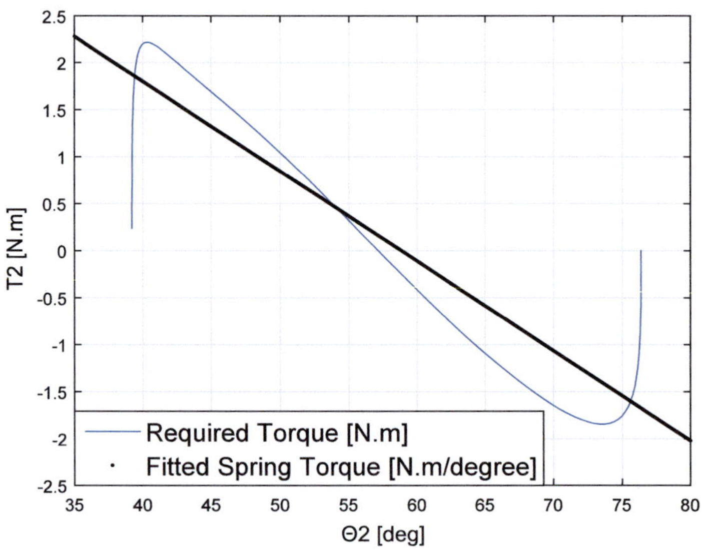

Fig. 10 Required input torque T12 versus approximated linear torque

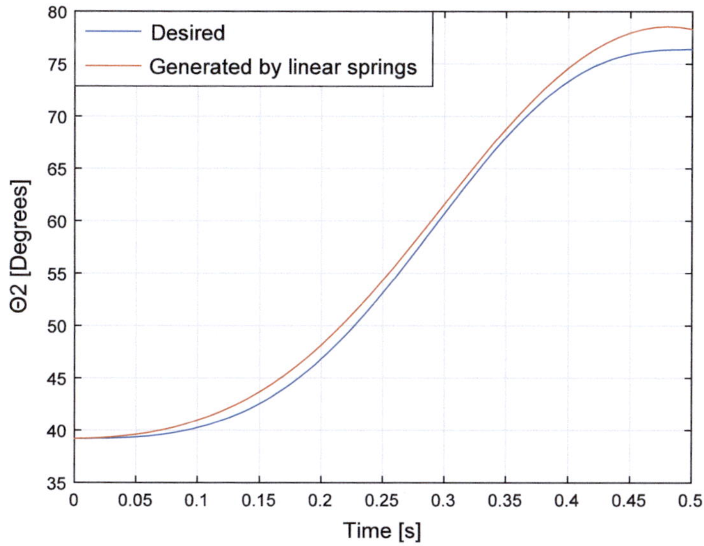

Fig. 11 Comparison of desired temporal orientation of link 2 and orientation generated by applying a linear input torque

shown. This is for the mechanism with the same inertial and geometrical characteristics as in Sect. 2.3.

The linear torque function that is shown in Fig. 10 is generated numerically with the use of the MATLAB function 'fit'. It can be approximated by two linear torsional springs. The respective equation of the linear torque is:

$$T_{12} = -0.09552\Theta_2 + 5.623\ (\mathrm{N\,m}) \tag{6}$$

The calculated linear torque is applied in a forward-dynamics model in Alaska software and the resulting temporal rotation of the input link is compared to the one gained in the kinematic analysis. The comparison is depicted in Fig. 11. The resulting curves in Fig. 11 suggest that with the use of two opposing linear springs the natural motion of the mechanism can be generated without an external power source. Note that this is the response of a mechanism without user-force. In Sect. 4 the external torque requirement with the presence of user force is investigated.

3.2 Linear Springs with Nonlinear Kinematics

The requirement is to determine two linear springs, one for acceleration and one for deceleration that can move the mechanism under the required input torque T_{12}. The principle is shown in Fig. 12. The accelerating spring (red) will cause the whole mechanism to accelerate until the input link meets the decelerating spring (green).

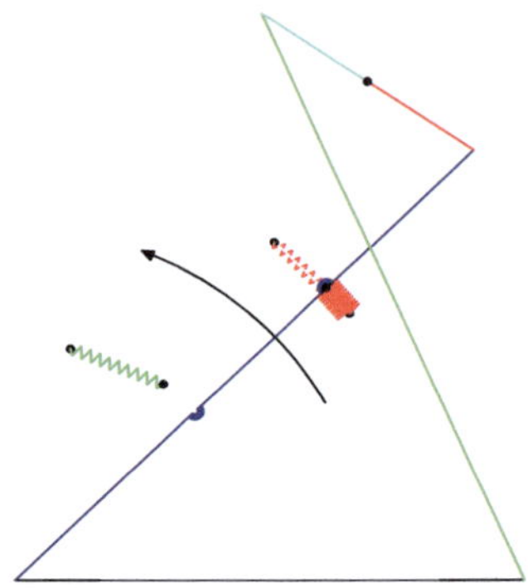

Fig. 12 The Chebyshev's mechanism at a random position with the accelerating spring (*red*) active

At that point, the accelerating spring will stop acting. Note that when the springs are in contact with the mechanism they can rotate around their fixed (ground) point.

Figure 13 shows the torque generated by two linear springs of arbitrary characteristics as compared to the required input torque (in this case without flywheel). The goal is to change the generated spring torque in order to approach the required torque. This is achieved by setting an optimization problem that minimizes the difference between the two torque profiles. There are many alternatives in calculating the difference, however, the overall difference throughout the operating range is selected, as it is calculated by a 2-norm. The design variables are the coordinates of the two attachment points of the spring's ends. The two distances of the attachment points, L_{S1} and L_{S2}, and the attachment angle, β, represent these points (a set for each spring). Thus the optimization problem has the form:

$$\min_{L_{s1},L_{s2},\beta} ||T_2 - T_{2S}|| \tag{7}$$

The optimization is performed using MATLAB and the fmincon function since the design variables are constrained. The optimization is performed with different

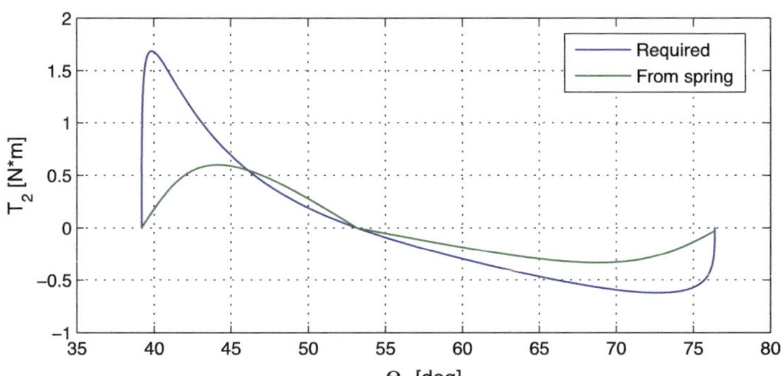

Fig. 13 Required torque and spring torque

Table 3 Optimized variables

Accelerating spring	Decelerating spring
$L_{s1} = 0.2547$ m	$L_{s1} = 0.1435$ m
$L_{s2} = 0.2549$ m	$L_{s2} = 0.1472$ m
$\beta = 39.18°$	$\beta = 76.72°$

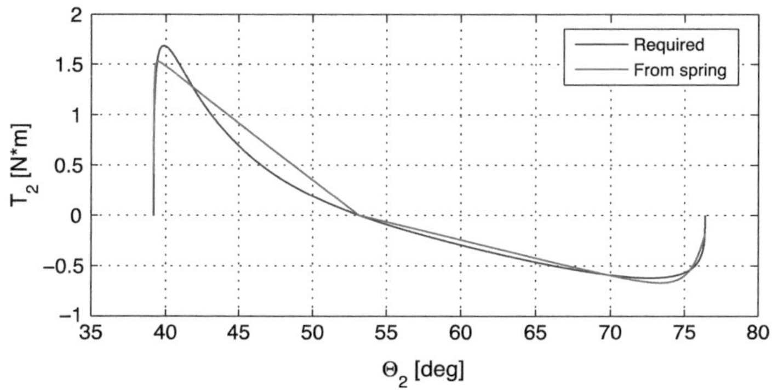

Fig. 14 Required torque and spring torque with the optimized variables

starting points in order to ensure that the optimum is found. The results of the optimization and optimum solution are given in Table 3.

The resulting spring torque for the optimized variables is then calculated by kinetostatic analysis and compared to the torque required to generate the MJM trajectory. The two torque profiles are shown in Fig. 14 where the optimized spring torque is close to the required torque.

Figure 15 shows the temporal orientation of link 2 that is generated with the use of the linear springs as compared to the required one. It can be seen that there is a zero difference that increases as the motion goes on. Also the spring-generated curve stops at 0.4 s. This is because as the spring rotates is almost aligns with the link and the generated torque tends to be zero.

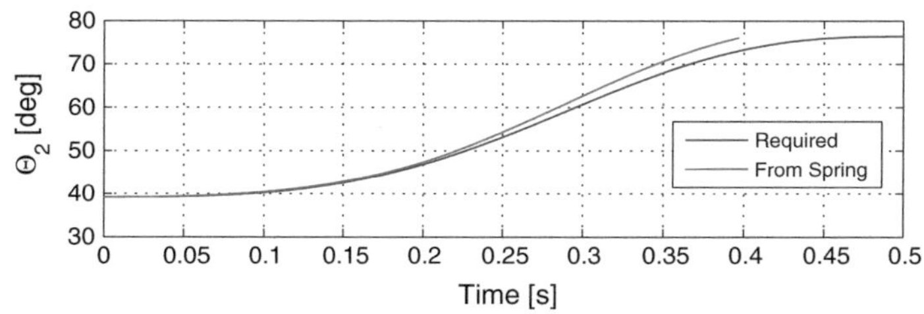

Fig. 15 Comparison of input link angle Θ_2 generated from forward dynamics versus the required Θ_2

4 Simulation Results

In the simulation environment two different cases are considered. In both cases the impaired user force (Fig. 5) is active while the torsional springs are active only in the first case. A motor is present at the input (pivot O_2) that is set to generate the required angular velocity ω_2 so that the MJM profile is generated at point 'P'. Angular velocity, ω_2 can be seen in Fig. 7. Figure 8 shows the simulated mechanism.

Figure 16 shows the resulting motor torque for the active and non-active springs case respectively. Figure 17 shows the corresponding power and energy, which are significantly reduced with the addition of the springs.

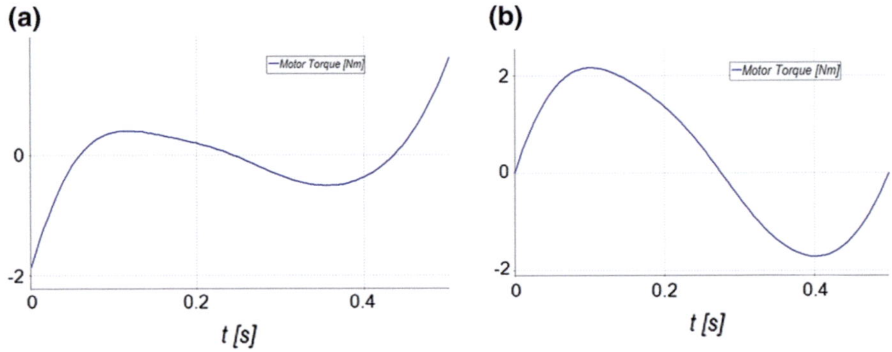

Fig. 16 Motor torque: **a** including torsional spring, **b** no attached torsional spring

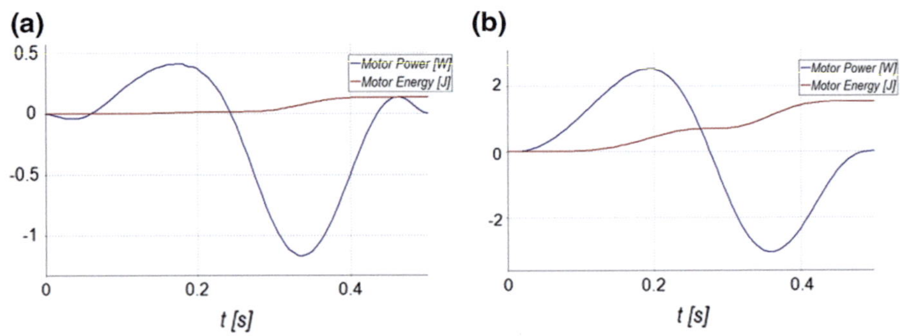

Fig. 17 Energy consumption and power of the external motor: **a** torsional spring, **b** no spring

5 Discussion and Conclusions

It is shown that the proposed design method can potentially lead to a low-cost rehabilitation mechanism that retains a number of characteristics and responses of high end systems. With the passive elements present, the motor size that provides the external torque can be significantly reduced and further analysis can establish the optimum mechanism geometry, inertial characteristics and active-passive control characteristics. These can lead to a design which will be effective in practice as a less expensive substitute of multi-DOF rehabilitation robots, but yet, as equally effective as possible.

References

1. Xydas, G.E., Louca, S.L., Mueller, A.: Analysis and passive control of a four-bar linkage for the rehabilitation of upper-limb motion. In: ASME 2015 Dynamic Systems and Control Conference, DSCC 2015, Columbus, OH, USA (2015)
2. Xydas, G.E., Mueller, A.: Minimally actuated 4-bar linkages for upper limb rehabilitation: performance analysis with forward and inverse dynamics. In: 39th Mechanisms and Robotics Conference (MR), ASME IDETC/CIE, Boston, MA, USA (2015)
3. Xydas, G.E.: Synthesis and analysis of a Chebyshev's straight line four-bar linkage for generating a minimum-Jerk velocity profile. In: 38th Mechanisms and Robotics Conference (MR), ASME IDETC/CIE, Buffalo, New York, USA (2014)
4. Xydas, G.E., Louca, S.L., Mueller, A.: Design of a minimally actuated mechanism for upper-limb rehabilitation: performance optimization via center of mass position variation. In: MEDICON 2016, Limassol, Cyprus (2016)
5. Berkelman, P., Rossi, P., Lu, T., Ma, J.: Passive orthosis linkage for locomotor rehabilitation. In: IEEE International Conference on Rehabilitation Robotics (2007)
6. Alam, M., Choudhury, I.A., Mamat, A.B.: Mechanism and design analysis of articulated ankle foot orthoses for drop-foot. Sci. World J. Article ID 867869 (2014)
7. Amirabdollahian, F., Gradwell, E., Loureiro, R., Collin, C., Harwin, W.: Effects of the gentle/s robot mediated therapy on the outcome of upper limb rehabilitation post-stroke: analysis of the battle hospital data. In: 8th International Conference on Rehabilitation Robotics, pp. 55–58 (2003)
8. Krebs, H.I., Hogan, N., Aisen, M.L., Volpe, B.T.: Robot-aided neurorehabilitation. IEEE Trans. Rehabil. Eng. **6**(1), 75–87 (1998)
9. Nef, T., Mihelj, M., Colombo, G., Riener, R.: ARMin—robot for rehabilitation of the upper extremities. In: Proceedings of the 2006 IEEE International Conference on Robotics and Automation Orlando, Florida (2006)
10. Lum, S.P., Burgar, G.C., Van der Loos, M., Shor, C.P., Majmundar, M., Yap, R.: MIME robotic device for upper-limb neurorehabilitation in subacute stroke patients: a follow up study. J. Rehabil. Res. Dev. **43**(5), 631–642 (2006)
11. Bardorfer, A., Munih, M., Zupan, A., Primozic, A.: Upper limb motion analysis using haptic interface. IEEE/ASME Trans. Mechatron. **6**(3), 252–260 (2001)
12. Flash, T., Hogan, N.: The coordination of arm movements: an experimentally confirmed mathematical model. J. Neurosci. **5**(7), 1688–1703 (1985)
13. Fitts, P.M., Peterson, J.R.: Information capacity of discrete motor responses. J. Exp. Psychol. **67**(2), 103–112 (1964)

14. Soechting, F.J., Terzuolo, A.C.: Organization of arm movements in three-dimensional space is piecewise planar. Neuroscience **23**(1), 53–61 (1987)
15. United Nations Factsheet on Persons with Disabilities. http://www.un.org/disabilities/documents/toolaction/pwdfs.pdf. Accessed 11 Nov 2016
16. Thomas, M.A.: Discussion on the shifts and changes in community based rehabilitation in the last decade. Neurorehabil. Neural Repair **13**(3), 185–189 (1999)
17. World Health Organization: Community-based rehabilitation guidelines (2010). ISBN 978 92 4 154805 2
18. World Federation for Neurorehabilitation: Position Statements: Neurorehabilitation in Developing Countries, Time for Action. http://wfnr.co.uk/education-and-research/position-statements/ (2015). Accessed 16 Nov 2016
19. Norton, R.L.: Design of Machinery: An Introduction to the Synthesis and Analysis of Mechanisms and Machines, 4th edn. McGraw-Hill (2008). ISBN: 978–0-07-312158-1
20. Freudenstein, F.: An analytical approach to the design of four-link mechanisms. ASME Trans. **76**(3), 483–492 (1954)
21. Alaska 4.0: Institut für Mechatronik. https://www.tu-chemnitz.de/ifm/ (2012)
22. Xydas, E.G., Louca, L.S.: Upper limb assessment of people with multiple sclerosis with the use of a haptic nine-hole peg-board test. In: Proceedings of the 9th Biennial ASME Conference on Engineering Systems Design and Analysis (2008)
23. Xydas, E.G., Louca, L.S.: Force control algorithm for robotic rehabilitation in generic reaching tasks for people with multiple sclerosis: development and preliminary experiments (under review)
24. Zilles, B.C., Salisbury, K.J.: A constraint-based god-object method for haptic display. In: Proceedings of the International Conference on Intelligent Robots and Systems (1995)
25. Xydas, E., Louca, S.L.: Design and development of a haptic peg-board exercise for the rehabilitation of people with multiple sclerosis. In: Proceedings of the 2007 IEEE 10th International Conference on Rehabilitation Robotics, June 12–15, Noordwijk, The Netherlands (2007)

Inter-individual Differences in Conscious and Unconscious Processes During Robot-Child Interaction

I. Giannopulu and T. Watanabe

Abstract The aim of the present study is to analyse conscious and unconscious processes using the paradigm of listener-speaker in neurotypical children aged 6 and 9 years old. The speaker was always a child; the listener was a human or a robot, i.e., a small robot which reacts to speech expression by nodding only. Physiological data, i.e., heart rate, as well as behavioral data, i.e., number of words in addition with reported feelings, were considered. The results showed that (1) the heart rate was higher for children aged 6 years old than for children aged 9 years old when the listener was the robot; (2) the number of nouns and verbs expressed by both age groups was higher when the listener was the human. The results are consistent with the idea that conscious and unconscious development would not only depend on natural environments but also on artificial environments represented by robots.

Keywords Paradigm of listener-speaker · Cardiovascular activity · Children · Conscious/unconscious processes

1 Introduction

Without doubt consciousness is one of the complex process facing the scientific perspective. According to one of the existing theories consciousness is correlated with DNA molecule. DNA molecule is thought to be responsible for advancing to

The original version of this chapter was revised: New figures have been updated. The erratum to this chapter is available at 10.1007/978-3-319-59972-4_24

I. Giannopulu (✉)
Bond University, Gold Coast, Australia
e-mail: igiannop@bond.edu.au; igiannopulu@psycho-prat.fr

T. Watanabe
Okayama Prefectural University, Okayama, Japan
e-mail: watanabe@cse.oka-pu.ac.jp

M. Husty and M. Hofbaur (eds.), *New Trends in Medical and Service Robots*,
Mechanisms and Machine Science 48, DOI 10.1007/978-3-319-59972-4_11

cellular and human consciousness, and has a kind of proto-consciousness which leads to higher degree of consciousness [1]. When DNA gives rise to human consciousness, three gene-based neurogenetic phases take place: the emergence of consciousness, the continual of human consciousness [2] and the neurodegeneration [3]. Following this approach, human consciousness is not only related to neurons and regions of the brain but also to a specific neurogenetic ground. In this theory, neurons are considered as the "fragments" of consciousness. A prerequisite for the emergence of consciousness is the development of thalamocortical fibers [4]. With the exception of olfactive tractus, the neurons from the sensory organs (e.g. visual, haptic, acoustic, vestibular, proprioceptive) reach the subplate of the cortex before about the 25 weeks of gestational age. The subplate serves as a waiting area and as a guidance hub for the afferents from the thalamus and the other areas of the brain. The expansion of thalamocortical axis in the somatosensory, auditory, visual and frontal cortices starts however, the corticocortical neuronal circuits develop late during infancy [4]. Following the human development, minimal consciousness [5] is associated with the first signs of communication with the external world: newborns' capacity to analyse facial expressions and voice [6, 7]. By the age of 4 months, babies seem to be able to discriminate negative from positive emotions [8, 9]. A positive correlation exists between the degree of emotional expression and the various types of smiles [10]. It is therefore accepted that perception is a prerequisite of human language [11, 12]. After 8 months, children are able to mentally represent the basic emotions and learn to relate nonverbal and verbal expressions [13, 14]. The use of language to name the emotional feeling and expression whatever their nature occurs between 2 and 10 years [14]. There are different levels of maturity in consciousness: young children use a relatively smaller number of words for naming emotions than old children [13]. As humans develop and mature language is considered to be the core nucleus of conscious process [15]. Indeed, what is at the origin of one of the trademarks of human development is the capacity to generate thoughts and concepts for ourselves and for the others which can be verbally expressed with the aim to communicate [8, 16]. In that context, conscious process necessitates the elaboration of coherent (grammatical and syntactically) sentences. In the opposite, unconscious process takes the form of nonverbal communication that can also be expressed by head nods, heart rate variation and/or contrasting facial and gestural expressions. Unquestionably, the ability to understand and share the referential statement of others and to express their own states consciously and/or unconsciously depends on the cerebral maturity [1]. Conscious and unconscious development emerges from the neural connections distributed across many cortical and sub-cortical regions respectively [17]. The cortical maturation associated with the evolution of consciousness gradually increases from early childhood to midchildhood, i.e., from 5 years to i.e., 9–11 years. The emergence of the three important cortical regions is sequential: temporal poles, the inferior parietal lobes and the superior and dorsolateral frontal cortices [18]. Sub-cortical regions develop in combination [19]. As a consequence, conscious as well as unconscious processes gradually follow that evolution, which is naturally characterized by intra and inter-individual differences.

With the aim to compare conscious expressions, reflected by the number of the produced nouns and the verbs and by the reporting feeling, as well as unconscious expressions given by the heart rate, we used the paradigm of "speaker-listener" [20] in children aged 6 and 9 years old. Given the fact that at both intra-individual and inter-individual levels, maturational differences characterize children aged 6 and 9 years old, our general hypothesis was that their conscious and unconscious expressions would differ. A recent study has shown that young children of 6 years old of developmental age who present less brain activity because of ASD, i.e., Autistic Spectrum Disorder, showed more important unconscious reactions, when the listener was the robot than when the listener was the human [16, 20]. By transposing to neurotypically developing children and given the cortical maturational differences, the general hypothesis is that the children aged 6 years old would have more unconscious reactions than the children aged 9 years old. In the previous study the interpretation was that ASD children were more interested in the robot because of its simplicity, nodding when the child speaks. As such, we expect that neurotypical children of the present study would be more interested in the human complexity. Finally, given the fact that conscious and unconscious processes are interwoven, inter-individual differences would exist in conscious and unconscious expressions.

2 Method

2.1 Participants

Children aged 6 and 9 years old participated in the study. Twenty children (10 boys and 10 girls) composed the group of 6 years old; twenty children (10 boys and 10 girls) composed the group of 9 years old. The developmental age of the first group ranged from 6 to 7 years old (mean 6.3 years; sd 4 months). The developmental age of second group ranged from 9 to 10 years old (mean 9.2 years; sd 5 months). Children attended regular schools and had no learning disorders, ADHD, neurodevelopmental, cardiac or psychiatric diseases as reported by their teachers. Their academic achievements were standard in their school. The study was approved by the local ethic committee and was in accordance with the Helsinki 2.0 convention. Anonymity was guaranteed.

2.2 Robot

A small toy robot, was used as a listener [21]. The robot is shaped like a bilobed plant and its leaves and stem make a nodding response based on speech input and supports the sharing of mutual embodiment in communication (Fig. 1). It uses a material called BioMetal made of a shape-memory alloy as its driving force. The

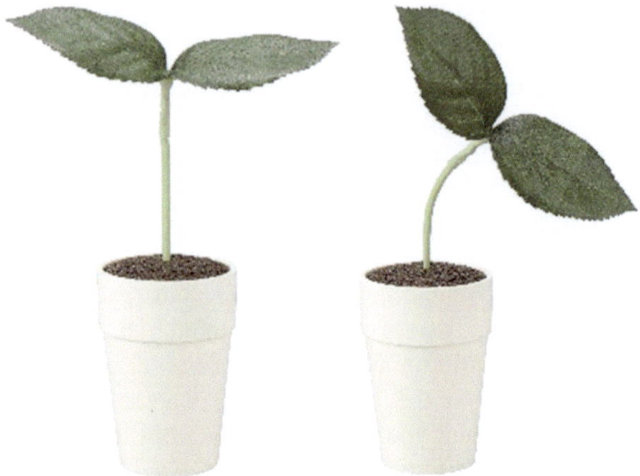

Fig. 1 The toy robot

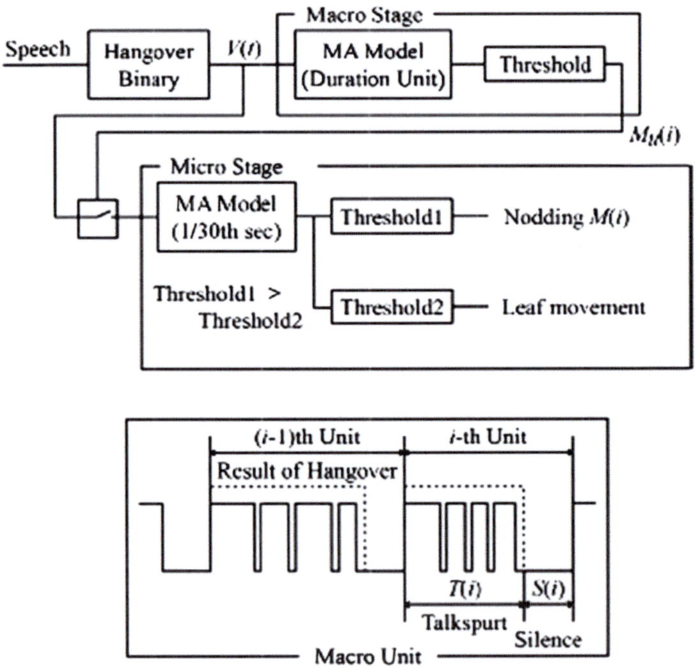

Fig. 2 Listener's interaction model

timing of nodding is predicted using a hierarchy model consisting of two stages: macro and micro (Fig. 2). The macro stage estimates whether a nodding response exists or not in a duration unit, which consists of a talkspurt episode T(i) and the following silence episode S(i) with a hangover value of 4/30 s. The estimator Mu(i) is a moving-average (MA) model, expressed as the weighted sum of unit speech activity R(i) in (1) and (2). When Mu(i) exceeds a threshold value, nodding M(i) also becomes an MA model, estimated as the weighted sum of the binary speech signal V (i) in (3). The robot demonstrates three degrees of movements: big and small nods and a slight twitch of the leaves by controlling the threshold values of the nodding prediction. The threshold of the leaf movement is set lower than that of the nodding prediction.

$$M_M(i) = \sum_{j=1}^{i} a(j)R(i-j) + u(i) \tag{1}$$

$$R(i) = \frac{T(i)}{T(i) + S(i)} \tag{2}$$

$a(j)$ linear prediction coefficient
$T(i)$ talkspurt duration in the i-th duration unit
$S(i)$ silence duration in the i-th duration unit
$u(i)$ noise

$$M(i) = \sum_{R=1}^{k} b(j)V(i-j) + w(i) \tag{3}$$

b(j) linear prediction coefficient
V(i) voice
w(i) noise

2.3 *Procedure: The Paradigm of Listener-Speaker*

For both groups of age, the study took place in a room which was familiar to the children. We defined three conditions: the first one was called “rest condition”, the second was named “human listener” and the third one was called “robot listener”. The second and third conditions were counterbalanced across the children. The duration of the “rest condition” was 1 min; the second and third conditions each lasted approximately 7 min. The inter-condition interval was approximately 30 s [20]. For each child, the whole experimental session lasted 15 min (Fig. 3).

In order to neutralize a possible “human impact” on children’s behavior, the experimenter was the same person for each child in each condition and group. At the beginning of each session, the experimenter presented the robot to the child explaining that the robot nods whenever the child speaks. Then, the experimenter hid the robot. The session was run as follows: during the “rest condition”, the heart rate of each child was measured in silence. At the end of that condition, the child was also asked to estimate her/his own emotion on a scale ranging from 1 (the

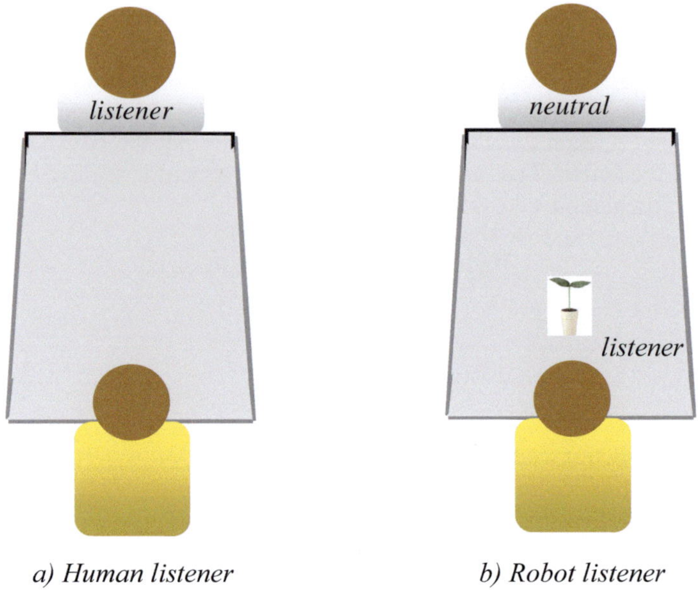

Fig. 3 Paradigm of listener-speaker

lowest score) to 5 (the highest score) [15]. During the "human listener" condition, the child was invited to discuss with the experimenter. The experimenter initiated discussion and after listened to the child acting as the speaker by nodding only. The heart rate, as well as the frequency of words and verbs expressed by each child was measured. During the "robot listener" condition, the robot was set to nod movements; the experimenter gave the robot to the child inviting the child to use it as it has been explained before. The robot was the listener, the child was the speaker and the experimenter remained silent and discreet. The heart rate and the frequency of words and verbs expressed by the child was recorded once again. At the end of the session, the child was invited to estimate the degree of its own emotion on the same aforementioned scale [15].

2.4 Dependent Variables and Analysis

The analysis was based on the following dependent variables (a) the heart rate, i.e., unconscious nonverbal emotional expression (b) the number of nouns and verbs expressed by each child, i.e., conscious verbal expression and (c) the degree of feeling, i.e., conscious verbal emotional expression [20]. The data analysis was performed with SPSS Statistics 17.0 [22].

3 Results

First, we present results for heart rate comparisons of both groups in three conditions: "rest", "human listener", "robot listener". After, we examine the number of nouns and verbs expressed by 6 years and 9 years old children in "human listener" and "robot listener" conditions. Finally, we give the emotional state reported for each group "before" and "after" the interaction with the robot listener.

Figure 4 gives the mean heart rate of both age groups inter-individually and intra-individually.

Intra-individually, it is shown that the mean heart rate of 6 years old children was higher when the listener was the robot ($\chi^2 = 6.68$, $p < 0.01$) than when the listener was the human ($\chi^2 = 4.09$, $p < 0.05$) both relative to the "rest condition". In the contrary, the mean heart rate of children didn't significantly differ when the listener was the human or the robot ($\chi^2 = 2.83$, $p > 0.05$). In the same vein, the mean heart rate of 9 years old group was higher when the listener was the robot ($\chi^2 = 3.90$, $p < 0.05$) than when the listener was the human ($\chi^2 = 3.54$, $p > 0.05$) relative to the "rest condition". However, for the same age group, the mean heart rate didn't significantly differ when the children were with the listener robot or with the human ($\chi^2 = 3.10$, $p > 0.05$).

Inter-individual, the mean heart rate of 6 years and 9 years old children was very similar ($\chi^2 = 3.43$, $p > 0.05$) in the "rest condition". Analogously, the mean heart rate of 6 years old and 9 years old group didn't statistically differ, when the listener was the human ($\chi^2 = 3.78$, $p > 0.05$). Conversely, the mean heart rate of 6 years old children was higher from the heart rate of 9 years old children when the listener was the robot ($\chi^2 = 6.78$, $p < 0.01$).

Fig. 4 Heart rate (bpm)

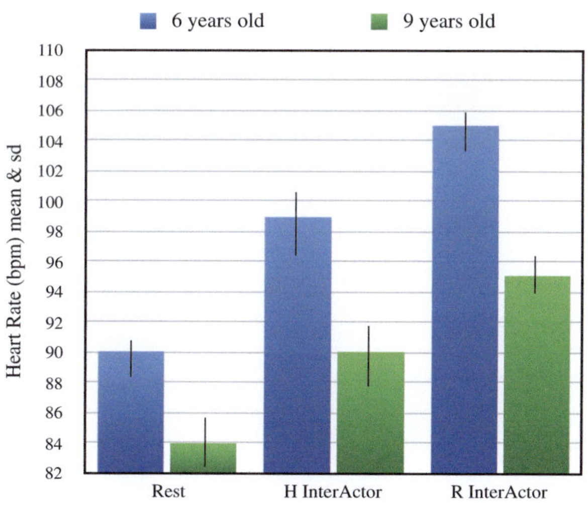

The number of nouns and verbs for each child in both age groups and in each experimental condition, i.e., "human listener" and "robot listener" was completed by two independent judges unfamiliar with the aim of the study. For that purpose, both judges performed the analyses of audio sequences. Inter-judge reliability was assessed using intra-class coefficients to make the comparison between them. The inter-judge reliability was good (Cohen's kappa = 0.79).

As shown in Fig. 5, intra-individually and for both age groups, the mean number of nouns and verbs was higher when the children have the human than when they have the robot as listener ($\chi^2 = 4.78$, $p < 0.05$ for the 6 years aged children and $\chi^2 = 7.78$, $p < 0.01$ for the 9 years old children). Inter-individually, the mean number of words was lower in "human listener" condition for the children aged 6 years than for the children aged 9 years ($\chi^2 = 5.22$ $p < 0.025$). In "robot listener" condition the mean number of words was higher for the group of 6 years than for the group of 9 years old ($\chi^2 = 4.03$, $p < 0.05$).

Intra-individually, as illustrated by the Fig. 6, the degree of feeling reported is very similar for both 6 and 9 years old children within each condition: "before" and "after" the robot ($\chi^2 = 2.98$, $p > 0.05$ for the 6 years and $\chi^2 = 3.03$, $p > 0.05$ for 9 years children respectively). Inter-individually, the feeling reporting didn't differ between 6 and 9 years old children before and after the interaction with the robot ($\chi^2 = 2.08$, $p > 0.10$ for the 6 years and $\chi^2 = 2.56$, $p > 0.10$ for 9 years children respectively).

Fig. 5 Number of words (nouns and verbs)

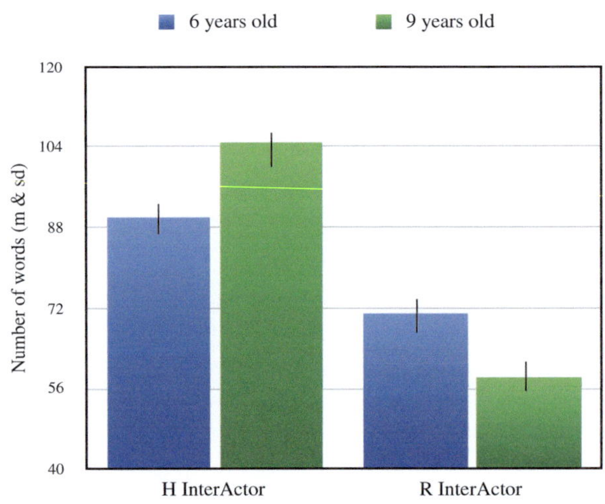

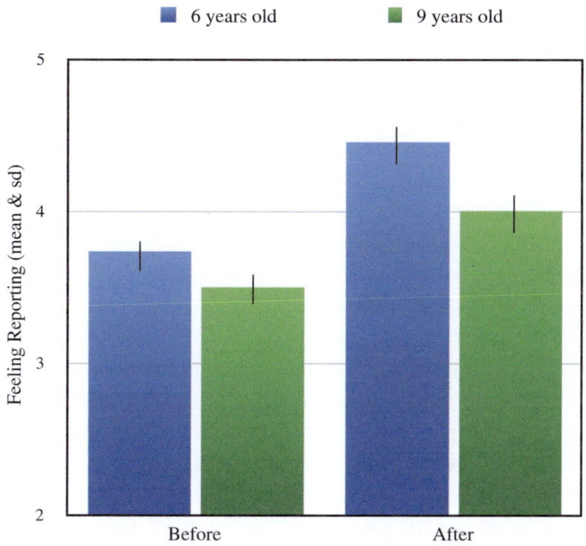

Fig. 6 Degree of feeling reported

4 Discussion

To our knowledge, this study is the first study, which analyzes both conscious and unconscious processes in neurotypical children using a toy robot in a listener-speaker situation. In the present situation, the speaker was always a child aged 6 or 9 years; the listener was a human or a robot. We have considered physiological data, i.e., heart rate which is associated with unconscious process as well as behavioural data, i.e., number of words and verbs as together with the verbal expression of emotional feeling which is linked with conscious processes. The results revealed that (1) the heart rate was higher for children aged 6 years old than for children aged 9 years old when the listener was the robot; (2) the number of nouns and verbs expressed by both age groups was higher when the listener was a human with significant differences between the groups: it was lower for the children aged 6 years than for the children aged 9 years; (3) the feeling reported before and after the contact with the robot it's similar for both age groups.

Our study provides two kinds of results. On the one hand, the unconscious expression differs between the children aged 6 and 9 years when the listener is the robot. It was more important for children aged 6 years old than for children aged 9 years. For both groups, conscious expression was higher when the listener was the human than when the listener was the robot. Such results are coherent with our hypothesis following which there would be inter-individual differences on unconscious and conscious expressions between children aged 6 years and 9 years. On the other hand, and for both age groups, the conscious feeling reported did not differ before and after the interaction with the robot. This latter result is incoherent with our hypothesis.

With regard to the unconscious expression, these findings clearly indicated that similar patterns of heart rate activities exist for both age group both in the "rest condition" and in the human listener condition. However, the children aged 6 years exhibited higher heart rate than children aged 9 years, when the listener was the robot. Such results cannot be attributed to an order effect as the "human listener" and the "robot listener" conditions have been randomised across the children. The heart rate variations we recorded likely reflect the activity of the autonomous nervous system: orthosympathetic and parasympathetic. Such a system is dynamically and bidirectionally connected to the central nervous system [20]. Physiologically speaking, the inter-individual differences of heart rate between 6 and 9 years old children in the condition where the robot was the listener would reveal differential peripheral action of the myelinated vagus nerve [23, 24], i.e., a differential degree of unconscious maturation. It would indicate neural inter-individual differences in temporal cortex (included internal and external areas), in the cingulate cortex and in the prefrontal cortex [25]. Developmentally speaking, the activity of the central nervous system increases to improve greater control over peripheral system. Indeed, both systems mature in combination and authorize the developing brain to become independent in the environment. These systems are still in development in children 6 and 9 years old [26, 27]. Following the results, the heart rate of 6 years old children is higher than the heart rate of 9 years old children when the listener is the robot. Literally, this seems to express that children aged 6 years old are more reliant on the robot than children aged 9 years old. Interestingly, even if all children reported a better emotional feeling after than before the interaction with the InterActor robot, but this difference was not statistically significant. Such a result would signify the emergence of a verbal statement, i.e., conscious expression, from a nonverbal emotion such given by the heart rate, i.e., unconscious expression. Consistent with the physiological data [25], our findings suggest that an important difference exists between level of consciousness among young children aged 6 years and old children aged 9 years: the lesser the brain development, the more the unconscious expression.

When the conscious verbal expression is taken into consideration, the data indicate that in the human listener condition, the number of words expressed by the children, whatever their age, was more important than the number of words the children express in the robot listener condition. In addition, children aged 6 years old less expressed themselves than children aged 9 years old. Given the differential degree of consciousness and the associated brain maturation, this difference can be considered as in accordance with a constant developmental observation following which the verbal functions continue to mature at 6 and grow up to adulthood [13, 19]. When the robot was the listener the young children, i.e., children aged 6 years, more expressed themselves than the old children, i.e., children aged 9 years old. Once again as referenced above, the children aged 6 years old seemed to be dependent on the environment, i.e., the robot. All in all, for both age groups, conscious verbal expression is more important when the listener is the human, likely because of human complexity.

Following a recent study a robot characterized by a simple predictable nonverbal behavior, namely nodding when the child speaks, better facilitate unconscious nonverbal emotional and conscious verbal expressions of children with autistic spectrum disorders [20]. With this new study, we have demonstrated that neurotypical children aged 6 years old better express unconscious behavior when the listener was the robot and conscious behavior when the listener was the human. Opposed to children with ASD, neurotypical children would prefer to interact with humans verbally, probably because human complex verbal and nonverbal behavior does not constitute an obstacle for them in communication.

5 Conclusion

The findings would be linked to the development of conscious and unconscious processes. In that way, nonverbal behavior expressed by the heart rate, which is an unconscious automatic activity would depend on a specific artificial environment: the robot. Analogously, verbal behavior given by the nouns and verbs pronounced by the children, which is a conscious activity would depend on a natural environment: the human listener. Specifically, conscious and unconscious processes would not only depend on natural environments but also on artificial environments [28].

Acknowledgements We are grateful to all the participants and their parents, the Major, the Pedagogical Inspector, the director and the team of principal elementary school of the first district of Paris, the National Department of Education and Research. The research is supported by the Franco-Japanese Foundation of Paris.

References

1. Grandy, J.K.: Consciousness. In: The Encyclopedia of Anthropology, vol. 1, pp. 563–566 (2006)
2. Grandy, J.K.: The three neurogenetic phases of human consciousness. J. Consc. Evol. **9**, 1–14 (2013)
3. Grandy, J.K.: The neurogenetic substructures of human consciousness. Essays Phil. **15**, 266–278 (2014)
4. Lagercrantz, H.: The emergence of consciousness: science and ethics. Semin. Fetal Neonatal Med. **19**, 300–305 (2014)
5. Zelazo, P.D.: The development of conscious control in childhood. Trends Cogn. Sci. **8**, 12–17 (2004)
6. Bowlby, J.: Attachement et perte: l'attachement. PUF, Paris (1978)
7. Main, M.: Introduction to the special section on attachment and psychopathology: 2. Overview of the field of attachment. J. Consult. Clin. Psychol. **64**, 237–243 (1996)

8. Garin, N., Moore, C.: Complex decision-making in early childhood. Brain Cogn. **55**, 158–170 (2004)
9. Russell, J.A.: Culture, scripts, and children's understanding of emotion. In: Saarni, C., Harris, P.L. (eds.) Children's Understanding of Emotion, pp. 293–313. Cambridge University Press, Cambridge (1989)
10. Messinger, D.S.: A measure of early joy? In: Ekman, P., Rosenberg, E.K. (eds.) What the Face Reveals: Basic and Applied Studies of Spontaneous Expression Union the Facial Action Coding System (FACS), pp. 350–353. Oxford University Press, Oxford (2005)
11. Giannopulu, I.: Multimodal interactions in typically and atypically developing children: natural vs. artificial environments. Cogn. Process. **14**, 323–331 (2013)
12. Gray, J.: Consciousness. Creeping of on the Hard Problem. Oxford University Press, Oxford (2004)
13. Bloom, L.: Language development and emotional expression. Pediatrics **102**, 5 (1998)
14. Baron-Cohen, S., Leslie, A.M., Frith, U.: Does the autistic child have a theory of mind? Cognition **21**, 37–46 (1985)
15. Giannopulu, I., Sagot, I.: I Positive emotion in the course of an experimental task in children (Ressenti émotionnel positif dans une tâche expérimentale chez l'enfant). Med.-Psychol. **168**, 740–745 (2010)
16. Giannopulu, I., Watanabe, T.: Give Children Toy Robots to Educate and/or to NeuroEducate. In: New Trends in Medical and Service Robots, pp. 205–216. Springer Book (2015)
17. Lagercrantz, H., Changeux, J.P.: The emergence of human consciousness: from foetal to neonatal life. Pediatr. Res. **65**, 3 (2009)
18. Schmitt, J.E., Neale, M.C., Fassassi, B., Perez, J., Lenroot, R.K., Wells, E.M., Gilded, J.N.: The Dynamic Role of Genetics on Cortical Patterning During Childhood and Adolescence. PNAS, Early Edition (2014)
19. Porges, S.W., Forman, S.A.: The early development of the autonomic nervous system provides a neural platform for social behavior: a polyvagal perspective. Infant Child Dev. **20**, 106–118 (2011)
20. Giannopulu, I., Montreynaud, V., Watanabe, T.: Minimalistic toy robot to analyse a scenery of speaker-listener condition in autism. Cogn. Process. **17**, 195–203 (2016)
21. Watanabe, T.: Human-entrained embodied interaction and communication technology. Emo Eng. 161–177 (2011)
22. SPSS STATISTICS 17.0: Python Software Foundation (2008)
23. Barres, A.B., Barde, Y.: Neuronal and glial cell biology. Curr. Opin. Neurol. **10**, 642–648 (2000)
24. Servant, D., Logier, R., Mouster, Y., Goudemand, M.: Heart rate variability. Applications in psychiatry. Encéphale **35**, 423–428 (2009)
25. Portes, S.W.: The polyvagal perspective. Bio Psychol. **74**, 116–143 (2007)
26. Manta, S.: Effets Neurophysiologiques de la stimulation du nerf vague: implication dans le traitement de la dépression résistante et optimisation des paramètres de stimulation. Thèse de Doctorat, Université de Montréal, Canada (2012)
27. Tomoko, T., Yoshimi, K., Sayaka, I., Kakuro, A., Fumikazu, S., Hideaki, K., Kanji, S., Masao, A.: Developmental changes in frontal lobe function during a verbal fluency task: a multi-channel near-infrared spectroscopy study. Brain Dev. **36**, 844–852 (2014)
28. Giannopulu, I.: Enrobotment: toy robots in the developing brain. In: Nakatsu, R., Rauterberg, M., Ciancarini, P. (eds.) Handbook of Digital Games and Entertainment Technologies, pp. 1–29. Springer Science, Singapore (2016)

Surgical Robotics—Past, Present and Future

F. Graur, E. Radu, N. Al Hajjar, C. Vaida and D. Pisla

Abstract Robotic surgery is in continuous development proving to be not only a better therapeutic option in certain procedures but also a pioneer field in which research occupies a very important role. The history of robotic begins with science-fiction literature, but it profiles the industrial and also health robots that are nowadays used. Robotic surgery begins later on with modified industrial robots, but from that point it has its own development. This article is a short history of surgical robotics, continued with the presentation of some surgical robots currently used. At the end, the characteristics of the future surgical robot are discussed, as well a proposal for a minimally invasive SILS robot.

Keywords Surgical robot · Minimally invasive · SILS robot · Robotic surgery

1 Introduction

Development of general surgery in recent decades was centered on minimally invasive procedures. This term refers to any procedure less invasive than open surgery used for the same pathology and was introduced by E. John A. Wickham, a promoter of this type of surgery [10]. The old assumption that "a big surgery requires a big incision" is no longer true for a long time [4]. In minimally invasive surgery as the access ports and incisions became smaller and smaller, the same size tools are developed [4], aiming not only to provide smaller dimensions but also enhanced functionality [30].

F. Graur · N. Al Hajjar (✉)
University of Medicine and Pharmacy "Iuliu Hatieganu", Cluj-Napoca, Romania
e-mail: na_hajjar@yahoo.com

F. Graur · E. Radu · N. Al Hajjar
Regional Institute of Gastroenterology and Hepatology "Octavian Fodor", Cluj-Napoca, Romania

C. Vaida · D. Pisla
CESTER, Technical University of Cluj-Napoca, Cluj-Napoca, Romania

M. Husty and M. Hofbaur (eds.), *New Trends in Medical and Service Robots*, Mechanisms and Machine Science 48, DOI 10.1007/978-3-319-59972-4_12

Surgical robots were introduced in mid-century when science fiction became reality. Surgical robot is defined as a machine that perform complex surgical tasks in master-slave configuration system [4]. In the last 3 decades surgical robots have experienced geometrical evolution and development, reflected on an extended number of robotic solutions reaching experimental stages and demonstrated by the growing number of articles published in scientific magazines and because of the growing interest in this field [6, 17]. If at first surgical robots were used to support, move and orient the camera in the operating field, subsequently it came to complex surgical robots in which the surgeon operates from a remote console far from the patient.

As in the case of industrial robots, in surgery were introduced robots in areas where accuracy and better precision were needed (Neurosurgery), to perform repetitive tasks (Urology) and higher speed compared to manual labor performed by humans. The desired shortening of surgical procedures time performed by robots has not yet been achieved in most areas where they are used [10].

In order to develop and implement into practice new surgical techniques with a shorter time, with a quicker recovery of the patient, with increased efficiency, it is mandatory to use advanced computer technologies: surgical robots, 3D imaging, augmented reality and surgical simulators (to shorten the learning curve of the new techniques) [16]. Development of surgery, which led to the surgical robots, developed new fields as: minimally invasive surgery, fetal surgery, virtual reality surgery, neuro-informatics surgery and today appeared the term of non-invasive surgery [3, 14].

2 Evolution of Surgical Robotics

2.1 History of Robotics in Surgery

Robotics started in 1921 with the play "Rossum's Universal Robots" by Karel Čapek, in which we find for the first time the word "robot", derived from the Czech word "robota" which means forced labor. Irony is that although the play was a satire on the industrialization of Europe, in the century that followed robots led to explosive industrialization of the entire planet [1, 2, 7, 8, 19].

The term "robotics" was introduced by Isaac Asimov in 1938 in his short story "Runaround" published in the magazine Super Science Stories, followed in 1942 by publishing of a collection of short stories "I Robot" in which robots coming into conflict with their owners are described. Asimov was the one that described also the first 3 Laws of Robotics, laws that govern the behavior of robots [1, 19]:

1. A robot may not injure a human being, or, through inaction, allow one to come to harm.
2. A robot must obey all orders given to it from humans, except where such orders would contradict the First Law.

3. A robot must protect its own existence, except when to do so would contradict the First Law or the Second Law.

From Capek and Asimov, many famous works of science fiction appeared and popularized the notion of "robot". In the George Lucas's series "Star Wars" they were friends with the people but in the movie series Terminator, they were people enemies [5].

The 3 Laws of Robotics remained actual and ethically acceptable in the development of surgical robots today [5].

Starting with the 2nd half of the twentieth century robots imagined by Capek and Asimov became reality, first in the industry, being used for mechanical work in factories to increase productivity, minimizing human error and accidents at work [11, 17]. General Motors was the first company that made the transition from fiction to reality in the field of robotics by introducing the Unimate robot in the assembly line in 1958 and it was first used in 1961.

2.2 *Current Use of Robots*

After that start point of robotics, the use of robots has experienced explosive development. They are used in a variety of applications, including space exploration, military field, medicine, etc. [17, 32].

Robots can be represented in the form of automatic arms, mobile devices or telerobotic systems. Regarding robots taxonomy they can be active, semi-active or passive. Semi-active and passive robots transmit the operator's commands and movements to the arms of the robot. Active robots are those who have a pre-defined schedule and runs on a computer algorithm, without the need for real time operator's intervention [17].

Robots have several advantages over humans, including the accuracy and repeatability of movement, which is why they get so extensively in industrial field, but the medical field is not as accurate and structured as industry. Such robots have several disadvantages in this area: low adaptability and a low level of applied force feedback (haptic). Regarding these considerations it is ideal and simple to use a robotic system to prepare the femoral head prosthesis (RoboDoc is a surgical robot used in orthopedic arthroplasty of the hip, a robot imaging guided after a plan drawn up by the surgeon before the operation on CT examinations, thus establishing the exact place and position of the prosthesis), but it is hard to imagine a robot that autonomously perform a cholecystectomy [5, 26].

The first use of a robot surgery was in 1985 at Memorial Medical Center, Long Beach, CA, USA, when an adjusted industrial robotic arm (Unimation PUMA 200) allowed a CT-guided stereotactic biopsy of brain, with an accuracy of 0.05 mm, being the prototype for Neuromate robot (which received approval from the Food and Drug Administration—FDA in 1999) [10, 31].

There was a gap for 6 years before the next stage in robotic surgery development. In 1991 in London, UK a surgical robot was first used (Probot—developed at Imperial College London) for the autonomous removal of a significant amount of tissue during a TURP (transureteral resection of prostate) [10].

In 1992 another industrial robot was adjusted for surgery in Japan: SCARA robot, with 5 degrees of freedom. It was used for total hip arthroplasty. A similar robotic system, Robodoc, was developed in Sacramento, CA, USA by Integrated Surgical Systems ISS. Robodoc system was first used on humans in 1992 as an autonomous robot for total hip arthroplasty (THA), and received FDA approval in 1998 and for TKA (total knee arthroplasty) in 2009 [10].

A few years later, in 2000, in Germany was used for the first time a robotic system similar to Robodoc called CASPAR—Computer Assisted Surgical Planning And Robotics. This is actually an industrial PUMA robot adapted for THA, TKA and to repair the anterior cruciate ligament [10].

The first class of surgical robots are based on autonomous industrial robots, or with an autonomous approach, which means that the robot will enable the fulfillment, at a certain point, of a lower or higher degree task without the intervention of the surgeon [10].

A second class of surgical robots is represented by those robots that are designed to assist the surgeon and work with it during interventions being capable to move autonomously, but are not scheduled in this regard but are programmed to replicate surgeon movements in a master/slave configuration of the system (such as da Vinci or Sensei).

Visionaries in telepresence surgery and its benefits were Scott Fisher, Ph.D.—NASA scientist and Joe Rosen, MD—plastic surgeon at the University Palo Alto, CA, USA. They have imagined this virtual presence of the surgeon in the operating field via remote manipulation of robotic arms. Their project, in collaboration with Phil Green, Ph.D. Stanford Research Institute and the Pentagon was to create a device to rescue the wounded person on the battlefield and giving them first aid by a surgeon from a remote console [3, 11, 12].

Some robots are designed to move the laparoscope during minimal invasive abdominal interventions. The surgeon commands such robots either by voice or by head movements. The first such prototype of voice commanded robotic arms is AESOP developed by Intuitive Surgical Inc. [20] followed by others like Viky or EndoAssist.

In this field the, a joint team of from CESTER, Technical University of Cluj-Napoca and Surgical Clinic III, University of Medicine and Pharmacy Cluj-Napoca, achieved a series of national premieres, Pisla et al. [13, 22, 23, 28, 29]:

- PARAMIS—the first Romanian parallel robot with voice control for laparoscope positioning in minimally invasive surgery (2009), presented in 2011 at the Congress of the European Association of Endoscopic Surgery as an oral presentation [27] and included as one of the acknowledged solutions in a "review" published in 2010 by a group of Japanese researchers, entitled "Classification,

Design and Evaluation of Endoscope Robots", which presents the 27 robotic structures developed worldwide for endoscopic surgery [25];
- PARASURG–5M—the first Romanian parallel robot for active instruments positioning in minimally invasive surgery (2011),
- PARASIM the first Romanian robotic surgical active instrument with enhanced dexterity (2012),
- HEPSIM the first Romanian liver surgery pre-planning and virtual training simulator [9].

Zeus robotic system (developed by Computer Motion Inc.) consists of three robotic arms—one handles the laparoscope and the other two are the active arms replicating surgeon's movements from a remote console, moving specially developed surgical instruments [24].

The da Vinci Surgical System created by Intuitive Surgical Inc. and launched in 1999 consists of 1 or 2 working console for surgeons with 3D visualization system of the surgical field and a cart placed near the operating table that has three or four robotic arms for endoscopic visualization system and special tools. Da Vinci transmits movements of the surgeon hands, wrists and fingers to the instruments in the surgical field, in real time, with tremor filtration [10] (Fig. 1).

Sculptor Acrobat (acronym for Active Constraint Robot) is also a synergistic robotic system, but with "hands-on" control. It was first used in 2001 for a series of

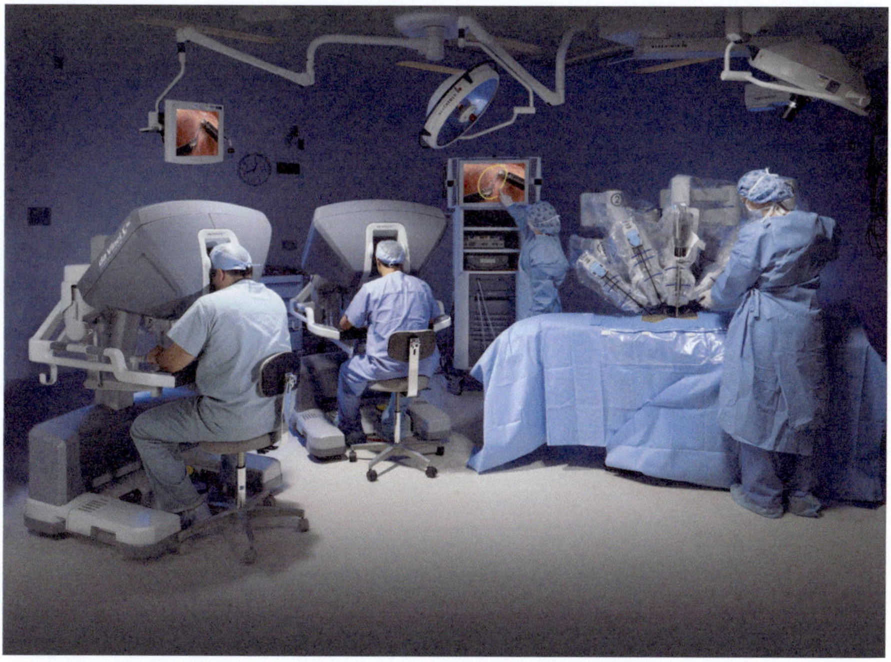

Fig. 1 Da Vinci Si system. © 2009 Intuitive Surgical, Inc

seven TKA. Another "hands-on" device, similar to Acrobot used in orthopedic surgery for hip and knee joints plasty is RIO (Robotic arm Interactive acronym for Orthopaedic system), produced by Mako Surgical, Florida, USA. The latter one got FDA approval in 2005 [10].

2.3 Future Robots

A third group of surgical robots has to be defined in the future. It will include intelligent miniature robotic devices and perhaps even disposable or resterilizable. A good example could be HeartLander—a miniature mobile robot, designed to be disposable and developed by Carnegie Mellon University and is designed to perform invasive targeted therapy on the surface of a beating heart. Therefore, while "nano-robots" or "micro-robots" capable of being injected into the bloodstream, or to be swallowed to make targeted therapy (even gene therapy or repair tissue at the cellular level), are just fantasy today. Mini-robots, like HeartLander are in the process of development and in the next decade will likely be part of surgical therapeutics [10].

Surgical robots can be divided into two categories: autonomous or teleoperated robots. Another less commonly used classification is that of the medical branch where the robots are used: urology, neurosurgery, orthopedics, general surgery, etc. [26].

A better and more useful classification of surgical robots was proposed by Camarillo et al. [5]. This classification is based on the role that the robot has during surgery and has been compared to the professional evolution of a surgeon from student (smaller responsibilities—low risk), then resident (responsibilities and risk are medium) and eventually specialist (full responsibility and maximum risk). Such surgical robots are classified by their active or passive role during surgery, being grouped in three categories: the passive robots that perform low-risk maneuvers, simple and precise tasks; active robots, which are deeply involved into the intervention; and a last category, restricted role robots, which includes robots performing tasks and invasive maneuvers with higher risk than those with passive role, but lower than active role. According to this classification, we can conclude that as robot autonomy grows, the role of the robot goes from active to passive. Therefore computer tomography and CyberKnife are the most passive robots used for medical purposes, having a much greater autonomy and also a very low risk during usage, and da Vinci and the surgical robots having an active role during the procedure, yet the slightest autonomy, in direct correlation with an increased risk during the procedure. RoboDoc, Acrobot and NeuroMate are classified on intermediate positions [5].

Camarillo et al. highlight that robots with active role seem to be superior to the passive ones, but the situation is contrary because the active ones, execute high risk tasks that require human supervision and significant human intervention during surgery, compared to those with passive role, which are autonomous and can perform tasks without supervision, these tasks having a very low risk or no risk [5].

Another classification of surgical robots could have three categories: internal, external and mixed robots:

1. External robots: those who perform surgical maneuvers on the body surface (Acrobot, RoboDoc, CT-scanners, CyberKnife);
2. Mixed robots: during the procedure have a segment located inside the patient and one outside the patient (NeuroMate, da Vinci, PARASURG-9M);
3. Internal robots: during the procedure they are entirely located inside the patient's body (endoscopic capsule, surgical robots of the future: miniature and easily managed from outside the body).

Da Vinci robotic system is the most versatile master/slave system existing at the moment. The system consists of 3 main components: 1–2 surgeon consoles, surgical robotic cart placed near the operating table with 3–4 robotic arms and Visual System, which features a 3D endoscope. It has 2 high resolution digital cameras with dual lens and three chip technology, each one recording the operating field from different angles and provides a different image to each eye, which is why the image formation on the cerebral cortex appears in 3D. The system also benefits from a flexible endoscope with 3 degrees of freedom, allowing much better synchronization of the image to surgeon eye and working tools [15, 16, 21].

Working console is actually a workstation from which the surgeon performs the entire surgery. It can be located up to 10 m far from the operating table. At the system console, besides 3D visualization of the surgical field there are also the 2 controllers from where the surgeon handles the tools in operatory field. The controllers are equipped with motion scaling and tremor reduction functions [4].

Tools tip of the instruments used by da Vinci robot are identical to that of conventional instruments used in open surgery, since these instruments are the result of over 150 years of evolution and experience in handling different types of dissection and tissue suture. The remaining components are entirely technically new. Thus the surgeon can transmit to the instruments the same movement as in the case of open surgery, thanks to the joints that mimics the joints of the fingers and wrist (EndoWrist robotic joint). These tools have the advantage of multiple use and sterilization and the possibility to be interchanged during the operation [5]. However there is still a limited number of available instruments in robotic surgery, this topic being an open field of research where the scientific community can contribute.

The reason for which da Vinci robotic system is the most efficient master/slave is because these technologies give the surgeon the feeling of presence in the surgical field, its immersion in the surgical field.

The future of robotic surgery will consist primarily in miniaturization of surgical robots as much as possible [17]. Also offering the surgeon the ability to use more than 2 arms while working, to be its own aid is a very important element that will be enhanced more and more in the future [5]. Decreasing scale to which the surgeon operates in the present and offering the opportunity to perform procedures at millimeter, using miniature robots that have multiple sensors (tactile, chemical, pressure, ultrasound etc.) that can provide the surgeon with valuable information in real-time, which may have an important role in surgery.

Recent research in the field Microelectromechanical systems (MEMS) opens the horizons in miniaturization. Ability to create miniature robots with multiple sensors (optical, pressure, accelerometer, chemical, force feedback sensors etc.) of multipurpose therapeutic robotic catheters, implantable mini-robots to measure real-time of the blood pressure in conjunction with the patient effort, to release the exact dose needed for antihypertensive necessary under the circumstances, or to release insulin dose, in diabetics patients. We can also go further and imagine nano-robots or micro-robots to be injected into the bloodstream or be swallowed and act at the cellular level and repair the destruction cell, particularly the brain cells, or to repair genetic mutations [5].

There are proposals of intelligent robots, stick to the section of spinal cord and leading to nerve fibers and thus restore their continuity and lead to the recovery of patient mobility. Earlier this new era in robotic surgery was done with the advent of endoscopic capsules that can be called the "bioMEMS" device.

2.4 Proposal of SILS Robot

SILS (Single Incision Laparoscopic Surgery) developed few years ago, introducing the concept of no-scar surgery. This, in combination with NOTES (Natural Orifice Translumenal Endoscopic Surgery) lead to the development of specific surgical instruments. We propose a concept of a new robot for the use in these types of surgeries.

The intervention begins with the patient in dorsal decubitus and in general anesthesia with oro-tracheal intubation. A skin incision is placed at the level of umbilicus. The pneumoperitoneum is created with the help of a Veres needle, used to introduce the carbon dioxide inside the abdominal cavity. The entrance place inside the abdominal cavity is the umbilicus (through a small hole of 10–15 mm in diameter) where a 10–15 mm trocar is inserted. Through this trocar the robotic arms, shaped after the SILS and NOTES instruments are inserted. This robot should be small and versatile, being capable to be used in different abdominal interventions. At the beginning we propose a mixt robot with the instruments tips inside the human body (into the abdomen) and the active parts (motors) outside the body. With the future miniaturization of the motors, the robot could became totally intracorporeal, inserted through the umbilicus or even through natural orifices.

In the lists below are the main characteristics of the both models:

A. Robot's specifications and performance—mixt robot, intra and extracorporeal parts;

1. Curved robotic arms to overcome the spatial limitation of the small access port;
2. 3–5 mm laparoscope with cold light and enhanced optical characteristics—for surgical field visualization;
3. Electrocautery at the tip of scissor or surgical hook;
4. Carbon dioxide insufflation port;
5. Motor hub outside the patient to control the robotic arms either by rigid transmission or by wires;
6. Surgeon's console with 3D visualization, adapted joysticks with haptic feedback;
7. Easy to use;
8. The dynamic range of force compatible to tissue resistance;
9. Low price and the possibility of being disposable or multiple sterilization;
10. Biocompatibility;
11. Multiple safety measures that can lock the robot's action in case of faults or inability to be controlled safely by the surgeon.

One model of such adaptation of Da Vinci robot was developed recently by Intuitive Surgical Inc (Fig. 2).

B. Robot's specifications and performance—total intracorporeal robot

1. Maximum size 12–15 mm, to be swallowed or inserted into the peritoneal cavity region through a trocar—"pil like" or "snake like";
2. Ability to travel within the peritoneal cavity and reach the target organ with or without being coordinated from a console outside of the body;
3. Multiple optical drive for an overview of the surgical field, including cold light (Fig. 3);
4. Optical Drive working with high power magnification for precise interventions;
5. Ability to analyze the surrounding tissue through ultrasound or even be able to puncture or biopsy the target lesion under ultrasound guidance;
6. Ability to have at least two miniature working arms, providing high accuracy in the execution of movements;
7. Minimum 5 degrees of freedom for working arms;
8. The possibility of achieving a work space
9. Possibility to suture the hollow organs wall hole after exiting the peritoneal cavity—in cases with NOTES robot
10. The dynamic range of force compatible to tissue resistance;
11. Easy to use;
12. Low price and the possibility of being disposable or multiple sterilization;

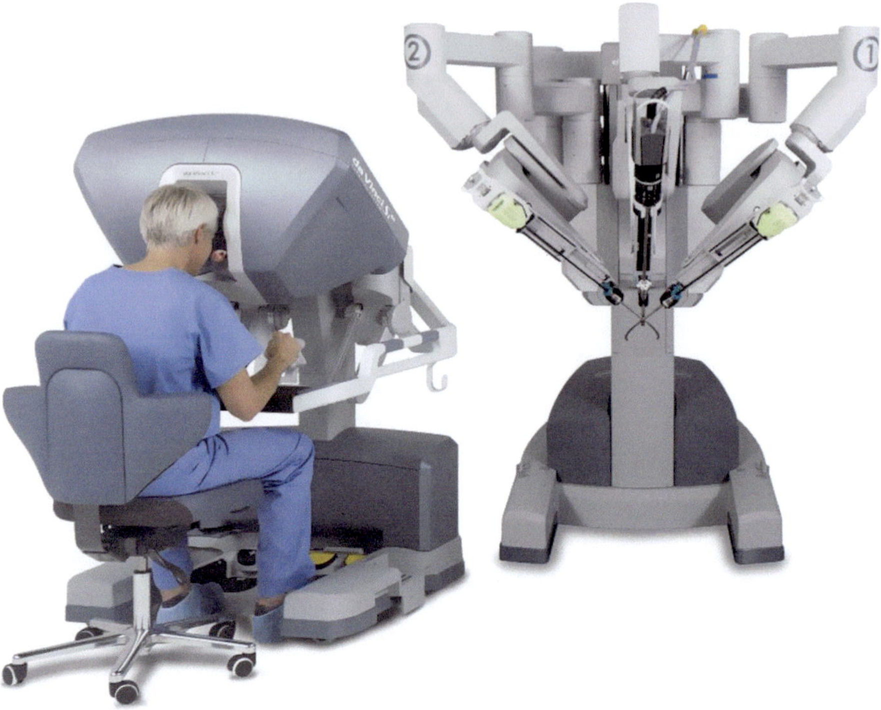

Fig. 2 Da Vinci Si system with Single-Site™ instruments. © 2009 Intuitive Surgical, Inc

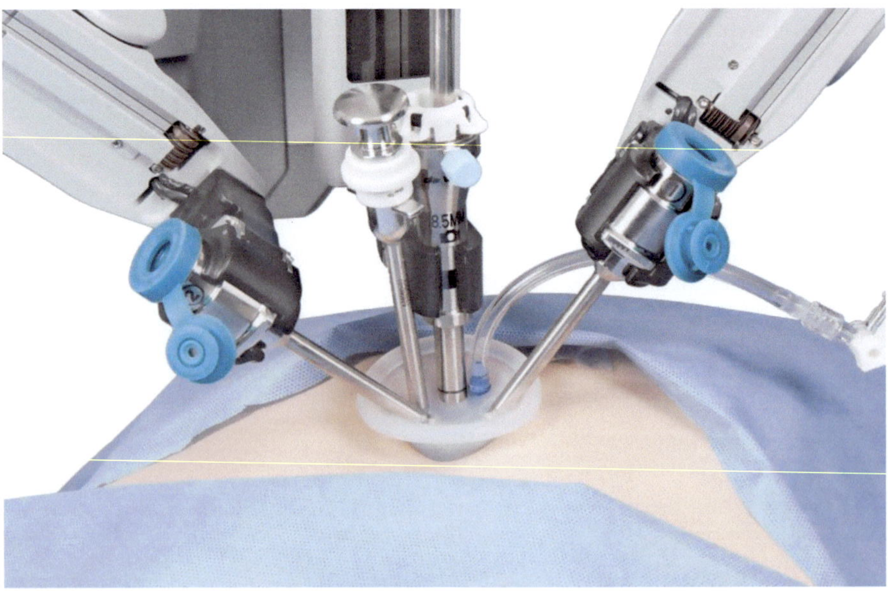

Fig. 3 Da Vinci Si system with Single-Site™ instruments—docked position. © 2009 Intuitive Surgical, Inc

13. Biocompatibility;
14. Multiple safety measures that can lock the robot's action in case of faults or inability to be controlled safely by the surgeon;

The robots, which play now a crucial role in our everyday life, appeared as a science fiction concept at first [17]. However robots can currently be seen rather as an extension and intensification of human capacities, than as theirs replacement. Not the same thing can be said, however, about the industrial field [18].

Now we can say that seems feasible to perform major surgery without incisions in the skin, surgery performed using natural orifices as access ports. Thus it can truly be "the Holy Grail" of "keyhole" surgery, given that MIS uses today smaller and smaller skin incisions [10].

A new field totally different is nanorobotics. All known structure are modified at this level, the motors are replaced with enzymes and proteins, assembled as molecular macro-aggregates capable to perform different tasks: transport chemotherapy in specific places, to deliver drugs in the cancerous cells; transport DNA or RNA sequences to replace the altered parts; cut or link proteins or other molecules; etc. They have to have sensors and also motion possibilities; to be biocompatible or biodegradable; to produce no or minimal harm to the host.

3 Conclusions

The future of surgical robots is definitely toward miniaturization. There is a problem whether to develop specific robots for each organ or pathology, or to develop very versatile robots able to operate on various tissues. The miniaturization toward nanorobots, is the field of molecular engineering and could offer the possibility of corrections at cellular, molecular and even genetic level. But these fields will not be in competition at least in the future decades, because various types of interventions will be needed at all levels, from microsurgery to nanoscale corrections.

Acknowledgements The authors are grateful for the financial support from the Romanian National Authority for Scientific Research UEFISCDI for project no. PN-II-RU-TE-2014-4-0992 and Iuliu Hatieganu University of Medicine and Pharmacy, 3rd Department Of Surgery, Cluj-Napoca, Romania, internal grant no. 4945/14/08.03.2016.

References

1. Asimov, I.: Runaround. In: Astounding Science Fiction. Street & Smith Publication Inc., New York (1942)
2. Asimov, I.: Robot. Fawcett Publications Inc., Greenwich, CT (1950)
3. Ballantyne, G.H.: Robotic surgery, telerobotic surgery, telepresence, and telementoring. Review of early clinical results. Surg. Endosc. **16**(10), 1389–1402 (2002)

4. Bozovic, V.: Medical Robotics. I-Tech Education and Publishing (2008)
5. Camarillo, D.B., Krummel, T.M., Salisbury Jr., J.K.: Robotic technology in surgery: past, present, and future. Am. J. Surg. **188**(4), 2–15 (2004)
6. Capek, J.: Opilec, in Lelio A Pro Delfina. Aventinum, Prague (1925)
7. Capek, K.: The Meaning of R.U.R.. Saturday Rev. **136**(79) (1923)
8. Capek, K.: Rossum's Universal Robots. Penguin Group USA, New York (2004)
9. Furcea, L., et al.: Avantajele implementãrii unei platforme de e-learning pentru chirurgia laparoscopicã hepaticã. Chirurgia **106**, 799–806 (2011)
10. Gomes, P.: Surgical robotics: Reviewing the past, analysing the present, imagining the future. Robot. Comput.-Integr. Manuf. **27**(2), 261–266 (2011)
11. Gourin, C., Terris, D.: History of robotic surgery. In: Russell, A.F. (ed.) Robotics in Surgery: History, Current and Future Applications. Nova Science: New York (2006)
12. Gourin, C.G., Terris, D.J.: Surgical robotics in otolaryngology: expanding the technology envelope. Curr. Opin. Otolaryngol. Head Neck Surg. **12**(3), 204–208 (2004)
13. Graur, F., et al.: Experimental laparoscopic cholecystectomy using paramis parallel robot. In: 21st International Conference of Society for Medical Innovation and Technology (2009)
14. Hashizume, M., et al.: A new era of robotic surgery assisted by a computer-enhanced surgical system. Surgery **131**(1, Supplement 1), S330–S333 (2002)
15. Hashizume, M., et al.: Early experiences of endoscopic procedures in general surgery assisted by a computer-enhanced surgical system. Surg. Endosc. **16**(8), 1187–1191 (2002)
16. Hashizume, M., Tsugawa, K.: Robotic surgery and cancer: the present state, problems and future vision. Jpn. J. Clin. Oncol. **34**(5), 227–237 (2004)
17. Hockstein, N.G., et al.: A history of robots: from science fiction to surgical robotics. J. Robot. Surg. **1**(2), 113–118 (2007)
18. Howe, R.D., Matsuoka, Y.: Robotics for surgery. Annu. Rev. Biomed. Eng. **1**, 211–240 (1999)
19. Kalan, S., et al.: History of robotic surgery. J. Robot. Surg. **4**(3), 141–147 (2010)
20. Kraft, B.M., et al.: The AESOP robot system in laparoscopic surgery: increased risk or advantage for surgeon and patient? Surg. Endosc. **18**(8), 1216–1223 (2004)
21. Lobontiu, A.: The da Vinci surgical system performing computer-enhanced surgery. Osp. Ital. Chir. **7**, 367–372 (2001)
22. Pisla, D., et al.: PARASURG hybrid parallel robot for minimally invasive surgery. Chirurgia (Bucur) **106**(5), 619–625 (2011)
23. Pisla, D., et al.: PARAMIS parallel robot for laparoscopic surgery. Chirurgia (Bucur) **105**(5), 677–683 (2010)
24. Sawa, Y., Monta, O., Matsuda, H.: Use of the Zeus robotic surgical system for cardiac surgery. Nihon Geka Gakkai Zasshi **105**(11), 726–731 (2004)
25. Taniguchi, K., et al.: Classification, design and evaluation of endoscope robots. In: Baik, S.H. (ed.) Robot Surgery. InTech (2010)
26. Taylor, R.H.: Robots as surgical assistants: Where we are, wither we are tending, and how to get there. In: Keravnou, E., et al. (eds.) Artificial Intelligence in Medicine: 6th Conference on Artificial Intelligence in Medicine Europe, AIME'97 Grenoble, France, March 23–26, 1997 Proceedings, pp. 1–11. Springer, Berlin, Heidelberg (1997)
27. Vaida, C., et al.: Voice-controlled parallel robot for minimally invasive surgery. In: 17th International Congress of the European Association for Endoscopic Surgery (EAES) Prague, Czech Republic, 17–20 June 2009 (2010)
28. Vaida, C., et al.: Development of a Voice Controlled Surgical Robot. In: Pisla, D., et al. (eds.) New Trends in Mechanism Science: Analysis and Design, pp. 567–574. Springer, Dordrecht (2010)

29. Vaida, C., et al.: Development of a control system for a parallel robot used in minimally invasive surgery. In: Vlad, S., Ciupa, R.V., Nicu, A.I. (eds.) International Conference on Advancements of Medicine and Health Care through Technology, 23–26 September 2009, Cluj-Napoca, Romania, pp. 171–176. Springer, Berlin, Heidelberg (2009)
30. Vaida, C., et al.: Orientation module for surgical instruments—a systematical approach. Meccanica **48**(1), 145–158 (2013)
31. www.biomed.brown.edu
32. www.robothalloffame.org/

Robotic System Navigation Developed for Hip Resurfacing Prosthesis Surgery

P.M.B. Torres, P.J.S. Gonçalves and J.M.M. Martins

Abstract This paper discusses the design of a navigation system developed to assist surgeons in the procedures of Hip Resurfacing prosthesis surgeries. In conventional surgery, mechanical jigs are used to obtain a correct alignment for the metal prosthesis, however it is a very time consuming process. In order to solve this problem emerges a new robotic system, named *HipRob*. The system is composed by a pre-operative sub-system for planning the prosthesis correct alignment and a flexible robot to be co-manipulated by the surgeon during the drilling procedures on the femur head. The real-time navigation of this robotic system is based on the registration between the femur model, constructed from the CT scan, and the surface constructed with ultrasound images, acquired during the surgical procedures. Experimental results, performed in a femur phantom, show that the robot location errors are around 2 mm.

Keywords Hip resurfacing · Medical robotics · Surgical navigation · Computer-assisted surgery

1 Introduction

The significant improvements of the life quality over the years are only achieved because there are researchers that constantly seek new solutions and new innovative methods to assist clinicians in the diagnosis and procedures. The use of new technologies in medicine allows to improve classical techniques and develop new solutions. These technologies can be used in the clinical diagnosis or in clinical

---

P.M.B. Torres (✉) · P.J.S. Gonçalves
Instituto Politécnico de Castelo Branco, Castelo Branco, Portugal
e-mail: pedrotorres@ipcb.pt

P.J.S. Gonçalves
e-mail: paulo.goncalves@ipcb.pt

P.M.B. Torres · P.J.S. Gonçalves · J.M.M. Martins
LAETA, IDMEC, Instituto Superior Técnico, Universidade de Lisboa, Lisboa, Portugal
e-mail: jorgemartins@tecnico.ulisboa.pt

M. Husty and M. Hofbaur (eds.), *New Trends in Medical and Service Robots*, Mechanisms and Machine Science 48, DOI 10.1007/978-3-319-59972-4_13

procedures such as surgery. In order to reduce the patient's trauma and recovery times, the traditional open surgery is being replaced by minimally invasive techniques in different surgical procedures. In the other hand, the image-guided navigation systems provides to the surgeons the possibility to tracking surgical instruments based on medical images. It is important to identify the anatomical structures during surgery, understand the target's movements and consequently use these informations in the control loop of the medical robotic systems. These techniques improves the accuracy and reduces the risks of surgical procedures.

This paper is focuses in a new navigation technique for medical robotic systems, developed to assist surgeons in the fields of orthopaedics, in particular to be used in the Hip Resurfacing (HR) prosthesis surgery. The system it was developed to solve a current problem identified by the orthopaedic surgeons who perform HR surgeries. The problem consists in the amount of time spent, during surgery, to obtain the correct alignment to perform an implant in the femur head, with the current techniques. The surgical navigation is based on the patient's Computed Tomography (CT) imaging data, to prepare surgical procedures before operation, i.e., to obtain the desired drilling point needed to implant the initial guide wire. During surgery, to achieve an accurate system to drill the femur head, the robot's surgical drill and the femur movements must be tracked. The surgical drill is tracked through a localizer system, while the femur movements are tracked also using Ultrasound (US) images. This real-time feedback allows to compensate the femur movements, during the bone drilling with the robot, without incisions in the femur.

Much research has been carried out in the fields of medical navigation systems for real time applications. Currently the ultrasound imaging modality has gained a special importance in the intra-operatory scenario due to its portability and the capability to produce images in real time. It is very useful to identify regions of interest and the movements of the anatomical structures that aims to track.

In [1] the US images are used in the guidance of a robotic system in the liver tumor treatment. It is discussed a medical robot guidance system based on ultrasound images to track the target automatically. The precise localization assists the surgeon and improves the surgery success. [2] presents a surgical navigation system based on the IGSTK (Image- Guided Surgical Toolkit) that guides medical robots to drill pedicle screws into vertebra. A Client-Server based architecture supported by OpenIGTLink protocol is used to realize the data transfer between navigation system and a KUKA robot. In [3], the authors present a review of surgery navigation system based on ultrasound guidance. In [4] an ultrasound diagnostic system is used as the navigation system for movable and deformable organs in the abdomen or chest. The authors developed a real-time updated navigation system using 3D ultrasound imaging for laparoscopic surgery. In [5] is presented an investigation to evaluate a new method to digitize pelvic bony landmarks using the ultrasound technology. An imageless Computer-Assisted Navigation System in Total Hip Arthroplasty (THA) has been shown to help increase the accuracy of cup placement. In [6] the authors investigated if a surgical navigation system using intraoperative ultrasound improves the outcomes of lumpectomy and if such a system can be implemented in the clinical environment. In [7] is presented an ultrasound-based navigation procedure for the head-neck-surgery. To conclude, in [8] it is presented a robotic motion compensation system for bone movement, using ultrasound images.

The remaining structure of the paper is organized as follows: Sect. 1 motivates the purpose of this project. Section 2 describes the materials and methods. The third section describes the experimental results, and the paper finished with a section about conclusions and future work.

1.1 Motivation

An high number of patients with damaged hip have degenerative joint disease (osteoarthritis rheumatoid arthritis and traumatic arthritis) avascular necrosis or developmental hip dysplasia [9]. In most cases, the patient's quality of life improves significantly with an hip surgery.

Total Hip Replacement (THR) is one of the most successful orthopaedic interventions used nowadays. The femoral head is removed and replaced by a prosthesis. According to the surgeon McMinn [10], the THR procedure is reasonably successful in elderly, relatively inactive patients. However, replacement hip joints wear out quickly in younger, more active patients, leading to the revision surgery and associated complications.

HR is a bone preserving alternative method to THR [11], which maintains the anatomical loading situation of the hip almost unaffected. It is viewed as an alternative to traditional THR for helping patients return to their active lifestyles. Observing Fig. 1, significant differences are noted between the prostheses used in HR and THR. HR is a bone-conserving hip procedure contrary to THR. However, the HR surgical technique is considerably more demanding than THR. Retaining the neck and head of the femur, for instance, makes it much harder for the surgeon to expose the socket. Shaping the femoral head appropriately also takes practice and if the surgeon does that poorly, the patient is far more likely to suffer a femoral neck fracture.

In the Birmingham Hip Resurfacing surgery (designed in Birmingham by Derrek McMinn), the implant alignment is the most important pre-operative consideration for correct implant positioning. According to the surgical procedures, described in [12], and illustrated in Fig. 2, the correct positioning is obtained pre-operatively

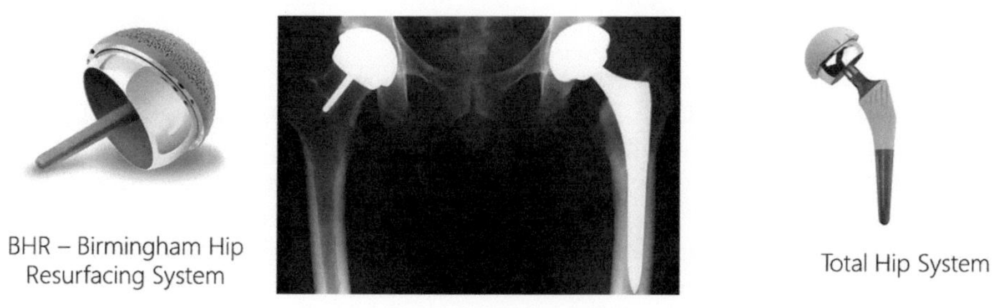

Fig. 1 Prosthesis used in hip resurfacing and total hip replacement

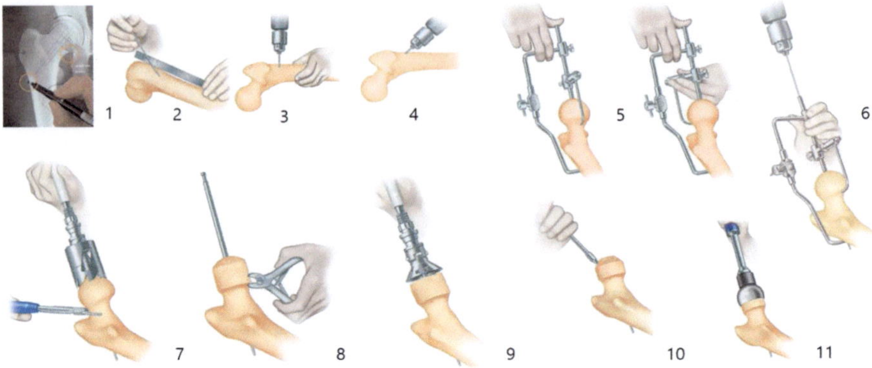

Fig. 2 *smith&nephew*, BIRMINGHAM HIP resurfacing system (extracted from [12])

(step 1), and intra-operatively, the alignment is made from a very time consuming mechanically procedure (step 5), through a alignment guide (named McMinn Alignment Guide). A guide wire is inserted when the desired position of the alignment guide has been achieved (step 6). The guide wire ensures that the spherical metal cap is positioned correctly on the femoral head. The success of the surgery depends on the correct positioning of the guide wire.

Several studies have identified the malpositioning as a risk factor for femoral neck fracture after HR [13–16]. Computer navigation systems, are an increasingly alternative to allow accurate placement of the femoral implant. Several studies comparing HR procedures performed using mechanical jigs and computer navigation systems, demonstrate that the computer navigation systems allows more accuracy [17–20]. Improve the navigation systems and assist surgeons in the HR procedures is the greatest motivation of this project, i.e., to find a robotic solution that increase the accuracy and reduce post-operative complications associated with the technique.

2 Materials and Methods

2.1 Navigation System

Pre-operatively, during the surgery planning, the surgeon defines the correct position and orientation for drill the femur head in order to implant the initial guide wire. Inside the operating room, during surgical procedures, pre-operative (CT) and intra-operative (US) image space must be registered, such that image space can be related directly to the real world coordinate system of the patient. For this reason, registration is the fundamental task in image guided surgery. Figure 3 shows the different coordinate systems of our navigation system. Pre-operatively it is known the target in the CT coordinate system. Intra-operatively there are four different

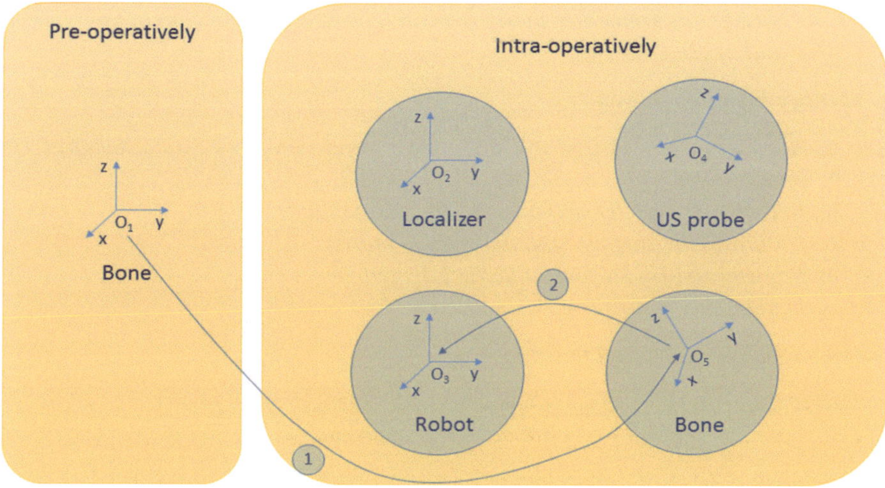

Fig. 3 Coordinate systems, involved in the navigation system

coordinate systems, the referential of the robot, of the bone, of the localizer and of the US probe.

Steps to identify the femur position and orientation inside the operating room:

1. ***Pre-calibration of the system to localize the femur:***
   a. ***Pre-operatively:***
      - *Do a CT scan of the femur;*
      - *Process the CT images;*
      - *Construct a volume with the 2D image slices;*
      - *Extract the bone point cloud (This point cloud is the bone model);*

   b. ***Acquiring data intra-operatively:***
      - *Perform a scan with the US probe on the femur;*
      - *Synchronize the image plane with the opto-tracker system;*
      - *Define a region of interest (ROI) in the first image acquired;*
      - *Cleaning the ROI with denoising methods;*
      - *Perform the bone contour segmentation;*
      - *Extract the points of the bone upper surface in the opto-tracker's reference frame;*
      - *Construct a 3D surface with the point cloud of each 2D slice;*

   c. ***Registration:***
      - *Reduce the OUTLIERS in both datasets, CT and US through the RANSAC algorithm;*
      - *Perform a global rigid registration through the ICP algorithm (Target: CT, Moved Points: US);*
      - *Perform a locally rigid registration through the ICP algorithm to refine the results;*

- *Obtain the transformation matrix that relates the US data in the referential of CT* (${}^{CT}T_{NDI}$);

2. ***Identify the bone movements:***

   a. *Acquiring, processing and extract the point cloud of 10 consecutive US image slices*;
   b. *Reconstruct the 3D surface with the point cloud*;
   c. *Calibrate the surface with the* ${}^{CT}T_{NDI}$ *matrix*;
   d. *Register the US surface with the CT model*;
   e. *Update the femur pose*;

Steps to update the robot position:

1. *Define the setpoint* (${}^{CT}P_{drill}$) *pre-operatively (ideal drilling point)*;
2. *Calculate the setpoint in the robot reference frame*;

   - *Measure the drill pose with the localizer* (${}^{NDI}T_{ROB}$);
   - *Calculate the drill point in the robot reference frame* ${}^{ROB}P_{drill}$, *knowing the calibration matrix* ${}^{CT}T_{NDI}$ *and the femur movements through the on-line registration* (*TR*);

3. *Perform the trajectory planning for the movements between consecutive setpoints*;
4. *Safeguard that the movements are smooth, don't update points above a certain threshold*;
5. *Move the robot for the new pose*;

As was written earlier, the ideal drilling point is estimated pre-operatively but needs to be spatially located within the intra-operative scenario, in order to be updated in case the femur moves. The drilling point in the CT reference frame is calculated at the beginning of the surgery, performed after the intra-operative calibration (${}^{CT}T_{NDI}$), and the drilling point position in the NDI referential frame (${}^{NDI}P_{drill}$), according to Eq. (1).

$$ {}^{CT}P_{drill} = {}^{CT}T_{NDI} \times {}^{NDI}P_{drill} \tag{1} $$

The new drilling point, calculated in the robot reference frame, considering the movements that may exist in the femur is given by Eq. (2). The update is sent to the robot controller in order to follow the femur movements, if they exist. The robotic system works on variable impedance control for physical surgeon-robot interaction.

$$ ({}^{ROB}P_{drill})_k = ({}^{NDI}T_{ROB})^{-1} \times ({}^{CT}T_{NDI})^{-1} \times (T_R)_k \times {}^{CT}P_{drill} \tag{2} $$

where, $(T_R)_k$ is the homogeneous matrix that represent the transformation obtained in the on-line local registration, which updates the calibration to compensate for femur movements.

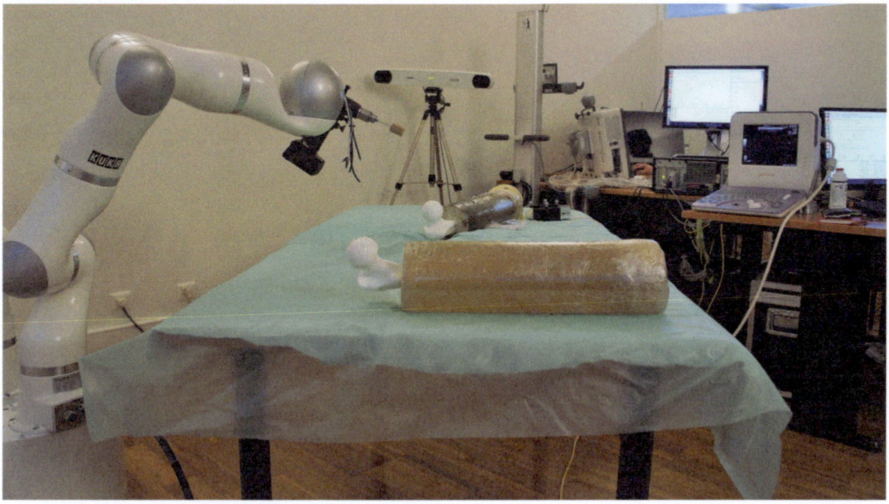

Fig. 4 Experimental apparatus

2.2 Experimental Apparatus

Figure 4 shows the experimental apparatus created in the developments of HipRob navigation system. This system consists of three workstations, an optical measurement system (NDI Polaris Spectra), a portable ultrasound system (Aloka prosound 2), with a 5 MHz linear probe and a USB video frame grabber. The vision-oriented software for bone tracking has been developed in C++ on NetBeans environment running under OS X operating system. This computer, responsible for the Bone Tracking, is connected to the NDI Polaris and frame grabber by USB. The calibration, registration and Navigation applications, run on another computer under Ubuntu Linux operating system. Both applications, calibration and Navigation, have been developed in C++ using the PCL [21], for 3D point cloud processing, registration and visualization. The third computer receives the updates obtained from the navigation system and implements the trajectory planning [22], for real-time robot control. All computers are connected by Ethernet and communicate via UDP Protocol. To perform experiments of robot positioning in real scenario, it was constructed a femur phantom, visible in the figure, with similar characteristics to a human femur.

3 Experimental Results

Several experiments were performed in order to validate this navigation system. The experiments were made in a femur phantom, constructed to simulate the drilling procedure. Figure 5 shows the bone tracking during on-line experiments. The red points correspond to the contour resulting of segmentation during the bone tracking. The ROI it is marked in the first acquired image and the algorithm, follows the

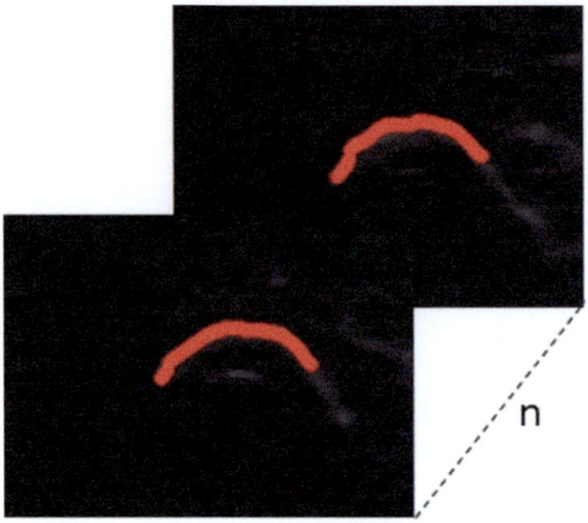

Fig. 5 Bone's contour tracking results obtained during on-line experiments

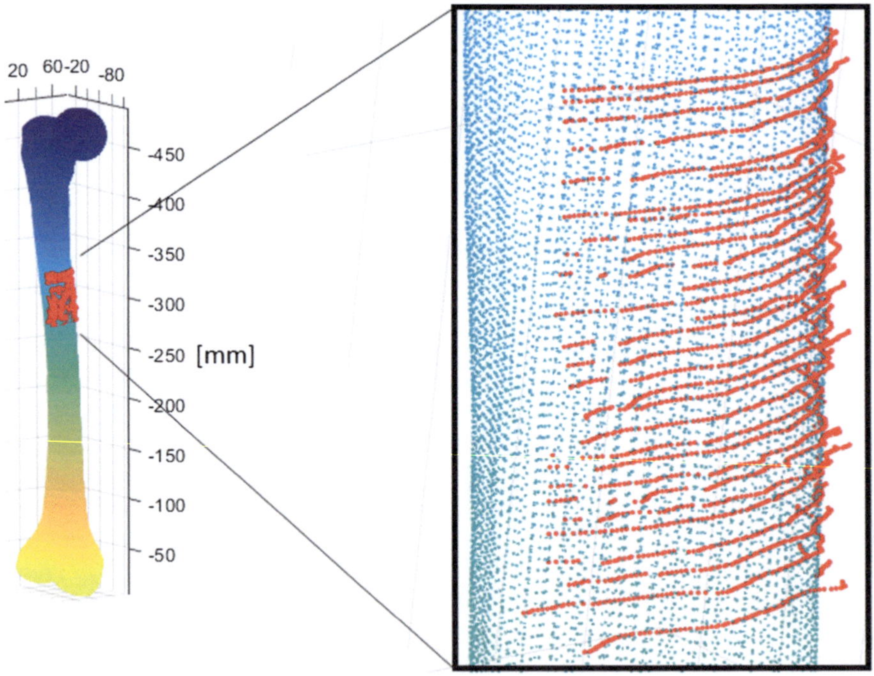

Fig. 6 Bone surfaces after registration. The femur model constructed with the CT point clouds, and the US surface (*red*) after aligned with the model

bone contour during the US scans. In Fig. 6 are depicted the registration result of an experiment. The surface model it was constructed with the CT point cloud and the red points correspond to the US point cloud after registration.

Table 1 Errors chain

Acquisition	Segmentation	Calibration	On-line registration	Tracking
1.33 mm	1.17 mm	0.76 mm	0.68 mm	2 mm

Table 1 present the errors obtained in each task that influence the system accuracy. The acquisition errors are particularly associated to wear of the opto-tracker reflective balls. The segmentation it is other task that influences the final result, however in this system it is obtained good results taking into account the type of images. The registration errors are distributed by the calibration and on-line process. Finally the tracking error it is the global navigation system error and the accuracy of the system. The robotic system can compensate the bone movements with errors around 2 mm. This error can be improved, if the errors of the previous tasks decrease.

4 Conclusions

The solution developed to track femur bones was successfully applied in a femur phantom. The system can also be adapted to other bone surgeries, that need a precise navigation of the surgical tools. The developed robotic system can compensate for femur movements, during bone drilling procedures. It is useful to ensure the drill desired positioning in order to perform a hole in the femur head, necessary to implant the initial guide wire, which ensures the correct implant's alignment. The robot's navigation system is based entirely on the information extracted from images obtained from CT (pre-operatively) and US (intra-operatively). Contrary to current surgical systems, it does not use any type of implant in the bone, to track the femur movements. The intra-operative bone tracking is performed in real time by registration of 3D US points with the femur 3D model (CT).

A KUKA lightweight robot was used to validate the applicability of the bone tracking system in the experimental tests carried out on a femur phantom. During the experiments the drilling point update was validated, with errors less than 2 mm/3°. This accuracy values are in line with the current conventional alignment systems, which demonstrates that the solution found in this project, is valid and have applicability. The drilling point update, calculated in the reference frame of the robot, is obtained at each 6 seconds.

As future work, the study could be improved if optimized the image acquisition and processing tasks.

Acknowledgements This work was partly supported by the Strategic Project, $PEst-OE/EME/LA0022/2013$, through FCT (under IDMEC-IST, Research Group: IDMEC/LAETA/CSI), FCT project $PTDC/EME-CRO/099333/2008$ and $EU-FP7-ICT-231143$, project ECHORD.

References

1. Qinjun, D.: The robot system of radio frequency ablation based on ultrasound navigation. In: 2010 2nd International Conference on Advanced Computer Control (ICACC), vol. 4, pp. 542–546 (2010)
2. Luo, H., Jia, F., Zheng, Z., Hu, Q., Xu, Y.: An igstk-based surgical navigation system connected with medical robot. In: 2010 IEEE Youth Conference on Information Computing and Telecommunications (YC-ICT), pp. 49–52 (2010)
3. Chen, X., Bao, N., Li, J., Kang, Y.: A review of surgery navigation system based on ultrasound guidance. In: 2012 International Conference on Information and Automation (ICIA), pp. 882–886 (2012)
4. Otsuka, R., Sato, I., Nakamura, R.: Gpu based real-time surgical navigation system with three-dimensional ultrasound imaging for water-filled laparo-endoscope surgery. In: 2012 Annual International Conference of the IEEE Engineering in Medicine and Biology Society (EMBC), pp. 2800–2803 (2012)
5. Shang, P., Bai, X.: An ultrasound approach to digitizie bony landmarks in navigation assisted total hip arthroplasty. In: 2013 6th International Conference on Biomedical Engineering and Informatics (BMEI), pp. 342–346 (2013)
6. Ungi, T., Gauvin, G., Lasso, A., Yeo, C.T., Pezeshki, P., Vaughan, T., Carter, K., Rudan, J., Engel, C.J., Fichtinger, G.: Navigated breast tumor excision using electromagnetically tracked ultrasound and surgical instruments. IEEE Trans. Biomed. Eng. **63**(3), 600–606 (2016)
7. Brennecke, T., Woern, H.: Support and imaging tasks using an ultrasound-based navigation procedure for minimally invasive neck surgery: experiments and analyses. In: 2015 IEEE 24th International Symposium on Industrial Electronics (ISIE), pp. 584–589 (2015)
8. Torres, P.M.B., Gonçalves, P.J.S., Martins, J.M.M.: Robotic motion compensation for bone movement, using ultrasound images. Ind. Robot: Int. J. **42**(5), 466–474 (2015)
9. Berry, D., Lieberman, J.: Surgery of the Hip. Elsevier (2013)
10. McMinn, D.J.W.: Modern Hip Resurfacing. Springer Science & Business Media (2009)
11. Muirhead-Allwood, Sarah, Sandiford, Nemandra, Kabir, Chindu: Total hip resurfacing as an alternative to total hip arthroplasty: indications and precautions. Seminars Arthroplast. **19**(4), 274–282 (2008)
12. Smith& Nephew: Smith and Nephew Birmingham hip resurfacing. Surgical Tech. (2008)
13. Shimmin, A.J., Back, D.: Femoral neck fractures following Birmingham hip resurfacing: a national review of 50 cases. J. Bone Jt. Surg. **87-B**(4), 463–464 (2005)
14. Shimmin, A.J., Bare, J., Back, D.L.: Complications associated with hip resurfacing arthroplasty. Orthop. Clin. North Am. **36**, 187–193 (2005)
15. Tapaninen, T., Kroger, H., Jurvelin, J., Venesmaa, P.: Femoral neck bone mineral density after resurfacing hip arthroplasty. Scand. J. Surg. **101**, 211–215 (2012)
16. Matharu, Gulraj S., McBryde, Callum W., Revell, Matthew P., Pynsent, Paul B.: Femoral neck fracture after Birmingham hip resurfacing arthroplasty: prevalence, time to fracture, and outcome after revision. J. Arthroplast. **28**, 147–153 (2013)
17. Davis, E.T., Gallie, P., Macgroarty, K., Waddele, J.P., Schemitsch, E.: The accuracy of image-free computer navigation in the placement of the femoral component of the Birmingham hip resurfacing. Bone Jt. J. **89**(4), 557–560 (2007)
18. Hodgson, A., Helmy, N., Masri, B.A., Greidanus, N.V., Inkpen, K.B., Duncan, C.P., Garbus, D.S., Anglin, C.: Comparative repeatability of guide-pin axis positioning in computer-assisted and manual femoral head resurfacing arthroplasty. Proc. Inst. Mech. Eng. **221**(7), 713–724 (2007)
19. Ganapathi, Muthu, Vendittoli, Pascal-André, Lavigne, Martin, Gunther, Klaus-Peter: Femoral component positioning in hip resurfacing with and without navigation. Clin. Orthop. Relat. Res. **467**(5), 1341–1347 (2009)
20. Bailey, Chris, Gul, Rehan, Falworth, Mark, Zadow, Steven, Oakeshott, Roger: Component alignment in hip resurfacing using computer navigation. Clin. Orthop. Relat. Res. **467**(4), 917–922 (2009)

21. Rusu, R.B., Cousins, S.: 3d is here: point cloud library (pcl). In: 2011 IEEE International Conference on Robotics and Automation (ICRA), pp. 1–4 (2011)
22. Pires, P.M.S.: Position and Force Control of Lightweight Robot Manipulators for Orthopedic Surgery. PhD thesis, Instituto Superior Técnico, Universidade de Lisboa (2014)

HiBSO Hip Exoskeleton: Toward a Wearable and Autonomous Design

R. Baud, A. Ortlieb, J. Olivier, M. Bouri and H. Bleuler

Abstract HiBSO is an active orthosis designed to assist the hip flexion-extension of the elderly. A fully autonomous system with untethered power electronics and energy supply is now available. Going beyond the restricted walking conditions of a treadmill unveils many opportunities for the understanding of human-robot interaction. Previous works have presented the mechanical design optimized for high transparency and light weight, while dedicated kinematics allow high torque for sit-to-stand transition and high speed for level walking. The control strategies are currently in the evaluation process. In this document, the recent improvements to the device will be described, from the mechanical design to the control electronics. Some specific aspects such as the remote communication for the controller are emphasized. The assessment of the power autonomy is addressed with two sessions of walking in different conditions, and revealed a maximum operating time of more than 80 min. In this context, the controller is based on adaptive oscillators for the gait detection and is combined with a 40% torque assistance based on biomechanics from the literature.

Keywords Exoskeleton · Active orthosis · Hip assistance · Wearable device

R. Baud (✉) · A. Ortlieb · J. Olivier · M. Bouri · H. Bleuler
Ecole Polytechnique Fédérale de Lausanne, Lausanne, Switzerland
e-mail: romain.baud@epfl.ch

A. Ortlieb
e-mail: amalric.ortlieb@epfl.ch

J. Olivier
e-mail: jeremy.olivier@epfl.ch

M. Bouri
e-mail: mohamed.bouri@epfl.ch

H. Bleuler
e-mail: hannes.bleuler@epfl.ch

M. Husty and M. Hofbaur (eds.), *New Trends in Medical and Service Robots*,
Mechanisms and Machine Science 48, DOI 10.1007/978-3-319-59972-4_14

1 Introduction

Assistive and wearable devices are an increasingly important field of research. Considering only the lower limb active robotic devices, Viteckova et al. [1] reported a number of 35 existing projects in early 2013, among which 7 were already commercialized. The number of publications in the domain also shows an exponential growth from 2002 to 2014 with a total amount close to 3000 scientific papers in 2014 [2]. While the field is largely covered, the broad range of applications and designs makes the number of devices per category relatively low. For example, the number of partial devices targeting the assistance of the hip flexion-extension to face ageing of the population or similar issues does not exceed five devices based on our knowledge. Some of these devices are quite advanced in their development such as the Honda Stride Assist [3] or the hip orthosis from the Cyberlegs project [4]. Other developments are still at research stage [5–7].

This paper will focus on the Hip Ball-Screw Orthosis (HiBSO), described in [8]. In this previous publication, tests have been performed to evaluate the influence of the device on healthy users walking on a treadmill, with all the electronics located in a desktop computer. While level walking on treadmill offers stable and controlled experimental conditions, it also constrains the user to follow a fixed pace regardless of the assistance level. As a consequence, it has been observed that the higher the level of assistance the more difficult it was for the user to stabilize her/his walking pace. For further investigations, but also for more mobility, the remotely located electronics of the device have been integrated into a compact and energetically autonomous wearable box fastened to the device.

The embedded electronics architecture and the different aspects of autonomy and wearability of the HiBSO will be presented. The physical interfaces and the mechanical optimizations of the mechanism are also described below. Considerations regarding the safety and the wireless communication between the embedded electronics and a remote computer are discussed. Finally, a first assessment of the power autonomy of HiBSO is realized under the performance of a continuous walking down to a minimal battery level. Two tests are performed, one indoor using a treadmill, the other outdoor in the street.

2 HiBSO

HiBSO is a partial assistive orthosis originally designed to assist people with muscular weaknesses such as elderly people. The particularities of the mechanical design, addressed in [5, 8], are a high transparency relatively to the power capacity, an optimized non-linear transmission ratio, an unconstrained motion of the hip adduction-abduction and of the internal-external rotation with nearly the full range of motion (ROM). The excavator-like kinematics of the mechanism can generate a nominal torque between 11 and 23 Nm in the typical walking range of motion, and a nominal torque of 25 Nm for larger flexion such as in sit-to-stand transitions and stairs ascent. An assistive controller based on adaptive oscillators as described by Ronsse et al. [9] was used with a predefined torque scheme [10] that is function of the user's weight, the gait cycle frequency and the specified percentage of assistance.

This design is targeting the elderly population, where a hip assistance is thought to improve the mobility of the user by reducing the risk of exhaustion and/or improving the walking velocity. While tests are undergoing with this active orthosis, the claimed objective of such assistive devices is the reduction of the required muscular power, considering a given activity. Two factors seem to be of main importance regarding this goal: the human-machine interaction and the added mass on the user. From several publications [11–13], it has been highlighted that decreasing the metabolic cost of healthy people using an active system is a very complicated task. As the assistive strategy i.e. the human-machine interaction, is not discussed in this paper, interesting characteristics of the device are its weight and its performances. In Table 1, these characteristics are given for three devices: Honda Stride Assist, hip orthosis from the Cyberlegs project and HiBSO.

The Honda device is very compact and light-weight but it has smaller torque capacity compared to the two other devices. The Cyberlegs hip orthosis has a large power density but there is no information on the operating time, and it has less degrees of freedom, so it needs a more careful adjustment to the user.

HiBSO is composed of three main parts: the physical interfaces with the body, the actuation mechanism and the control electronics. These elements are illustrated on Fig. 1. In the following, each parts are depicted and discussed in terms of wearability and autonomy with a particular focus on the control electronics.

2.1 *Physical Interfaces*

The physical interfaces have for function to transmit the assistive forces from the mechanism to the user limbs. They also allow to support the weight of the whole device. They should transmit as rigidly as possible the torque to the user to avoid

Table 1 Characteristics of different hip assistive devices

Device	Weight (kg)	Max. Torque (Nm)	Power autonomy	References
Honda stride assist	2.7	4	~60 min	[3]
Cyberlegs hip orthosis	8.5	35	–	[4, 15]
HiBSO	9.5	Continuous: 14–24 Short period (<3 s): 42–72	~80 min. with 40% assistance	

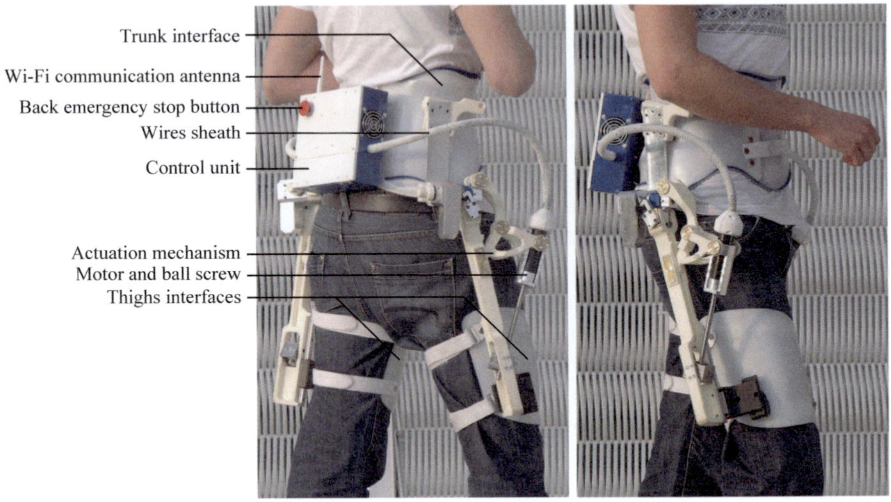

Fig. 1 Illustration of the different parts of HiBSO including the control box and embedded electronics, the actuation mechanism and the physical interfaces

parasitic movements that could lead to discomfort and hinder the controller stability. At the same time, the interfaces should minimize the pressure on the skin by enlarging the loading surface, and avoid shear stress on the skin that could lead to injuries. The interfaces elements used for HiBSO are highlighted on Fig. 2.

The trunk and the two thighs elements were realized from single person molding by an orthopedist. They are made of thick thermoplastic sheets, and include two Velcro straps for tightening. They are tailored for the person they were molded on.

Fig. 2 Physical interfaces including the trunk *upper part* and the two thighs *lower parts*

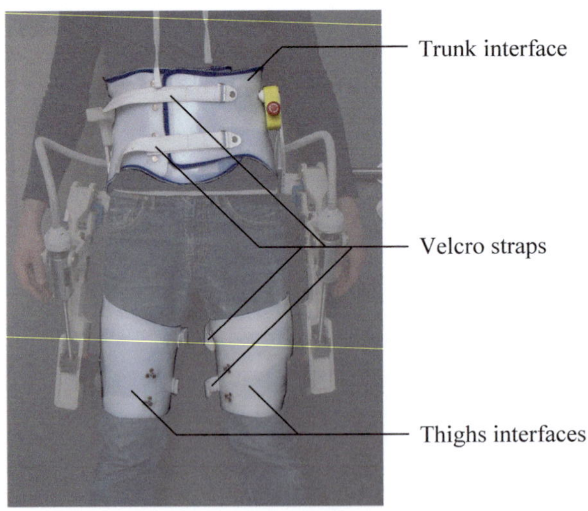

Other people can also wear them, but in this case, they may become uncomfortable when walking for an extended period of time.

The trunk interface is made of three elements. The side parts are linked to the back one by screws in slotted holes, which allows to adjust to the waist width of the user. Finally, the trunk interface has a thin foam layer inside to make the contact with the body more comfortable.

The thighs interfaces have little rubber studs inside to increase the friction with the user's cloths. However, due to the conic shape of the limbs and the muscle contraction-relaxation, the interfaces tend to slip gradually toward the knees. This is due to the fact that vertically, the orthosis structure cannot hold the interfaces, because of the linear bearings. A solution is to use short pants with suspenders, and neoprene bands stitched directly to the short. The interfaces shells have Velcro bands inside, to ensure adhesion without slip. Some work still has to be done toward a more flexible and user-friendly solution.

The interfaces are easy to don and doff. The typical suit-up time of the whole exoskeleton is 1–2 min.

2.2 Mechanical Design

The actuation mechanism has already been presented in [5, 8], however several modifications have been made to augment the wearability of the device and are described here. The design characteristics of the original design are summarized in Table 2. The modifications made concern the main material and the manufacturing process, the technology used to realize several pivots and some added/suppressed joints. Figure 3 illustrates both the original and the current version of the mechanism with their differences. First, the original structure was made completely from aluminum using conventional machining process (milling, turning, etc.). In order to reduce the manufacturing time and potentially the weight, rapid prototyping based on ABS selective laser sintering (SLS) has been used to realize most of the current mechanism. As the precision with rapid prototyping is not as good as conventional processes, joints where rigidity, high resistance to wear, and precision are required are locally realized by metallic parts. In the following, pivot joints that were all made from ball bearings have been mostly replaced by plain bearings (steel shaft in a brass housing) to reduce the complexity and the weight of the mechanism.

Finally, several modifications have been made on the architecture of the joints. The first improvement comes from practical issues. While the mechanism was worn, it has been noticed that it presented unwanted motions in several directions. The problems have been identified at the thigh interfaces where the large skin deformation can create a redundancy regarding a few DOFs. As a result, the three free rotations at the thigh level have been deleted and all the motions are still as unconstrained as before without observing any discomfort from the users.

The replacement of the aluminium body of the mechanism by an ABS structure makes it more flexible, especially in torsion (axis parallel to the thigh axis). The

Table 2 Characteristics of the original actuation mechanism

		Precisions
Actuated DOF(s)	Hip flexion-extension	ROM: −20° ext. to 110° flex
Free DOF(s)	Hip adduction-abduction Translation along the thigh axis 3 rotations of the thigh	ROM: Full motion about 0° of flex. and locked for flexion larger than 50°
Actuation	Maxon DC motor RE30 60 W	
Transmission	Maxon Spindle Drive, red. ratio 1:1	Ballscrew with 2 mm pitch
Weight	1.7 kg w/o actuator 2.5 kg w/o actuator	

DOF degree of freedom

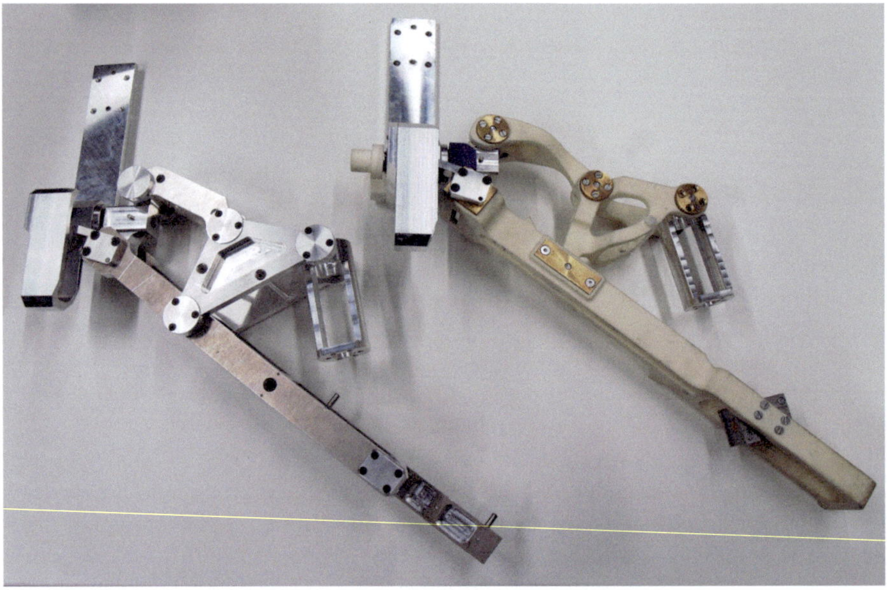

Fig. 3 Illustration of the original (*left*) and the current (*right*) actuation mechanisms. *On the left*, the body is fully made out of aluminium and has seven ball bearings pivot. *On the right*, the main body is made out of ABS and has seven plain steel-brass bearings pivot and one ball bearing joint (for the abduction)

stainless steel ballscrew is however much stiffer and then gets most of the torsion load, which leads to higher friction and unwanted lateral stress. In order to avoid such loading on the nut and the screw, the simple pivot is replaced by a universal joint to allow the transmission to follow the structure deformation without loading it (see Fig. 4).

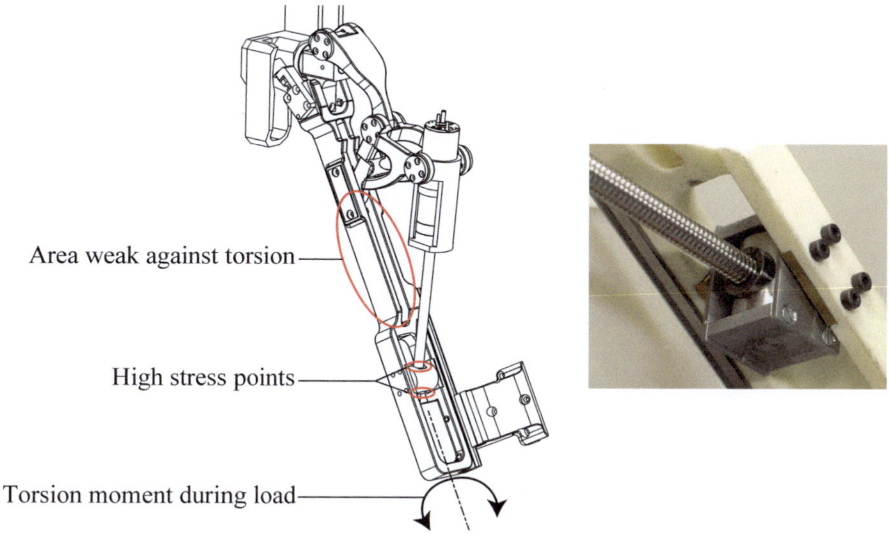

Fig. 4 *Left* Illustration of the problem of torsion with the over constrained assembly. *Right* Picture of the universal joint solution to avoid radial loads on the nut and the ball screw

3 Embedded Electronics

In order to make it autonomous, HiBSO is now untethered, and has a control box on the back. It contains an embedded computer, the power electronics, and the battery (Figs. 5 and 6). It was specifically designed for wearable assistive devices, so it is wireless and lightweight.

As HiBSO is an assistive device, and all its weight is carried by the user, the mass has to be kept very low, otherwise it hinders benefits from the active assistance. The proposed solution has a mass of 1.5 kg, including the battery, which represents approximately 16% of the full system mass.

The content is protected from shocks by a rigid aluminum case, and the motors and sensors wires are in a flexible polyamide sheath.

3.1 Embedded Computer

The embedded computer is built from the open-source BeagleBone Black single-board computer, running a soft real-time Debian Linux. Thanks to its ARM processor the power consumption is very low: 2.5 W. A custom daughterboard is providing an IMU (3-axis MEMS accelerometer and gyroscope) to estimate the pelvis orientation, and battery monitoring (voltage and current measurement). A Wi-Fi USB adapter is setup as an access-point, such that laptops and smartphones can connect remotely, for monitoring and high-level control. A Bluetooth USB

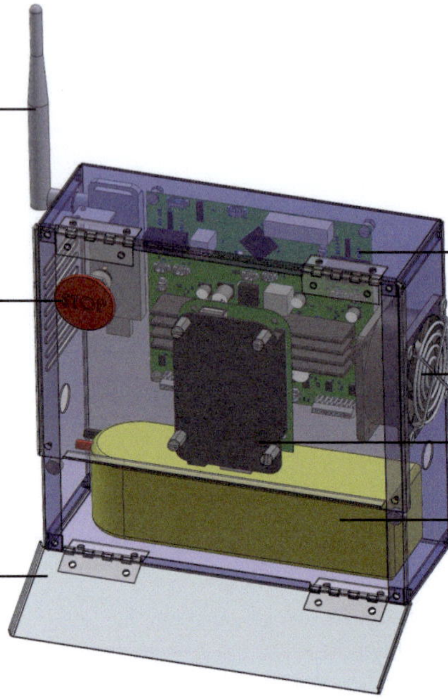

Fig. 5 Rendering of the components of the control unit, including: the embedded computer, the motors controller board, interchangeable battery, cooling fan, emergency button and communication antenna

adapter is also available, e.g. for communicating with a heartbeat sensor or any other device using this technology.

The software running on the BeagleBone Black controls the gait, collects the sensors data, and records them to a logfile on an SD card. This file can later be downloaded and analyzed offline. Losing the Wi-Fi link does not affect the gait assistance or the logging (which can then be used as a safety "black box"). As all the measurements are performed on the same machine, no manual synchronization is required. The assistance algorithm described in [14] was ported on the embedded computer.

The system is powered by a single 24 V Lithium-Polymer battery with a rated capacity of 5 A h, and a mass of 660 g.

3.2 Power Electronics

The motors controller board is a custom printed circuit board (PCB), with the STM32F7 microcontroller. It can regulate a torque, a position or a trajectory. A single board can control two motors. It is connected to the embedded computer with a differential serial transmission (RS-422). In order to increase the safety, the

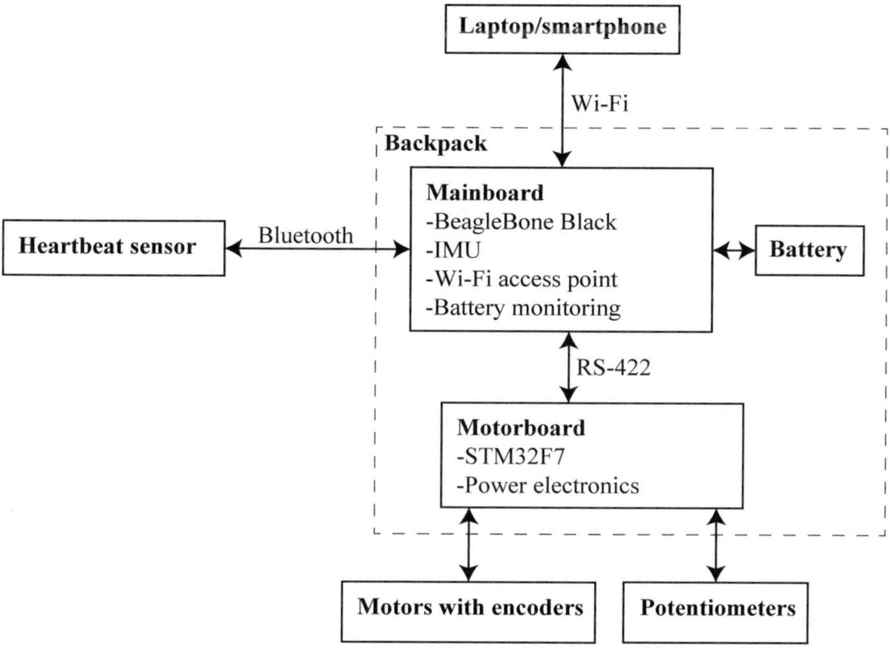

Fig. 6 Simplified schematic of the hardware architecture providing an overview of the sensors and communication environment

firmware is able to check the consistency of the redundant sensors readings (encoder and potentiometer), and trigger the emergency stop if they are incoherent. Two emergency stop buttons (at the front and back) can stop the power electronics. Note that in this case, the sensing and the computer remain functional.

3.3 External Devices

Desktop computers, laptops and tablets can connect to the embedded computer for remote supervision. A smartphone application is being developed to let the user choose the assistance level, check the battery remaining capacity, or select the assistance mode (walking, stairs climbing, standing up from a sitting position, etc.).

4 Wearability and Autonomy Assessment

The battery dimensioning is important, because while a large operating time is required, the orthosis will not be able to reduce the energy expenditure if the weight is too large.

A first test was performed on a treadmill. A healthy young subject (male, 25 years old, 183 cm, 70 kg) walked at a comfortable speed of 4 km/h, without interruption. The assistance rate was set to 40% relatively to the weight of the subject. The battery lasted 83 min before the embedded computer automatically triggered the emergency stop, because the minimum safe battery voltage was reached (3.7 V per cell). This represents a 5.5 km walking distance. The average pace was 102 steps per minute.

A second test was performed overground outdoor, and therefore at self-selected speed with a second subject (male, 27 years old, 202 cm, 95 kg). The assistance rate was set to provide the same assistive torque as the previous experiment (corresponding to 30% of assistance for the second subject). The total distance walked with active assistance was 6 km, at a mean speed of 5.1 km/h (duration: 71 min) with 96 steps per minute. The environment was varied, with flat sections and slopes. There was no remote monitoring during this experiment, the exoskeleton was fully autonomous.

5 Conclusion

The assistive hip orthosis described here is a fully operational device characterized by its easy wearability, great freedom of motion (without any restriction), adjustability and light weight. To our knowledge, it is among the devices of this type the closest to practical usability. This active orthosis will be further used for experiments in more various conditions, thanks to its wireless design and long operating time. Human-machine interaction such as presented by this device i.e. assistive strategies, is a very critical and complex approach. In fact, several searches revealed that the difficulty is to not actually increase the metabolic cost while providing power to an exoskeleton user. Building a fully autonomous wearable device such as the presented one will enable future experiments that will study the impact of different strategies on the energy expenditure of different activities. There is typically a need of research in tasks that can usually not be performed in laboratory using a remotely connected controller and power supply. Stairs ascending or descending, for example, is a major concern among the elderly population, however, very few assistive devices have carefully considered this issue.

While the potential of clinical assessment with this easy to wear and fully autonomous assistive orthosis is promising, some improvements will be proposed in parallel to these evaluations. The next revision of this exoskeleton will include a torque sensor to accurately measure the torque applied on the user thigh. This is expected to increase the transparency performance, especially for small forces, and remove the need for a friction model of the orthosis. The structure mass will also be optimized.

References

1. Viteckova, S., Kutilek, P., Jirina, M.: Wearable lower limb robotics: a review. Biocybern. Biomed. Eng. **33**, 96–105 (2013)
2. Young, A., Ferris, D.: State-of-the-art and future directions for robotic lower limb exoskeletons. IEEE Trans. Neural Syst. Rehab. Eng. 1–1 (2016)
3. Honda: Honda Worldwide|Walking Assist|Features. http://world.honda.com/Walking-Assist/features/index.html (2015). Accessed 25 Feb 2016
4. Giovacchini, F., Vannetti, F., Fantozzi, M., Cempini, M., Cortese, M., Parri, A., Yan, T., Lefeber, D., Vitiello, N.: A light-weight active orthosis for hip movement assistance. Robot. Auton. Syst. **73**, 123–134 (2015)
5. Olivier, J., Ortlieb, A., Bouri, M., Bleuler, H.: Mechanisms for actuated assistive hip orthoses. Robot. Auton. Syst. **73**, 59–67 (2015)
6. Lewis, C.L., Ferris, D.P.: Invariant hip moment pattern while walking with a robotic hip exoskeleton. J. Biomech. **44**, 789–793 (2011)
7. Ortlieb, A., Olivier, J., Bouri, M., Bleuler, H.: Series elastic actuation for assistive orthotic devices: case study of pneumatic actuator. Presented at MESROB, Nantes, France (2015)
8. Olivier, J., Ortlieb, A., Bouri, M., Clavel, R., Bleuler, H.: A ball-screw driven motorized hip orthosis. Trans. Control Mech. Syst. **3** (2014)
9. Ronsse, R., Vitiello, N., Lenzi, T., van den Kieboom, J., Carrozza, M.C., Ijspeert, A.J.: Human-robot synchrony: flexible assistance using adaptive oscillators. IEEE Trans. Biomed. Eng. **58**, 1001–1012 (2011)
10. Winter, D.A.: Kinematic and kinetic patterns in human gait: variability and compensating effects. Hum. Mov. Sci. **3**, 51–76 (1984)
11. Walsh, C.J., Endo, K., Herr, H.: A quasi-passive leg exoskeleton for load-carrying augmentation. Int. J. Hum. Rob. **04**, 487–506 (2007)
12. Gregorczyk, K.N., Hasselquist, L., Schiffman, J.M., Bensel, C.K., Obusek, J.P., Gutekunst, D. J.: Effects of a lower-body exoskeleton device on metabolic cost and gait biomechanics during load carriage. Ergonomics **53**, 1263–1275 (2010)
13. Ronsse, R., Lenzi, T., Vitiello, N., Koopman, B., van Asseldonk, E., De Rossi, S.M.M., van den Kieboom, J., van der Kooij, H., Carrozza, M.C., Ijspeert, A.J.: Oscillator-based assistance of cyclical movements: model-based and model-free approaches. Med. Biol. Eng. Comput. **49**, 1173–1185 (2011)
14. Olivier, J., Ortlieb, A., Bouri, M., Hannes, B.: Investigations on the Influence of an Assistive Hip Orthosis on Gait. Presented at EuroHaptics, London, England (2016)
15. Ruiz Garate, V., Parri, A., Yan, T., Munih, M., Molino Lova, R., Vitiello, N., Ronsse, R.: Walking assistance using artificial primitives: a novel bioinspired framework using motor primitives for locomotion assistance through a wearable cooperative exoskeleton. IEEE Robot. Autom. Mag. **23**, 83–95 (2016)

Balance Control for an Active Leg Exoskeleton Based on Human Balance Strategies

V. Huynh, C. Bidard and C. Chevallereau

Abstract This paper presents an open-loop balance control for an active leg exoskeleton based on human balance strategies, and how the machine can balance itself according to perturbations. The control is designed to balance the exoskeleton with a view to assist a well and able operator that leads the movements of the coupled system {operator+exoskeleton}. It is inspired by biomechanic works showing that human balance relies on three strategies: the displacement of the center of mass, the contribution of each leg to produce efforts and stepping. We assimilate the exoskeleton to a *Linear Inversed Pendulum* model to describe its global behavior, and we use its *capture point* to identify a loss of balance situation possibly caused by the operator and adapt the reaction of the machine. Thanks to *capture point*'s dynamics regarding to the *center of mass* and the *center of pressure*, we are able to control the machine and bring it back into a stable situation.

Keywords Balance control · Capture point · Exoskeleton

1 Introduction

Lower leg exoskeletons are more and more developed whether it be for medical applications such as carrying a paraplegic person and rehabilitation, or for industrial applications to enhance operator's skill [1–4]. In both case, balance control is essential for the coupled system. At present, for medical purposes, the balance of the system is managed by crutches (Rewalk), by the exoskeleton alone (Rex) or by

V. Huynh · C. Bidard (✉)
LIST, Interactive Robotics Laboratory, CEA, 91191 Gif-sur-Yvette, France
e-mail: catherine.bidard@cea.fr

V. Huynh
e-mail: vaiyee.huynh@cea.fr

V. Huynh · C. Chevallereau
Institut de Recherche en Communications et Cybernetique de Nantes, Nantes, France
e-mail: christine.chevallereau@irccyn.ecnantes.fr

M. Husty and M. Hofbaur (eds.), *New Trends in Medical and Service Robots*, Mechanisms and Machine Science 48, DOI 10.1007/978-3-319-59972-4_15

an external structure for rehabilitation (Lokomat). For load carrying exoskeletons (BLEEX, Hv3), devices where the operator is well and able, the lateral balance is assumed by the operator while the exoskeleton carrying its own weight and an additional load. In our works, we will only consider exoskeletons where the machine has to assist the operator in various ways, in particular, in balance recovery.

Balance control is one of the biggest issues of biped robotic or biomechanic works. Balance means that the system does not fall down and the feet are stationed. Therefore, we take inspiration from these researches [5–7] to design a balance control for an exoskeleton, without considering the entire coupled system, to react to external perturbations with a smooth action on the system. The objective is to have a balance control for the machine which will imitate human mechanisms in order to support the operator action and reduce his efforts while moving.

1.1 Human Balance Strategies

Balance control for us as humans seems to be simple and easy as we stand, walk and run everyday without falling down. Researchers in biomechanics reveal different strategies we employ to stay stable. *Winter* [5] studies human balance based commonly on inverted pendulum, in quiet standing (double support) and subjected to low perturbations. He shows the importance of center of pressure (COP) placement in the base of support shaped by the feet—the weighted average point of all the pressures over the contact area feet/ground—, directly linked to center of mass (COM) placement thanks to ankle and hip strategies in order to maintain COM in safe boundaries. He also shows the importance of load/unload mechanism of each leg to correct the postural sway. These two mechanisms involve different muscles and one prevails over the other depending on the posture. Supposing the ground is horizontal, they are summarized in this first equation:

$$\mathbf{X}_{COP,global} = \alpha_0 \mathbf{X}_{COP,0} + \alpha_1 \mathbf{X}_{COP,1} \tag{1}$$

with $\alpha_0 = \dfrac{R_{n,0}}{R_{n,0} + R_{n,1}}$, $\alpha_1 = \dfrac{R_{n,1}}{R_{n,0} + R_{n,1}}$ and $\alpha_0 + \alpha_1 = 1$, and where $\mathbf{X}_{COP,global} = \left[x_{COP,global}\ y_{COP,global}\ 0\right]^T$ is the Cartesian position of the global COP in double support, $\mathbf{X}_{COP,0} = \left[x_{COP,0}\ y_{COP,0}\ 0\right]^T$ and $\mathbf{X}_{COP,1} = \left[x_{COP,1}\ y_{COP,1}\ 0\right]^T$ are the Cartesian positions of left and right foot COP respectively, $R_{n,0}$ and $R_{n,1}$ are the normal reaction forces under left and right foot respectively and $R_{n,0} + R_{n,1}$ represents the total body weight. Equation (1) shows that we can modify COP location via the COP location of each contact area, left and right, or via normal forces distribution between the support zones.

To prevent falling from higher perturbations, a third mechanism is identified: stepping [5, 6] in order to have a new support polygon, new boundaries for COM to remain stable. Hof et al. [7] give a formulation of the equations of motion for balance in a very general form based on inverted pendulum model. These mechanisms, in particular the third one, are very efficient in sagittal plan but in frontal plan, they are limited. For instance, if we are highly pushed on the side, all the weight is transferred on the opposite leg, therefore we cannot move this leg to enlarge the base of support. To recover balance we need to jump on the side. The jump part will not be handled by our balance control.

For safety, it is important that the machine does not hurt the operator by applying efforts in the wrong way. We try to design the balance control in order to have strategies close to human's.

1.2 Instantaneous Capture Point

1.2.1 Definition

The condition of balance for static stability "the vertical projection of COM on the ground (GCOM) should be within the convex polygon shaped by the feet called support polygon" is valid only when dynamic effects can be neglected as velocity and acceleration are limited. A more important point called *instantaneous capture point* [8, 9] or *extrapolated center of mass* [10] is required inside the support polygon to allow the system to come to a stop. To make it easier to understand, it represents for a linear inverted pendulum model, the position that the inverted pendulum base needs to move instantaneously to stop and for a humanoid, it is the place that the step should be taken to come to a stop. The Cartesian position of the instantaneous capture point (ICP) is defined as (Fig. 1a):

$$\mathbf{X}_{ICP} = \mathbf{X}_{GCOM} + \frac{\dot{\mathbf{X}}_{GCOM}}{\omega_0} \tag{2}$$

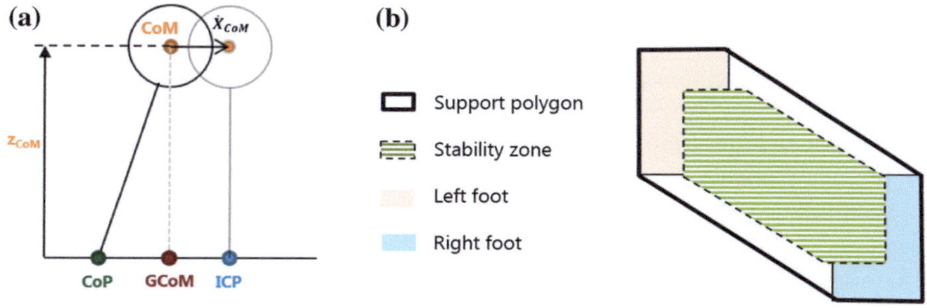

Fig. 1 **a** LIP model: Definition of ICP. **b** Stability zone

with $\omega_0 = \sqrt{\frac{g}{z_{COM}}}$ where $\mathbf{X}_{GCOM} = [x_{COM}\ y_{COM}\ 0]^T$ is the Cartesian position of the vertical projection of COM, $\dot{\mathbf{X}}_{GCOM} = [\dot{x}_{COM}\ \dot{y}_{COM}\ 0]^T$ is the Cartesian velocity of GCOM, g is the gravitational acceleration and z_{COM} is the height of COM.

1.2.2 Dynamics

To study human balance or control bipedal walking robots, the linear inverted pendulum (LIP) model from *Kajita* is widely used [11]. This model uses different assumptions such as:

- the system is modeled as a point mass corresponding to COM
- COM is kept at a constant height with a massless telescoping leg
- the base joint of the pendulum COP is torque free

For the horizontal acceleration of the COM, the equations of force equilibrium of LIP model give:

$$\ddot{\mathbf{X}}_{GCOM} = \omega_0^2(\mathbf{X}_{GCOM} - \mathbf{X}_{COP}) \tag{3}$$

By differentiating the definition of ICP and manipulating the equations, it leads to these two important equations [9, 12–14]:

$$\dot{\mathbf{X}}_{GCOM} = -\omega_0(\mathbf{X}_{GCOM} - \mathbf{X}_{ICP}) \tag{4}$$

and

$$\dot{\mathbf{X}}_{ICP} = \omega_0(\mathbf{X}_{ICP} - \mathbf{X}_{COP}) \tag{5}$$

Equation (4) shows that GCOM has a stable first-order open loop dynamics: GCOM converges toward ICP and (5) shows that ICP has an unstable first-order open loop dynamics, it illustrates ICP revulsion regarding to COP. Via its ICP, we are able to control GCOM movements and consequently, the machine's motion: we calculate a COP that creates the desired movement, this implies that ICP moves on a known straight line and GCOM simply follows.

In this paper, we consider a fully actuated exoskeleton standing on a flat ground without considering the whole coupled system {operator+exoskeleton} and we suppose the exoskeleton transparent, it means that it can be driven easily by an operator. In order to preserve balance, thus the safety of the operator, we will only focus on how the exoskeleton should react to perturbations, which can be from the operator. We present a balance control for an exoskeleton assisting well and able persons so we need to preserve their comfort to the maximum. Control ICP allows us to take advantage of the natural dynamics of LIP model and therefore to have a smooth control of system's COM. From now, we will only consider ICP instead of COM since we know that COM naturally converges toward it.

2 Balance Control

2.1 Strategies and Detection of a Loss of Balance Situation

If ICP exceeds the boundaries of the support polygon (SP), stability can no longer be maintained without stepping. In order to preserve the stability to the maximum, we do not let ICP to move close to SP boundaries except if the operator forces the exit. We define an area called *stability zone* (SZ) where no balance control is necessary, because ICP is far enough from limits to remain in a stable situation. We chose this zone such as it represents 70% of the support polygon (Fig. 1b).

To detect a loss of balance situation, we track ICP position and we consider, three different cases (Fig. 2):

- **ICP is inside SZ**: the system is stable, balance control is disabled.
- **ICP is outside SZ but inside SP**: the system is still stable but gets closer to an unstable situation, the balance control brings back ICP inside SZ.
- **ICP is outside SP**: the system is unstable, the system is going to fall if nothing is done. Human's reflex is to step in order to prevent from falling. We design the balance control to help him to balance and to reduce efforts he should produce to move.

In accordance with ICP position, the balance control will adapt to the situation.

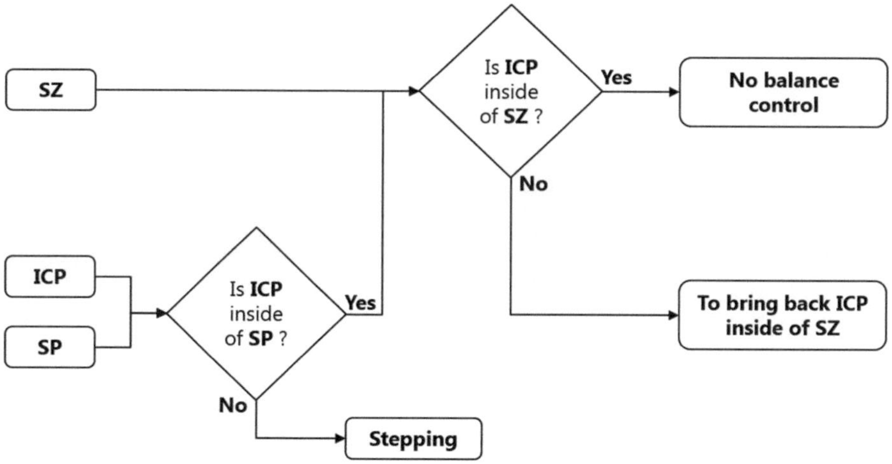

Fig. 2 Balance control logic diagram. (ICP = Instantaneous Capture Point, SP = Support Polygon, SZ = Stable Zone)

2.2 Balance Control for a Load Carrying Exoskeleton

To design a balance control for this kind of device that ensure human's movements freedom to the maximum in regard of the machine's transparency and limitations, we need to take into consideration operator's intentions. From the machine's point of view, the operator behaves like an external force applied at attached points that accelerates the exoskeleton's COM and implicitly moves its ICP and we try to assist the recovery of balance of the system. Consequently, we will only focus on how to control stance leg(s): we suppose that the operator will let himself be controlled by the machine for the stance leg and for the swing one, we suppose the exoskeleton is completely transparent and the movement is driven by the operator.

We suppose that the operator is well fastened to the exoskeleton so that he orders the velocity of the machine and we have $\dot{\mathbf{X}}_{GCOM,e} = \dot{\mathbf{X}}_{GCOM,op}$, we can write:

$$\mathbf{X}_{ICP,e} = \mathbf{X}_{GCOM,e} + \frac{\dot{\mathbf{X}}_{GCOM,op}}{\omega_{0,e}} \tag{6}$$

with $\omega_{0,e} = \sqrt{\frac{g}{z_{COM,e}}}$ where the subscripts $_e$ and $_{op}$ mean 'exoskeleton' and 'operator' respectively.

3 Capture Point Placement

One of the important part of the control is to regulate ICP location and keep it in a stable situation. Depending on the situation, we first determine a desired position for the ICP, then thanks to a simple first order control law and Eq. (4), a desired COP is calculated. The goal is to calculate the correction wrench that the actuators should produce to send the real COP to the desired one and therefore, to create the desired motion.

3.1 Desired Instantaneous Capture Point

The correction motion depends on the location of the desired ICP. The balance control idea is to keep ICP in SZ either by creating a correction motion that brings it back into SZ or by modifying the support polygon with a step to make it safe. The different cases are:

1. **ICP is inside of SP and inside of SZ**: There is no correction, $\mathbf{X}^{(d)}_{ICP} = \mathbf{X}_{ICP}$ where the superscript $^{(d)}$ means 'desired'.

2. **ICP is inside of SP and outside of SZ**: $\mathbf{X}_{ICP}^{(d)}$ is the projection of the current ICP on SZ based on a Euclidean heuristic.
3. **ICP is outside of SP**: We choose to trigger a step because we know the system is unstable and the single support phase can begin. To determine $\mathbf{X}_{ICP}^{(d)}$, we extrapolate the location of ICP. We integrate the Eq. 5 and given the current location of ICP, we can deduce the direction of the motion at time t_0 when ICP go out of SP for the first time. We calculate the location of ICP at t_s, minimal time to make a step, if nothing is done to correct or modify its trajectory:

$$\mathbf{X}_{ICP}(t = t_s) = \left(\mathbf{X}_{ICP}(t = t_0) - \mathbf{X}_{COP,0}\right)e^{\omega_0 t_s} + \mathbf{X}_{COP,0} \tag{7}$$

To maximize the stability margin at the end of single support phase, when the swing foot reaches the ground, ICP should be at the center of the support polygon, so $\mathbf{X}_{ICP}^{(d)} = \mathbf{X}_{ICP}(t = t_s) =$ center of the next double support polygon. Therefore, we can determine the ideal location of the step $\mathbf{X}_{step}$ and then, the ideal next double support polygon at $t = t_S$ (Fig. 4). As long as the swing foot does not reach the ground and the single support is not finished, t_0, and so $\mathbf{X}_{step}$, remains the same: $t_0 \leq t \leq t_{end}$. Note that the step has not to be made at $t = t_s$: the desired ICP indicates the direction of motion of the system. Our goal is to encourage the motion in a desired direction, not to force a movement (Fig. 3).

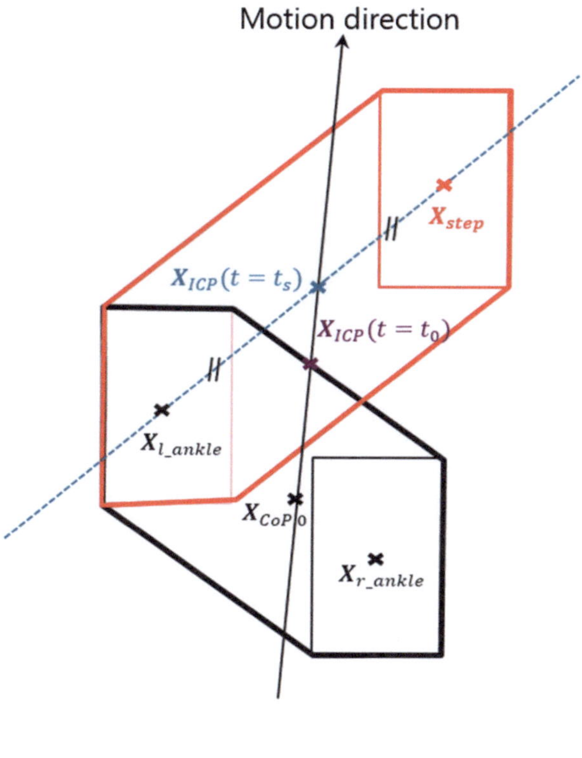

Fig. 3 Determination of the ideal next double support polygon

3.2 Desired Center of Pressure of LIP Model

Our objective is now to deduce articular torques that the legs should produce to reach the desired ICP. Torques will place COP at a specific location which will modify ICP velocity. We can write ICP velocity as:

$$\dot{\mathbf{X}}_{ICP} = K_{ICP}.\left(\mathbf{X}_{ICP}^{(d)} - \mathbf{X}_{ICP}\right) \tag{8}$$

where K_{ICP} is the proportional gain.

Basing on LIP model, we deduce COP position by equalizing Eq. (5) from equations of motion of LIP and (8):

$$\omega_0\left(\mathbf{X}_{ICP} - \mathbf{X}_{COP}\right) = K_{ICP}.\left(\mathbf{X}_{ICP}^{(d)} - \mathbf{X}_{ICP}\right) \tag{9}$$

$$\mathbf{X}_{COP} = \mathbf{X}_{ICP} - \frac{K_{ICP}}{\omega_0}.\left(\mathbf{X}_{ICP}^{(d)} - \mathbf{X}_{ICP}\right) \tag{10}$$

with $K_{ICP} > 0$ in order to preserve the direction of the motion, else K_{ICP} is not consistent with system dynamic. COP must be inside SP in other case, the stance feet will rotate. Therefore, COP can't physically be outside SP, if $\mathbf{X}_{COP}$ is outside, we use a heuristic to project it on SP.

3.3 Computation of Correction Wrench

This section deals with how to compute the correction wrench that allows us to reach our ICP objective. In the previous section, we determined the location of the COP that moves ICP to the desired ICP. It means that placing the current COP there creates an acceleration at COM as following (Eq. 3):

$$\ddot{\mathbf{X}}_{GCOM} = \omega_0^2(\mathbf{X}_{GCOM} - \mathbf{X}_{COP}) \tag{11}$$

So we can easily write the correction wrench that brings the system to a stable situation as:

$$\mathbf{W}_{corr,G} = \begin{bmatrix}\mathbf{F}_{corr}\\ \mathbf{M}_{corr,G}\end{bmatrix} = \begin{bmatrix}m\ddot{\mathbf{X}}_{GCOM}\\ \mathbf{0}\end{bmatrix} \tag{12}$$

with

$$\mathbf{F}_{corr} = m\ddot{\mathbf{X}}_{GCOM} = \frac{mg}{z_{COM}}(\mathbf{X}_{GCOM} - \mathbf{X}_{COP}) \tag{13}$$

where m is the mass of the system and $\mathbf{X}_{COP}$ is the one calculated previously. Note that the generated correction wrench is an horizontal force applied on COM and have zero moment around it.

So we can write the dynamic equation:

$$\mathbf{Ad}_G \mathbf{W}_{ground,P} + \mathbf{W}_{weight,G} - \mathbf{W}_{corr,G} = \mathbf{W}_{dyn,G} \tag{14}$$

where

- $\mathbf{Ad}_G$: adjoint transformation associated with COP to COM.
- $\mathbf{W}_{ground,P}$: wrench of ground reaction force applied at COP.
- $\mathbf{W}_{weight,G}$: wrench of gravity force applied at COM where m is the mass of the system.
- $\mathbf{W}_{corr,G}$: correction wrench applied at COM which we determined.
- $\mathbf{W}_{dyn,G}$: dynamic wrench applied at COM.

Now $\mathbf{W}_{corr,G}$ is known, we obtain the entire effort that the actuators need to produce. Let's:

$$\mathbf{W}_{act} = \mathbf{W}_{corr} - (\mathbf{W}_{weight,G} + \mathbf{W}_{dyn,G}) \tag{15}$$

$\mathbf{W}_{corr}$ is produced to help the operator and $(\mathbf{W}_{weight,G} + \mathbf{W}_{dyn,G})$ is necessary for the machine to care its weight and an additional load which is its first job before assisting.

4 Coefficient of LEG Contribution

Once $\mathbf{W}_{act}$ is known and to calculate joint torques, we adopt the intuitive strategy used by Pratt et al. [15] of distributing the forces between the two legs. The leg support fractions are two coefficients $(\alpha_0; \alpha_1)$ ($0 =$ left, $1 =$ right) describing the fraction of the desired wrench to be exerted by each leg with $\alpha_0 + \alpha_1 = 1$. $\alpha_i = 0$ means that leg i is the swing one. In [16] the forces are distributed according to the following geometric ratio:

$$\alpha_i = \frac{\|\mathbf{X}_{GCOM} - \mathbf{X}_{1-i}\|_2}{\|\mathbf{X}_0 - \mathbf{X}_1\|_2} \tag{16}$$

with $i \in \{0, 1\}$ and where $\mathbf{X}_0$ and $\mathbf{X}_1$ are respectively the center of left and right foot polygon. Expression (16) shows that if the mass gets closer to a foot, the related leg contribution increases to support it. In [14], Pratt et al. use the ratio of COPs distances but it supposed to know or estimate left and right COP position.

However these coefficients do not take into consideration perturbations. We propose a coefficient that takes into account the direction of perturbations using ICP, and the limits of SP to transfer the load from a leg to the other appropriately when needed.

4.1 Description of the Situation

Giving a feet configuration, we will resist to a perturbation by supporting more efforts on one leg than the other: if we are pushed on the right side, the contribution of the right leg will be higher than the one on the left. We introduce a first coefficient β which represents the proximity to a foot:

$$\beta_i = \frac{\|\mathbf{X}_{ICP}^{(p)} - \mathbf{X}_{1-i}\|_2}{\|\mathbf{X}_0 - \mathbf{X}_1\|_2} \tag{17}$$

with $i \in \{0, 1\}$ and where $\mathbf{X}_{ICP}^{(p)}$ is the projection of ICP on feet axe.

β indicates which leg should produce more efforts to resist the perturbation. However, taking into account the feet positions only is not enough: ICP can get closer to the support polygon's boundaries and still have a $\beta \simeq 0.5$. Indeed, when ICP leaves the polygon, a step is taken. To anticipate this action, we need to transfer the weight to the future support leg to allow swing foot take-off. Therefore, we introduce a second coefficient γ as following:

$$\gamma = \frac{\|\mathbf{X}_{ICP}^{(p)} - \mathbf{X}_{ICP}\|_2}{\|\mathbf{X}_{ICP}^{(p)} - \mathbf{X}_{bound}\|_2} \tag{18}$$

where $\mathbf{X}_{bound}$ represents the projection of ICP on the closer boundary. This way, we have all necessary information to describe the location of ICP in SP and determine the coefficients of leg contribution α (Fig. 4).

4.2 Stabilization

We build α in function of β and γ. Let's consider ICP on feet axe: we want $\alpha_0 = \beta_0$. However, if ICP moves away from the axe to join SP limits, α has to converge to 1 for the closest leg:

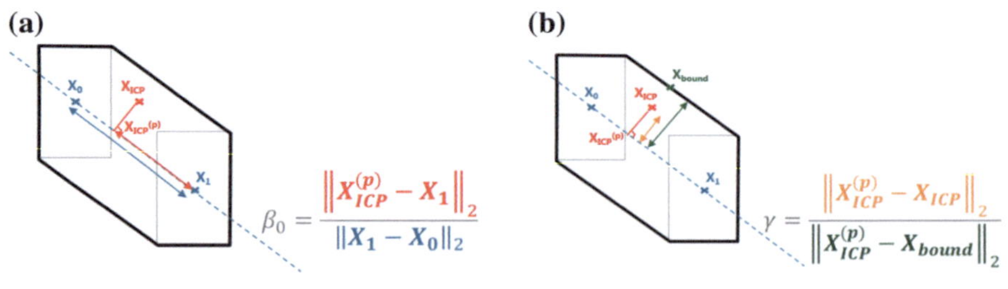

Fig. 4 **a** Definition of β. **b** Definition of γ

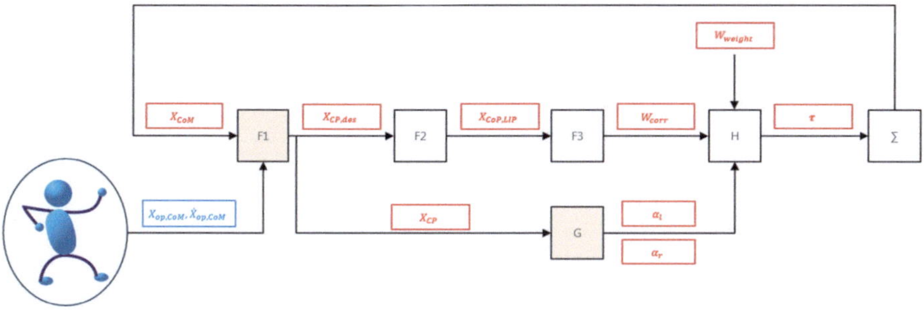

Fig. 5 Open-loop balance control scheme

$$\alpha_0(\gamma) = \begin{cases} 1 - exp\left(-\lambda(\gamma + \gamma_{\beta_0})\right) & \text{if } \|\mathbf{X}_{ICP} - \mathbf{X}_0\|_2 \leq \|\mathbf{X}_{ICP} - \mathbf{X}_1\|_2 \\ exp\left(-\lambda(\gamma + \gamma_{\beta_0})\right) & \text{if } \|\mathbf{X}_{ICP} - \mathbf{X}_0\|_2 > \|\mathbf{X}_{ICP} - \mathbf{X}_1\|_2 \end{cases}$$

$$\alpha_1(\gamma) = 1 - \alpha_0(\gamma)$$

where λ is the convergence velocity and γ_{β_0} is the necessary offset to have $\alpha_0(\gamma = 0) = \beta_0$. With this α, the weight transfer is handled and the leg is ready to anticipate the perturbation and stabilize the system.

At this point, we have the contribution of each leg to split the efforts in the following way:

$$\mathbf{W}_{act,i} = \alpha_i.\mathbf{W}_{act} \tag{19}$$

We develop this algorithm in order to implement it on a force controlled exoskeleton using screw cable system actuators [4]. This is why, we use the Jacobian matrix to calculate joint torques to apply to the machine (Fig. 5).

5 Simulations

We consider a fully-actuated exoskeleton of twelve degrees of freedom with six per leg: hip flexion/extension and abduction/adduction, thigh rotation, knee flexion/extension, ankle flexion/extension and prono-supination. Since we can't really simulate an autonomous operator, to overcome his presence in the simulator, we use a Cartesian external force $\mathbf{F}_{push}$ applied at the center of the phantom during t_{push} seconds to represent when he pulls the machine.

We test different situations with following parameters $t_s = 1\text{s}$, $K_{ICP} = 100$ (x points to the right, y forward and z up) with the feet configuration in Fig. 6:

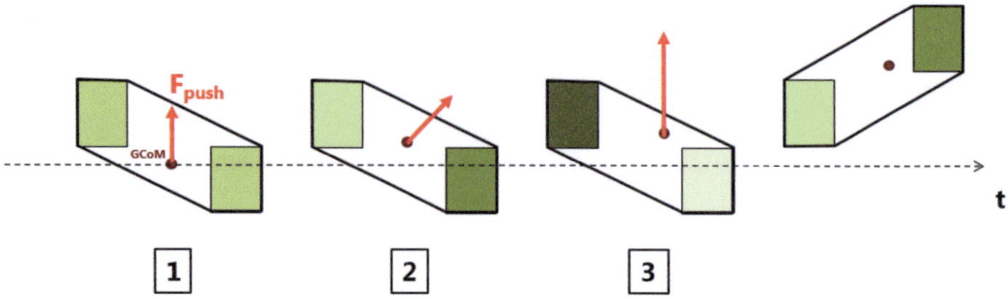

Fig. 6 The three steps of the simulation where perturbations are accumulated. The more the foot polygon is *dark green*, the more the leg contribution coefficient is close to 1

1. The operator moves forwards: ICP inside SZ, the balance control does not need to be active. $\mathbf{F}_{push} = \begin{bmatrix}0 \ 100\text{N} \ 0\end{bmatrix}$ and $t_{push} = 0.15\text{s}$.
2. He moves forwards and diagonally: ICP leaves SZ, the balance control brings ICP back into SZ. $\mathbf{F}_{push} = \begin{bmatrix}100 \ 100\text{N} \ 0\end{bmatrix}$ and $t_{push} = 0.15\text{s}$.
3. He moves faster forwards: he forced ICP to leave SZ and then SP, the balance control detects that a step will be taken to recover balance (left leg support). $\mathbf{F}_{push} = \begin{bmatrix}0 \ 350\text{N} \ 0\end{bmatrix}$ and $t_{push} = 0.075\text{s}$.

In the simulation, at $t = 0\text{s}$ we unlock exoskeleton's joints and the balance control is enabled and it converges toward an stable state: ICP inside of SZ and $(\alpha_0; \alpha_1) \approx (0.49; 0.51)$. On the graphs, dotted lines represents the beginning of each phase previously mentionned:

- Figure 7a, b highlight the perturbations shown on COM velocity graphs and the consequences on desired and current ICP trajectories. The most interesting is ICP trajectories: current ICP well tracks on desired ICP. At the first stage, ICP is inside SZ, therefore $\mathbf{X}_{ICP}^{(d)} = \mathbf{X}_{ICP}$. The second perturbation leads ICP to get out of SZ: the balance control brings it back in order to guarantee the stability. At the third stage, ICP exits SZ then SP. A step is taken. Current ICP converges toward desired ICP but we don't wait for its complete convergence to switch from single support phase to double support phase.
- Figure 7c represents the pursuit of COM for ICP in a natural convergence. It shows that our balance control regulates indirectly and smoothly COM trajectory in order to control the movement according to a direction.
- Figure 7d shows the evolution of leg contribution coefficients $(\alpha_0; \alpha_1)$. Magenta line represents left leg and yellow line, right leg. The first perturbation is forward: ICP get close to left foot, α_0 increases. The second one is forward and to the right: α_1 increases. Then, at the third stage, the system is pushed forward so ICP is close to left foot and reaches SP limits. All the weight is transferred on left leg, in order to trigger the swing phase.

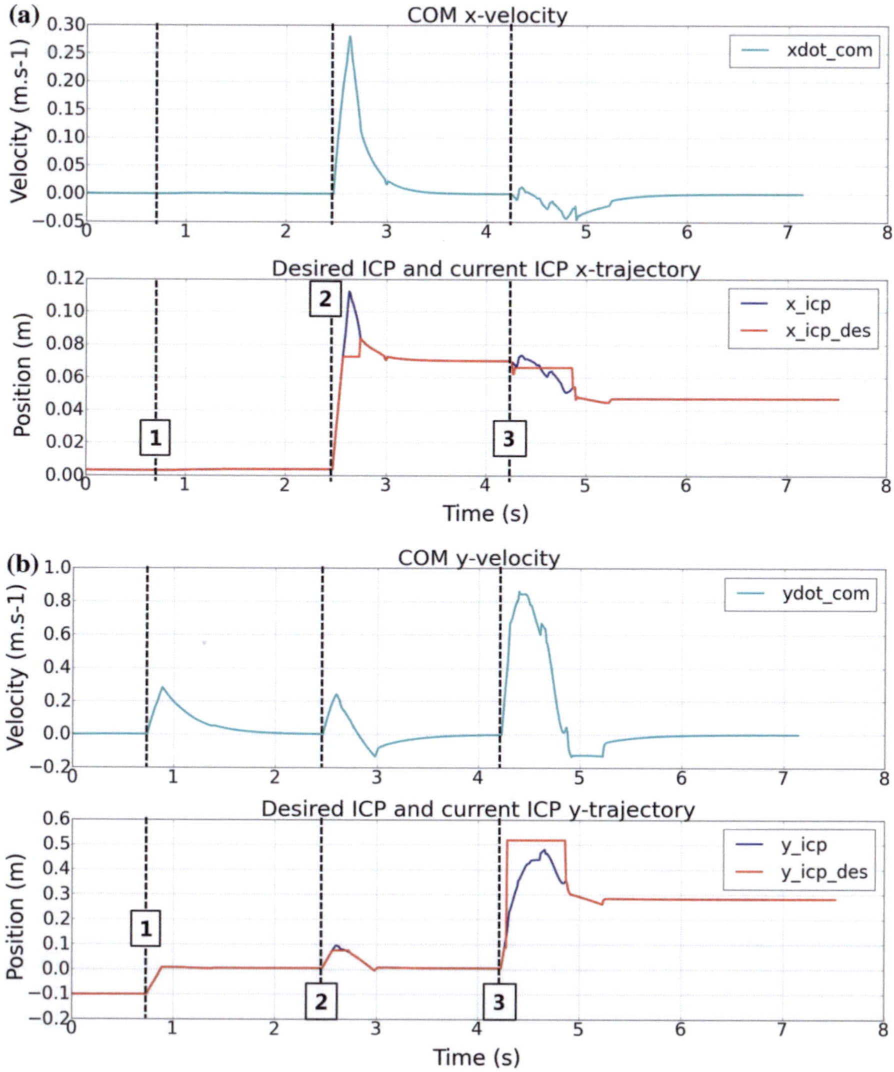

Fig. 7 **a** and **b** represent the desired and the current ICP position in function of the perturbations on COM represented by COM velocity. **c** represents the trajectory of COM and ICP. **d** represents the coefficients of leg distribution

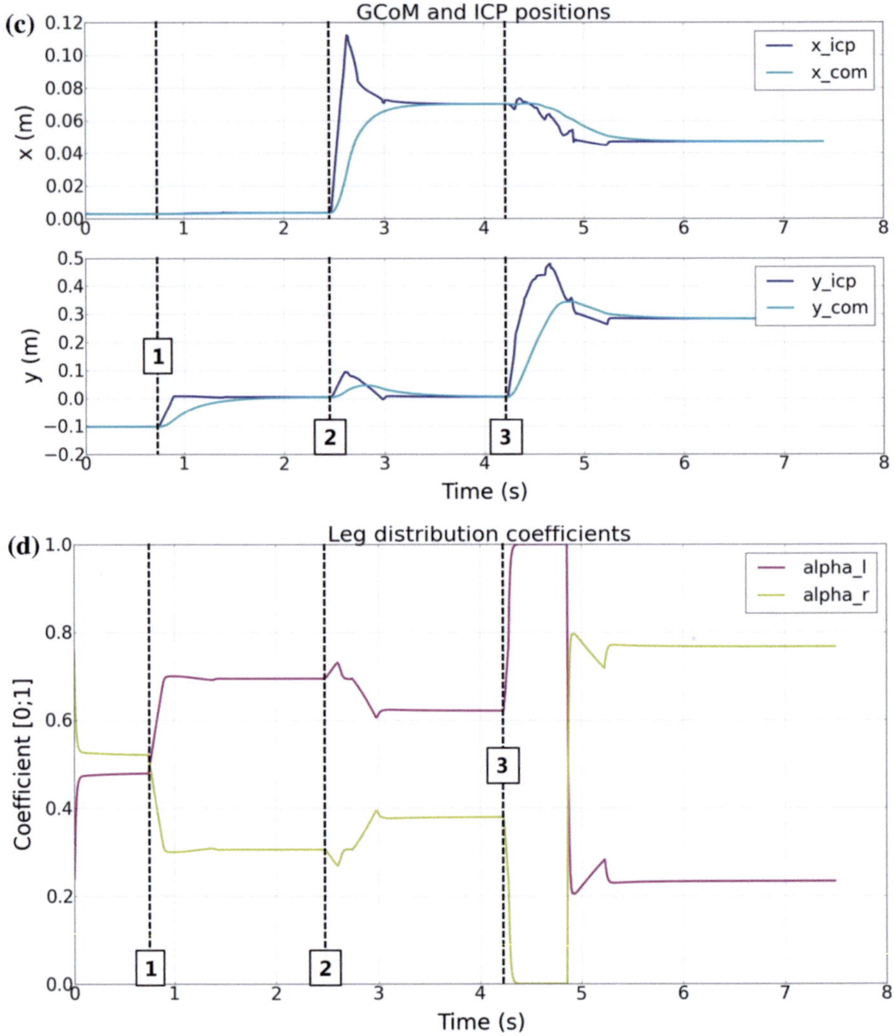

Fig. 7 (continued)

6 Conclusion

We presented a balance control based on the control of the instantaneous capture point of the exoskeleton. It allows the machine to detect a loss of balance situation and to imitate human mechanisms in order to help him to recover his balance. In this paper, we supposed a fully-actuated exoskeleton and we neglected the interaction with the operator. Undergoing works deal with underactuaction (lightening machines implies reducing the number of actuators) or overactuaction which leads to opposite efforts produced by both legs. Moreover, we need experiments to validate that our balance control is well accepted by the operator.

References

1. Dollar, A.M., Herr, H.: Lower extremity exoskeletons and active orthoses: challenges and state-of-the-art. IEEE Trans. Robot. **24** (2008)
2. Bogue, R.: Exoskeletons and robotic prosthetics : a review of recent developments. Ind. Robot.: Int. J. 421–427 (2009)
3. Moriniere, B., Verney, A., Abroug, N., Garrec, P., Perrot, Y.: EMY: a dual arm exoskeleton dedicated to the evaluation of Brain Machine Interface in clinical trials. In: IEEE/RSJ International Conference on Intelligent Robots and Systems (IROS), pp. 5333–5338 (2015)
4. Garrec, P., Kfoury, F.: Misalignment-tolerant cable actuator, Patent WO2014128178 A1 (2014)
5. Winter, D.A.: Human balance and posture control during standing and walking. Gait & Posture **3**, 193–214 (1995)
6. Horak, F.B., Nashner, L.M.: Central programming of postural movements: adaptation to altered support surface configurations. J. Neurophysiol. **55**(6), 1369–1381 (1986)
7. Hof, A.L.: The equations of motion for a standing human reveal three mechanisms for balance. J. Biomech. **40**, 451–457 (2005)
8. Pratt, J., Carff, J., Drakunov, S., Goswami, A.: Capture point: a step toward humanoid push recovery. In: Proceedings of IEEE International Conference on Humanoid Robotics, pp. 200–207 (2006)
9. Koolen, T., de Boer, T., Rebula, J., Goswami, A., Pratt, J.: Capturability-based analysis and control of legged locomotion, Part 1: theory and application to three simple gait models. Int. J. Robot. Res. (2012)
10. Hof, A.L., Gazendam, M.G.J., Sinke, W.E.: The condition for dynamic stability. J. Biomech. **38**, 1–8 (2004)
11. Kajita, S., Kanehiro, F., Kaneko, K., Fujiwara, K., Harada, K., Yokoi, K., Hirukawa, H.: In: Proceedings of the IEEE International Conference on Robots and Automation (2003)
12. Hof, A.L.: The 'extrapoled center of mass' concept suggests a simple control of balance in walking. Hum. Mov. Sci. **27**, 112–125 (2007)
13. Englsberger, J., Ott, C., Roa, M.A., Albu-Schffer, A., Hirzinger, G.: Bipedal walking control based on capture point dynamics. In: Proceedings of the IEEE International Conference on Intelligent Robots and Systems (2011)
14. Pratt, J., Koolen, T., de Boer, T., Rebula, J., Cotton, S., Carff, J., Johnson, M., Neuhaus, P.: Capturability-based analysis and control of legged locomotion, Part 2: application to M2V2, a lower-body humanoid. Int. J. Robot. Res. (2012)
15. Pratt, J., Pratt, G.: Intuitive control of planar bipedal walking robot. In: Proceedings of the IEEE International Conference on Robotics and Automation (1998)
16. Racine, J.L.: Control of a lower limb extremity exoskeleton for Human Performance Amplification, Ph.D. dissertation. University of California, Berkeley (2003)

First Investigations into Artificial Emotions in Cognitive Robotics

D. Moser, R. Thenius and Th. Schmickl

Abstract In nature, the combination of processes of emotion and cognition has a deep impact on type and quality of reaction to environmental stimuli. In this work, we want to test the feasibility of artificial hormones in artificial neural networks. We take a minimal evolving neural network and look into the implications and opportunities of extending this model of communicating nodes, with one virtual hormone gland. To explore the differences in behavior, that we expect to develop with this modification, we modify an already well established model, the Braitenberg Vehicle. These vehicles were faced with a simple energy gathering task. The behavior, efficiency and fitness of these vehicles in identical environment, with the artificial hormone active and inactive, is examined. It shows, that the implementation of artificial emotion leads to an increase in efficiency of the evolved solution.

Keywords Artificial emotions · Neural networks · Complex behaviors · Artificial evolution

1 Introduction

1.1 Motivation

To navigate in, and react to an immensely diverse and dynamically changing environment, is a challenging task for robots. As the challenges of mechanical nature in the field of robotics were often conquered with bio-inspired solutions, it is logical to look in the same direction when approaching cognitive problems.
Humans and other animals are quite versatile in these kind of tasks, so we propose to explore methods to implement bio-inspired approaches in artificial systems to close this gap. Further, it is paramount for agents in these environments, to fully function with the lowest possible expenditure of available energy, so efficiency is a key factor

D. Moser (✉) · R. Thenius · Th. Schmickl
Artificial Life Laboratory, University of Graz, Graz, Austria
e-mail: daniel.moser@uni-graz.at

M. Husty and M. Hofbaur (eds.), *New Trends in Medical and Service Robots*, Mechanisms and Machine Science 48, DOI 10.1007/978-3-319-59972-4_16

of success. This is true for power consumption as well as navigation and task fulfillment. The notion that cognition and emotion are closely linked is already well documented [21]. It is also suggested that experimental cognitive and emotional robotics can provide insights into emotion theory and neuroscience [4]. In this paper we define artificial emotion as a feedback-loop in the interconnected system of neurons, gland and artificial hormone. This self influencing cycle has simplified characteristics of the above mentioned natural systems, and as such is an bio-inspired extension to the already bio-inspired Artificial Neural Network (ANN), which is shortly described in Sect. 2.1.

What we expect to get from the exploration of this subject in the long run, is:

- A novel approach to cognitive adaptability and context dependent decision finding in agents.
- An increase in efficiency in the use of computing resources and in energy management.

1.2 The Questions

To start our investigation regarding the feasibility of implementing an artificial hormonal, we formulated three questions:

1. *Question Q.1* Can the efficiency of an artificial neural network be enhanced by a self-influencing, system-wide simulated neuromodulation with artificial hormones?
2. *Question Q.2* What increase in efficiency can we observe and possibly exploit for cognitive robotics?
3. *Question Q.3* Does evolution use and hold the features of artificial emotion?

1.3 The Hypothesis

Based on the above mentioned question *Q*.1 we formulated following hypothesis:

H0: The implementation of a hormonal system has no influence on the performance of an ANN.

H1: The implementation of a hormonal system has some influence on the performance of an ANN.

H1.a: The implementation of a hormonal system decreases the performance of an ANN for the tested task.

H1.b: The implementation of a hormonal system increases the performance of an ANN for the tested task.

Due to the fact that question *Q*.2 aims for the implementation in the context of a real-world robotic system, we decided to use descriptive formulations to answer this question, instead of formulating a hypothesis.

2 The Method

To test the above mentioned hypothesis and questions, we developed a simple multi-agent simulation, including artificial evolution. Inspired by previous work about artificial emotions and neuromodulation in ANNs [19], an experimental setup was chosen to test our hypothesis. Multiple agents, equipped with a simple neural-network, had to collect food and reproduced, given the reproduction threshold R was reached (see Table 1). The developed simulation environment was designed for fast testing of the hypothesis, and a minimum of parameters. This allowed for having a maximum of generality for the acquired insights into evolving ANNs and the influence of artificial emotion systems. The programming environment we chose was the NetLogo 5.3 simulation and modeling environment [20]. A more detailed description of the simulation processes, procedures and the simulation interface can be found in Sect. 2.2.

2.1 *The Artificial Neural Network*

Artificial Neural Networks are inspired by the biological brain and are in stark contrast to the functionality of the standart von Neumann model of modern computing machines [9]. First investigations have been published as early as 1943 [11] and renewed interest emerged with the advances in the development of back-propagation

Table 1 This table describes the constants and variables used in this paper in the context of the simulation environment

Variable	Explanation	Value	Unit	Constant	Evolving	Scope
A	Age	0	Time-steps	No	No	Agent
B	Agents in the simulation	100	Agents	Yes	No	Global
C	Energy after reproduction	40	Energy	Yes	No	Global
E	Initial energy on food-patches	100	Energy	No	No	Global
F	Food gathered	0	Energy	No	No	Global
H	Initial hormone level	0.3	–	Yes	No	Agent
M	Max energy gathered per time-step	10	Energy	Yes	No	Global
P	Food-source-patches in the simulation	50	Patches	Yes	No	Global
R	Reproduction threshold	100	Energy	Yes	No	Global
S	Max speed of agents	2	Patches	Yes	No	Global
U	Mutation factor	0.05	–	Yes	No	Global
w_1, w_2	Dampening or amplifying factor	$0, \ldots, 1$	–	No	Yes	Agent

learning algorithms in 1986 [13] and with advances in hardware, that made it possible to create more complex and complete models.
An ANN consists of a network of interconnected mathematical entities called neurons.
Each neuron calculates a sum of its weighted inputs. The weight on each input can be either inhibitory or excitatory and therefore influences the result of the calculation and the output of the neuron.
This setup allows for adaption and the ability to *learn*. In the context of ANNs, learning describes the reforming of connections and updating of the input-weights in each neuron to fit the task. An ANN can be trained with predefined examples of correct results to a specific task, without an explicitly given set of rules.
The calculations that happen in the neurons itself in combination with the topology of the network is of great importance for the functionality and many approaches and techniques have been proposed [18],[16] for different systems.
The network used in this experiment, exhibits all traits of an ANN. As Fig. 3 shows, the two Synapses and the Hormone Gland of the agents are a simple network of neurons with multiple connections (Figs. 1 and 2).

2.2 *Structure of the Simulation*

The setup for the conducted experiments in this simulation consisted of empty ground-patches and randomly scattered food-source-patches that initially contain *E* energy-points (see Table 1). An example of such a randomly generated world can be

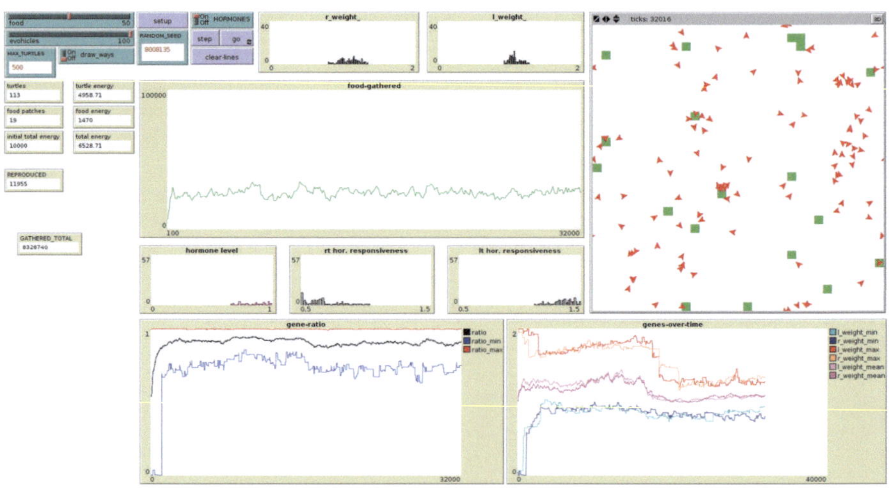

Fig. 1 Interface of the simulation environment developed to test how an artificial hormone system influences the efficiency of an ANN

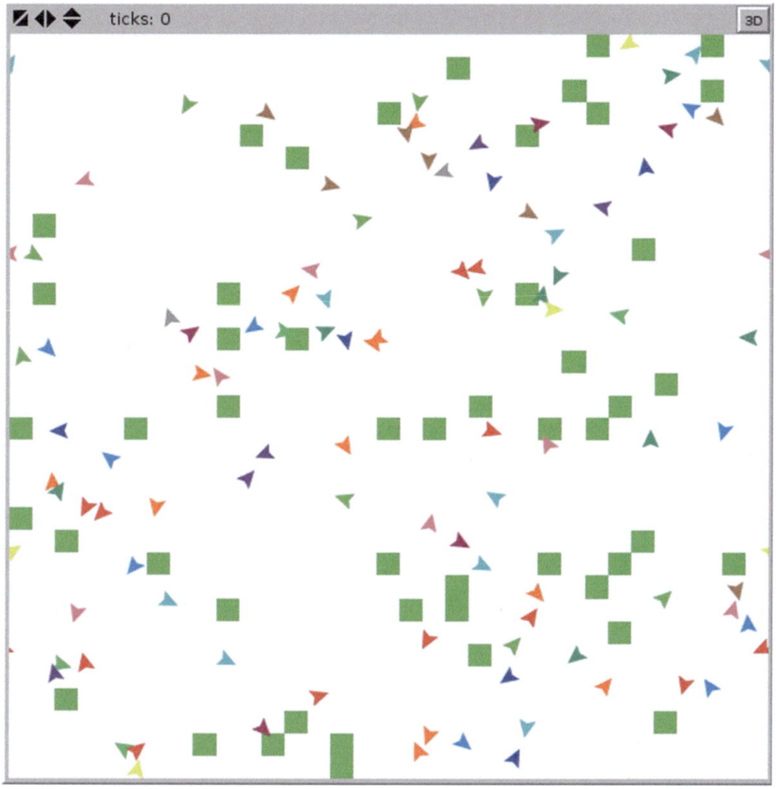

Fig. 2 The simulated world directly after setup and zero time-steps. The triangles represent the agents which can move around. The *green squares* are stationary food-source-patches

seen in Fig. 2. The amount of food-source-patches was set to a fixed value P. Values of P and other constants used in the presented experiments can be found in Table 1. The spawning agents were set to a fixed value B (see Table 1). The agents were then randomly placed on coordinates, which were not food-sources or already occupied by agents. The food-source patches regrowed on a random position if consumed, the detailed mechanics of this process are described in Sect. 2.6.2.

Besides the energy decreasing measure when reproducing, other inhibitory procedures against unregulated growth were set in place. The initial energy in the system, consisting of the energy-points abundant in food-resource-patches and agent-energy was logged and stored in a global variable.

Each time the *regrow* procedure was called, the total-energy in the system was calculated and only if the addition of another food-source would not have exceeded the initial total-energy, the food-source was created Further, the same calculation was done each time the *reproduction* procedure was called and if the limit was reached, the agents got capped at the reproduction-threshold until the system had leveled out again.

The authors are fully aware that this is an inaccurate depiction of energy flow in natural systems, but an adequate approximation, that fulfills the requirements to test the hypothesis mentioned in Sect. 1.3.

2.3 The Agents

In their basic abilities, all the agents were identical. They can sense food-sources, accelerate forward, decelerate, rotate on the spot, eat, reproduce and die. The quality of the sensory, eating and reproducing abilities was also identical in every agent, and described in detail in Table 1.

2.4 The Tested Networks

Figure 3 shows the schematics of an agent with the two sensors that were connected to the opposite motors through the weighted synapses. The hormone gland got activity signals from the right sensor. This influenced the outcome of the hormone-level calculation in Eq. 1 which in turn influenced on the calculation in the synapses as shown in Fig. 2.

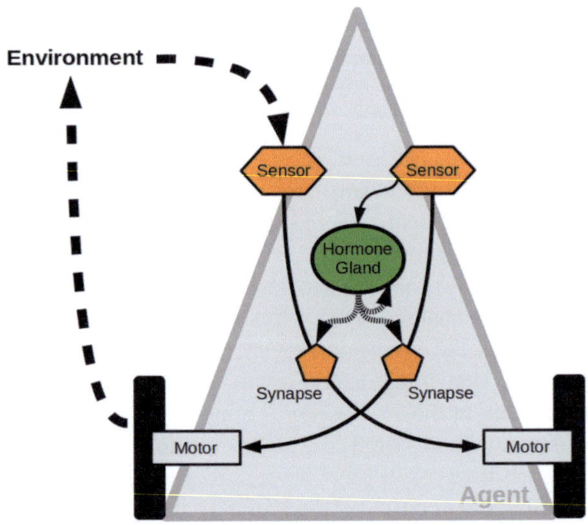

Fig. 3 A depiction of a Braitenberg vehicle of type 2b, extended with 2 synapses and a hormone gland. In the simulation the gland can be activated or deactivated

2.4.1 The Braitenberg Vehicle

The agents were a simple ANN-controled Braitenberg vehicles of type *2b* [3]. They had two wheels, actuators and motors on opposing sides that can be controlled independently. For further simplification of the navigation process, the movement was limited to forward and the maximum speed was set to S (see Table 1). By controlling the difference in speed of each motor, the direction and speed can be adjusted. In our design, the wheels were placed at a distance of two patches. The two sensors were placed on the axis of the wheels in a distance of one patch from each other, and connected to the opposite motor. At the start of each experiment these two connections, w_1, w_2 (see Table 1), were weighted. Evolving w_1 and w_2 (as described in the Sect. 3.1) lead to effective controllers emerging during the experiment run.

2.4.2 How Did We Implement Emotion

Contrasting to several experiments that have been conducted as to how artificial emotion or cognitive functionality could be implemented into ANNs [8, 10, 19], a novel approach was devised in this work. We diminished complexity to an absolute minimum, to reach general. but clear results. To implement the described functionality, we added a virtual gland to one of the sensors. Depending on the input of this single sensor, the level of one type of artificial hormone in the system is regulated. This process is shown in Eq. 1.

The initial value of the artificial hormone level at the beginning of each experiment was set to H (see Table 1). The level in the current time-step was influenced by the level in past time-step, allowing for prolonged effects of intense-input events and therefore a self influencing loop.

$$h_{level} = h_{level} \cdot 0.9 + sensor_{input} \cdot 0.1 \tag{1}$$

whereby h_{level} represents the current level of hormones in the system and $sensor_{input}$ represents the input from the connected sensor to the gland.

Each weight in itself is weighted by an evolving hormone-receptivity, that influences the input-output conversion as shown in Eq. 2.

$$sensor_{input} = sensor_{input} \cdot (responsiveness_{h,weight} \cdot h_{level}) \tag{2}$$

whereby $sensor_{input}$ represents the input from the respective sensor, $responsiveness_{h,weight}$ represents the responsiveness of the respective weight to the hormone level h_{level} in the system.

All experiments were conducted with hormone glands active, as well as with inactive glands. This allowed for direct comparison of efficiency and fitness of the agents in the two configurations (Fig. 4).

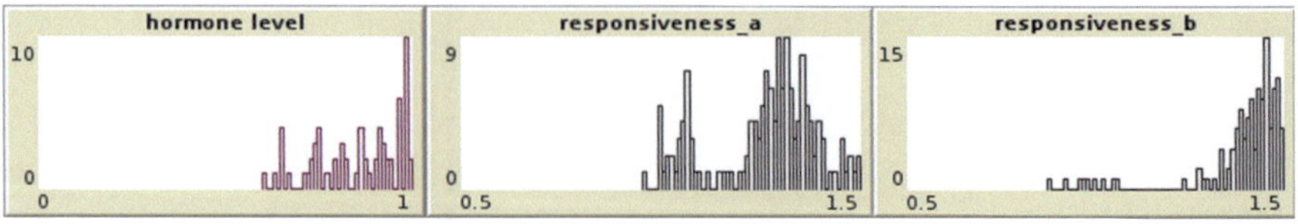

Fig. 4 The hormone levels in the agents and the respective receptivity weights in a population of 77 agents. The hormonal functionality was activated and 10,000 time-steps of a randomly chosen run had passed. The x-axis represents the different genes that influence the hormone level and responsiveness of the weights to these hormones. The y-axis represents the distribution of these genes in the population. This shows, that the hormone system had also a functioning evolutionary process, as the genes accumulated and were not distributed evenly across the spectrum

2.5 Evolution

On-board evolution in swarm robotics has proven to be effective in simulation as well as in real world applications [2, 15]. For this experiment, we chose a simple, two-weight system. The initial values for the weights were chosen as a random generated float between 0 and 2, and then applied to the sensory input signal as described in Eq. 3. These values were chosen after testing boundaries, and seemed feasible to the authors, since the behaviour of the evolutionary process is not influenced.

$$actuator_{output} = \frac{(weight \cdot sensor_{input})}{MS} \tag{3}$$

whereby $actuator_{output}$ represents the signals that were sent to the motor by the controller, *weight* represents the dampening or amplifying factor between sensor and actuator and S represents the maximal speed of an agent (see Table 1). The weights can therefore amplify or dampen the intensity of the communication between sensors and actuators. Was the random configuration of an agent advantageous in finding the food-resources, this agent was likely to reach the reproduction-threshold R (see Table 1) and hatch another agent with a mutated but similar genetic material. The details of the mutation process are described in Sect. 2.5.2.

2.5.1 Reproduction

As the agents evolved to navigate to food-sources and consume them, their energy-points exceeded the reproduction-threshold of R (see Table 1). As soon as this happens the *reproduction* procedure is called.
The procedure resets the energy-points of the reproducing agent to C and spawns an agent on the same patch. The reduction of energy represents the loss of energy due to the reproductive process. The hatched agent receives C initial energy-points. The *mutate* procedure is called, slightly changing the w_1 and w_2 of the controller. A detailed description of the mutation process can be found in Sect. 2.5.2.

2.5.2 Mutation

The mutation process applies to the weight parameters of the agents.

- *weight_a*, *weight_b* :
  Applied to the respective sensory input of the agent, this weight either amplifies or dampens the input signal that gets communicated to the opposite motor-actuator.
- *responsivity_a*, *responsivity_b* :
  If the hormone system is activated, these weights determine the rate of reaction of the above mentioned weights to the systems hormone level.

Every one of these parameters was randomly mutated by increasing or decreasing the float-value associated with it. The amount of mutation is determined by a random float between 0 and U (see Table 1), that was applied to each of the weights, as shown in Eq. 4.

$$weight = weight \pm rand(U) \tag{4}$$

whereby *weight* represents the dampening or amplifying factor between sensor and actuator, *rand*(U) represents a random float number between 0 and U (see Table 1). The results are limited inbetween 0 and 2 for the input weights, based on the chosen values described in Sect. 2.5. The limits for the hormone responsiveness weights were chosen between 0.5 and 1.5. The authors tested several ranges of responsiveness and concluded based on the simplicity of the model and the observed behaviour on these values.

The authors are fully aware that this is a very string simplification of the process of nature. We want to point out, that the process of mutation is simulated in such a way, that makes it possible to test the hypothesis mentioned in Sect. 1.3.

2.6 *The Experiment*

2.6.1 Overview

To test the hypothesis mentioned in Sect. 1.3, we ran several simulation experiments, as described in Sect. 2. One experiment run lasted for 10,000 time-steps. This value was chosen arbitrary after observing several runs and concluding the system has stabilised at this point. Each experiment was repeated twenty times. We measured how many energy-points were collected, and how much energy was invested into movement to collect energy-points.
The efficiency e of the population was calculated based on the collected energy c of all agents and the expended energy o of all agents, according to the Eq. 5.

$$e = o/c \tag{5}$$

whereby e represents an efficiency value, o the expended energy and c the gathered energy.
One set of experiments was done with classical Braitenberg vehicles, without a hormonal system included. A second set was performed including a hormonal system. The ability of the described system to evolve controllers, that were able to collect more energy than they consume was observed, as well as the efficiency e of agents with and without hormones.

2.6.2 The Task

Agents were confronted with the task to survive by finding and consuming food, that was randomly scattered in the world. The goal of each agent was to reach the reproduction-threshold of R (see Table 1) that lead to hatching offspring that carried similar genetic material that was defined by the weights, e.g. genes, in each system. This procedure is detailed in the Sects. 2.5.1 and 2.5.2.

In the given task more speed meant getting to food-sources faster, but also costed more energy. As more food can be consumed the longer the agent was in direct contact on a food-source, an optimal solution of dynamic movement had to be found. The fixed abundance of food was a challenge to the competing agents, as faster movement got the individual agent to the food-sources quicker, but also minimized the amount of food that can be consumed from the patch if the deceleration was not adequate. The evolved weights of successful agents were kept in the population pool and were amplified through asexual reproduction. Per default every food-source-patch spawned with E consumable energy-points on it, and every time-step an agent resided on one of these patches, this agent received M (see Table 1) energy-points. When the food-source was depleted, the regrow-food procedure is called. To not exceed the initial energy of the system, this function calculated the total energy in the system, and if another food-source would not have exceeded the initial energy, it created a randomly placed food-source on an empty patch.

3 Results

3.1 Evolutionary Process

Our system showed the evolution and persistence of successful traits as seen in Fig. 5. Both types of agents (with and without hormones) were able to evolve controllers, that were able to collect energy and "reproduce" in the simulated environment, as described above. Further the adaptation of the agents within the evolutionary process was observed. An exemplary result for the adaptation of the genes over time can be found in Fig. 6.

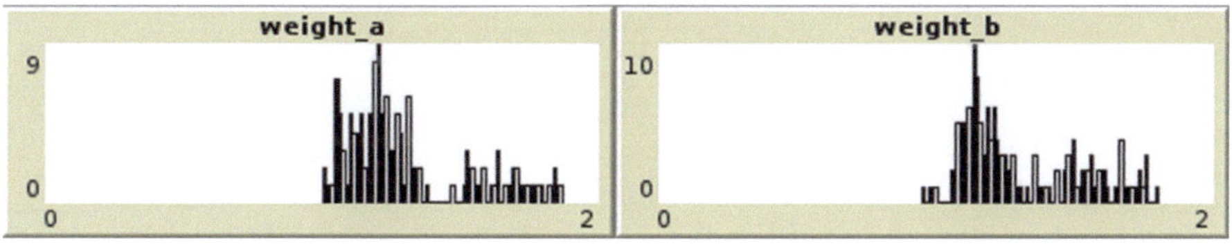

Fig. 5 The distribution of the evolved weights in the agent-set, after 10,000 time-steps in a randomly chosen run, and with hormonal effects activated. The *x*-axis represents the different genes that influence the factor that translates the sensory input signals to the actuators. The *y*-axis represents the distribution of these genes in the population. This shows an emerging evolutionary pattern in the controllers, as genes accumulate around advantagous values and are not evenly distributed

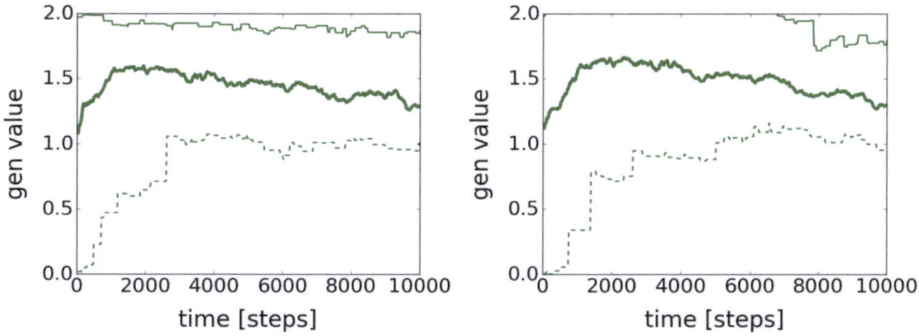

Fig. 6 Graphs of the maximum, minimum and mean values of the two weights over time, with hormonal functionality activated and after 10,000 time-steps. Whereby the solid thick line represents the mean of the maxima/minima of the two weights, the dashed line represents the maximum/minimum of the *right* weight, and the solid thin line represents the maximum/minimum of the *left* weight

3.2 Comparison of Efficiency

The comparison of the efficiency, as described in Eq. 5, showed, that agents evolved with a hormonal system had a higher performance for the given task as seen in Fig. 7. After 10,000 time-steps the agents with a hormonal system had evolved a controller that is significantly more efficient then agents without an hormonal system.

4 Discussion

4.1 General Outcome

With this work, we show that hormonal feedbacks have an influence on the ability of an artificial neural network to evolve an efficient controller for the given task

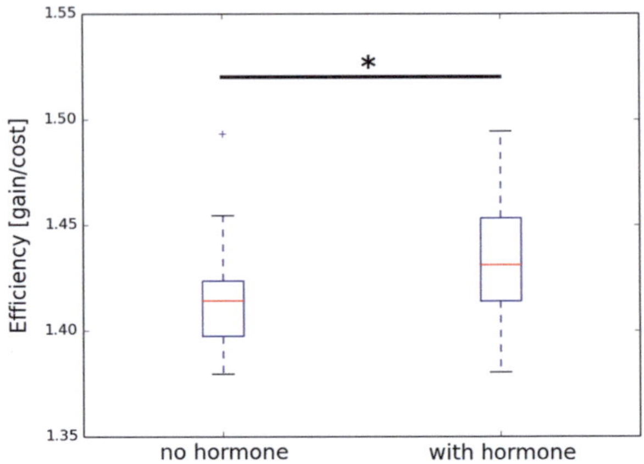

Fig. 7 Comparrison of the efficiency *e* of neural networks with and without hormonal modulation. It shows that the system with hormonal modulation has a significant higher efficiency. $N = 20$, *: $p \leq 0.05$, MannWhitneyWilcoxon-Test

described in Sect. 2.6.2. Both types of controllers (with and without hormones) were able to reproduce in the given environment, and, on a genetic level, adapted to the the given environment. Regarding the hypothesis presented in Sect. 1.3, it can be said, that $H0$ and $H1.a$ could be rejected. We could not reject Hypothesis $H1.b$ (including $H1$). Regarding the questions formulated in Sect. 1.2 we can conclude:

1. *Question Q.1* **Yes,** artificial neural networks efficiency can be enhanced by simulated neuromodulation with artificial hormones?
2. *Question Q.2* The implementation of a hormonal system significantly **increases** the efficiency for the given task, as seen in Fig. 7.
3. *Question Q.3* **Yes,** In all tested runs evolution found solutions that included the artificial emotions.

4.2 Limitations of the Presented Results

The results presented here are based on first experiments in an extremely simple environment, with a minimalistic neuronal controller, and a minimalistic hormonal controller. This design was necessary to test basic features of the system from a very general point of view. The authors are aware, that, although the insights into the described system are very general, the implementation into a more detailed simulation environment and into actual robots itself has to be done to fully support this claim. The interplay of neural networks and virtual hormone systems could be advantageous in complex and dynamic physical environments in the real world, given an appropriate complexity for the given task.

4.3 Comparison with Literature

As mentioned in the introduction, the inspiration for the theory behind this experimental approach, resulted from the study of some general work on artificial intelligence and emotion [1, 6, 7]. Research into the less artificial neurological aspects proved to be valuable and inspired the theory behind our approach [5, 14]. Especially the work by Fellous and Arbib on emotions from a purely functional viewpoint, seeing emotions not as emotional expression for communication and social coordination, inspired us to this approach. Prooving the feasibility of using emotions as a functional "tool" for organizing behavior, action, reaction and learning in an evolving system, has been tried before. But given the complexity of these processes in nature, simulations seem to have gotten rather complex as well. In contrast to this, an opposite approach was chosen in this work. The idea was to model the most simplified simulation environment, that allowed to conduct experiments on the impact of artificial emotions on a neuronal network. In [8] a very complex system with a distinctive seperation of sensations, feelings, emotions and hormones is proposed. This model has also some key functionality that we wanted for our work; The reaction to not only current sensory input, but an output that is strongly influenced by past sonsory or emotional events. The setup of the networks was rather complex as well, as a distinction between feelings and emotions was made. The authors of this work concluded, that the suggested artificial emotion modifications of their systems proved to have a slight improving impact on the systems performance. Extensive research on the topic neuromodulation in artificial systems has been conducted in a masterthesis by Lo [10], with a focus on implementation on different kind of ANNs and in an environment of T-maze navigation tasks. In contrast to these we wanted to implement a comparatively more realistic task than the former example, a simulation with more than one agent and theoretically indefinite runtime. We also wanted to reduce the complexity of the simulated emotions to reduce error and result-complexity.
This chosen approach allowed us the possibility to quickly estimate the real-world value of our findings.

5 Future Work

The work presented here is the first step on a research track investigating the usability of self-modulated artificial neural networks in robotics, as well as a tool in cognitive robotics in general. This system will be tested on both, actual robots and extensive simulations for feasibility. A challenge lies in the transfer of a neural network, that is in the state of adaptation from one robot to another, while deployed in various tasks. Major focus will be laid on underwater service robotics [12, 15, 17] and the usage of the presented adaptive system in highly dynamic underwater environments in interaction with eachother, the surrounding ecosystem and humans.

6 Conclusion

Summing up the results presented in this work, we conclude that the combination of hormonal and neuronal controller structures lead to a change of the dynamics in the described system. We plan to exploit this feature for robotic systems and their application. Especially the increase of movement dynamic based on the hormonal influence will be investigated in detail. To which extent these concepts of artificial evolution and emotion are directly applicable in scientific or technological scenarios is topic of ongoing discussions and investigations.

Acknowledgements This work was supported by: EU H2020 FET-Proactive project 'subCULTron', no. 640967.

References

1. Arbib, M.A., Fellous, J.M.: Emotions: from brain to robot. Trends Cogn. Sci. **8**(12), 554–561 (2004). doi:10.1016/j.tics.2004.10.004
2. Baele, G., Bredeche, N., Haasdijk, E., Maere, S., Michiels, N., Van de Peer, Y., Schmickl, T., Schwarzer, C., Thenius, R.: Open-ended on-board evolutionary robotics for robot swarms. In: Evolutionary Computation, 2009. CEC'09. IEEE Congress on, pp. 1123–1130. IEEE (2009)
3. Braitenberg, V.: Vehicles: Experiments in Synthetic Psychology. MIT Press (1984)
4. Cañamero, L.: Emotion understanding from the perspective of autonomous robots research. Neural Netw. **18**(4), 445–455 (2005)
5. Dolan, R.J.: Emotion, cognition, and behavior. Science **298**(5596), 1191–1194 (2002)
6. Fellous, J.M.: From human emotions to robot emotions. In: Hudlicka, E., Canamero, L. (eds.) Architectures for Modeling Emotion: Cross-Disciplinary Foundations, AAAI Spring 2004 Symposium, Stanford. American Association for Artificial Intelligence (2004)
7. Fellous, J.M., Arbib, M.A.: Who Needs Emotions?: The Brain Meets the Robot. Oxford University Press (2005)
8. Gadanho, S.C., Hallam, J.: Robot learning driven by emotions. Adapt. Behav. **9**(1), 42–64 (2002)
9. Jain, A.K., Mao, J., Mohiuddin, K.: Artificial neural networks: a tutorial. IEEE Comput. **29**, 31–44 (1996)
10. Lo, E.M.: Neuromodulation in artificial systems. Ph.D. thesis, University of Oklahoma, Department of Zoology (2012)
11. McCulloch, W.S., Pitts, W.: A logical calculus of ideas immanent in nervous activity. Bull. Math. Biophys. **5**(4), 115–133 (1943). doi:10.1007/BF02478259
12. Read, M., Möslinger, C., Dipper, T., Kengyel, D., Hilder, J., Thenius, R., Tyrrell, A., Timmis, J., Schmickl, T.: Profiling underwater swarm robotic shoaling performance using simulation. In: Towards Autonomous Robotic Systems, pp. 404–416. Springer (2013)
13. Rumelhart, D.E., McClelland, J.L., Group, P.R., et al.: Parallel Distributed Processing: Explorations in the Microstructure of Cognition, vol. 1–2. Cambridge, MA (1986)
14. Scherer, K.R.: Emotion serves to decouple stimulus and response. In: The Nature of Emotion: Fundamental Questions, pp. 127–130 (1994)
15. Schmickl, T., Thenius, R., Christoph, M., Timmis, J., Tyrrell, A., Read, M., Hilder, J., Halloy, J., Campo, A., Stefanini, C., Manfredi, L., Orofino, S., Kernbach, S., Dipper, T., Sutantyo, D.: Cocoro—the self-aware underwater swarm. In: 2011 Fifth IEEE Conference on Self-Adaptive and Self-Organizing Systems Workshops (SASOW), pp. 120–126 (2011). doi:10.1109/SASOW.2011.11

16. Stanley, K.O., D'Ambrosio, D., Gauci, J.: A hypercube-based encoding for evolving large-scale neural networks. Artif. Life **15**(2), 185–212 (2009). doi:10.1162/artl.2009.15.2.15202
17. subCULTron: Submarine cultures perform long-term robotic exploration of unconventional environmental niches (2015). http://www.subcultron.eu/
18. Thenius, R., Schmickl, T., Crailsheim, K.: Novel concept of modelling embryology for structuring an artificial neural network. In: Troch, I., Breitenecker, F. (eds.) Proceedings of the MATHMOD, pp. 1821–1831 (2009)
19. Thenius, R., Zahadat, P., Schmickl, T.: Emann—a model of emotions in an artificial neural network. In: Lio, P., Miglino, O., Nicosia, G., Nolfi, S., Pavone, M. (eds.) 12th European Conference on Artificial Life (ECAL 2013), pp. 830–837. MIT Press (2013). doi:10.7551/978-0-262-31709-2-ch122
20. Wilensky, U.: Netlogo. Center for Connected Learning and Computer-Based Modeling, Northwestern University. Evanston, IL (1999). http://ccl.northwestern.edu/netlogo/
21. Ziemke, T., Lowe, R.: On the role of emotion in embodied cognitive architectures: from organisms to robots. Cogn. Comput. **1**(1), 104–117 (2009)

Legal Frame of Non-social Personal Care Robots

E. Fosch Villaronga

Abstract This paper describes some relevant legal aspects concerning non-social robots. Special attention is drawn to Person Carrier Robots (PCaR) and Physical Assistant Robots (PAR). Although concrete legal binding regulations concerning these two sub-types of Personal Care Robots (PCR) are missing, the insertion of this assistive technology into the market arises some legal and ethical concerns. The main concerns include: cognitive aspects involved in the use of the technology; data protection matters: the way roboticists can make their technology comply with to the new European General Data Protection Regulation; liability contexts depending on their degree of autonomy; privacy and autonomy issued; as well as understanding how the decrease in the human-human interaction could undermine the dignity of the person.

Keywords Personal care robots · Privacy · Person carriers · Physical assistant · Non-social robots · Cognitive HRI

1 Introduction

In 2014, the Industrial Standard Organization released a set of standard safety requirements for Personal Care Robots for the activities of the daily living (ADL). These standard requirements were the first to address non-medical applications of these robots in terms of physical human-robot interaction (HRI). In particular, Personal Care Robots include two non-social robots: Person Carrier (PCaR) and Physical Assistant Robots (PAR); and one social robot: Mobile Servant Robots (MSR) (vid. Fig. 1) [1].

E. Fosch Villaronga (✉)
Joint International Doctoral (Ph.D.) Degree Erasmus Mundus in Law, Science and Technology Coordinated by CIRSFID, University of Bologna, Bologna, Italy
e-mail: eduard.fosch@unibo.it

E. Fosch Villaronga
IDT-UAB, Universitat Autònoma de Barcelona, Barcelona, Spain

M. Husty and M. Hofbaur (eds.), *New Trends in Medical and Service Robots*,
Mechanisms and Machine Science 48, DOI 10.1007/978-3-319-59972-4_17

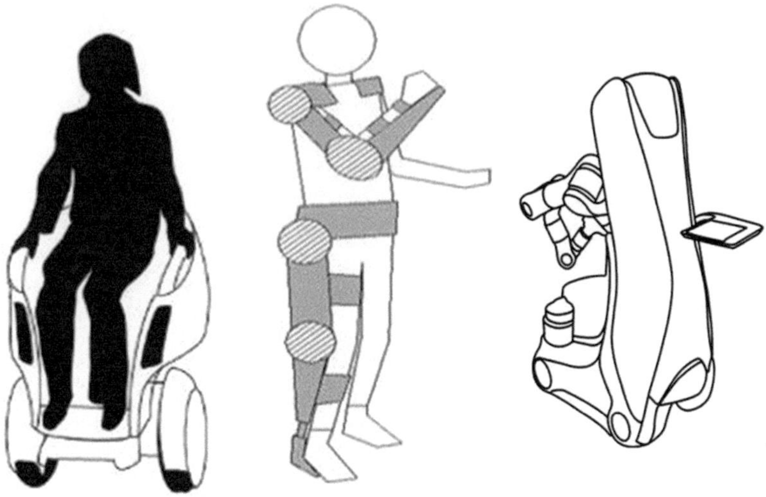

Fig. 1 Non-social and social personal care robots. Extracted from the pictures collected in this interview with Gurvinder Virk http://bit.ly/2eIUIV2

The first two are considered non-social technologies because they do not offer a two-way interaction, they do not express nor understand thoughts or feelings, they are not socially aware, they do not interact unpredictably or spontaneously, and they do not provide the feeling of companionship or of mutual respect [2]. Indeed, non-social robots interact physically with the user, i.e. with a "zero distance between the robot and an object in its external environment" assisting the user to perform tasks, without the need of responding empathically to their users. Non-social robots add only a simple presence to their user's life, and not a sophisticated presence as compared with MSR [3]. Moreover, while non-social robots usually help the user perform a task (supplementing force, restoring gait or simply conveying them from a place to another one), social robots normally perform tasks *for* the user.

The HRI also differs within the non-social robots identified by ISO. PAR normally work in a "seamless integration with the user's residual musculoskeletal system and sensory-motor control loops" to assist the user "with minimal cognitive disruption and required compensatory motion" [4]. They are normally fastened to the user's body, although there are restraint-free types. PCaR on the contrary just convey persons to an intended destination and their HRI varies depending on the user interfaces used to estimate the intention of movement.

ISO 13482:2014 addresses the engineering hazards concerning these non-social assistive technology, e.g. robot shape, emissions, electromagnetic interference, robot motion, localization and navigation errors; and also hazards relating to their use, e.g. stress, posture or usage. However, the use of these robots involves other hazards disregarded by the standard such as hazards due to unlawful processing of personal data, incorrect categorization [5], or occurrence of isolation scenarios or hazards due to the decreased human-human interaction.

This paper addresses legal and ethical concerns regarding the insertion of non-social assistive technology. These concerns include: relevant cognitive aspects involved in the use of the technology; data protection: the way roboticists make their technology comply with the new European General Data Protection Regulation; liability contexts depending on the robot's degree of autonomy; privacy and autonomy matters; and the issue of decreased human-human interaction, which can undermine the dignity of the person.

Four different use cases that will show the urgent need to incorporate other interdisciplinary hazards in industrial standards to address unanswered questions and protect the final user, which is the ultimate goal for the European Union. Section 2 will introduce two cases concerning PCaR: (1) the first case concerns data protection issues, mainly cognitive privacy, data portability and profile modules; (2) the second one refers to privacy and security issues in Internet of Things (IoT) environments, and liability in autonomous robots. Section 3 will include another two cases: (1) the first one will be about data protection, and will focus mainly on consent; and (2) the second one will be about the cognitive aspects of the use of robots, user's autonomy, free will and dignity of the person. Conclusions will be drawn in Sect. 4.

2 Pepa and Her Person Carrier

2.1 Privacy by Design and Data Portability

Consider the following use case:

> Pepa had always problems with her lower-limbs. She is old and she does not like the idea of driving an exoskeleton. The nursing home replaced the old manual wheelchairs with shared person carrier robots. They work in autonomous mode with obstacle recognition through cameras. She uses the carrier when she goes out with her family. The robotic person carrier breaks and she needs a new one, but the producer stopped producing it. Now she will have to use a new one from another producer.

A low-cost wheelchair with a pan-tilt camera inspired this case [6], the article 7 of the European Charter of Fundamental rights [7] and the article 20 of the recently approved General Data Protection Regulation (GDPR) [8].

In theory, privacy is not a major concern for PCaR as their primary use is not related to the invasiveness of the user's private life but rather to convey him/her to an intended destination. Depending on the technology applied to the robot however, this privacy could be undermined. For instance, obstacle recognition through cameras can pose privacy at risk if cameras record other things rather than the obstacles to avoid, especially if the user's private information or the data of third parties are recorded. Attention to data protection matters should be drawn as it the

GDPR will enter in force in 2018 and will oblige any data controller to fulfill several requirements, including embedding privacy into their systems from the design phase of the product. Yet, the provision of the so-called "privacy by design" is not very clear: does it refer to the use of a programming language that enforces privacy policies from the beginning (such as Jeeves does? [9])? Does it mean to anonymize data as soon as it collected?

Ann Cavoukian coined the privacy-by-design concept under the believe that mere compliance with regulations could not guarantee the protection of privacy. She suggested to include this philosophy in the organization's modus operandi. Although lacking of concrete guidance to the data controller, this principle obliges the data controller (and in this case the roboticists as the European Parliament draft report says) at the time of the determination of the means for processing and at the time of the processing itself, to implement appropriate measures for ensuring that all the requirements of the regulation are met. This implementation will need to be pro-active, as a default setting, embedded into the design, with a full functionality, offering a full lifecycle protection, open and user-centric [10].

Beyond the discussion of the feasibility of GDPR, the inclusion of person carrier robots available to the different patients in a nursing home will force the devices, the more and more, to incorporate profile modules to identify each user—for personalization purposes. This will raise some privacy concerns regarding other rights that will also enter in force with the GDPR, this is, the data portability right. Indeed, the person carrier will:

(1) First need to be protected against vandalism acts and include a password or some bionic identification system to avoid a possible misuse (as ISO 13482:2014 suggests). Attention should be drawn to recent stolen fingerprints in the United States Government [11].
(2) Second, the device should allow data-portability because if it breaks or the producer producing it (as happened with the iBot project) the users should have the possibility to easily transmit setting information and their preferences to a new carrier (it may be possible that when that happens, the user's impairment has worsened and cannot re-train the carrier as previously done with the prior wheelchair). The right to data portability stands for the right of the data subject "to receive the personal data concerning him or her, which he or she has provided to a controller, in a structured and commonly used and machine-readable format and have the right to transmit those data to another controller without hindrance from the controller to which the data have been provided" (*see* Art. 20 GDPR) [8].
(3) Third, all the information collected should be used only for the proper functioning of the device and not for other reasons (e.g. increasing the knowledge of the wheelchair provider to ameliorate the wheelchair, or other business related issues such as: selling new components to compensate some failures, selling some new gadgets to be incorporated to the wheelchair, etc.).

2.2 *Internet of Things and Responsibility*

Here follows the second case:

> The new person carrier works in an Internet-of-Thing (IoT) environment. Pepa enjoyed going outdoors with it until she ran over a child accidentally. The mother of the child sued Pepa. Pepa claimed the responsibility was of the nursing home; the nursing home argued in court that it was the carrier's fault because it is autonomous. The manufacturer of it said that the wheelchair works on cloud-robotics base and that, despite being autonomous, once sold to the nursing home it is their responsibility.

This case is inspired by the Dr. Hawking Connected Wheelchair Project [12], a lawsuit for damages caused by an autonomous ground vehicle, and the recent communication from the National Highway Traffic Security Agency (NHTSA) that will interpret the self-driving system of the Google car as the "driver" of it [13].

Data Protection in Internet of Things Environments

Although there is no general consensus on the definition, IoT refers to the "scenarios where network connectivity and computing capability extends to objects, sensors and everyday items not normally considered computers, allowing these devices to generate, exchange and consume data with minimal human intervention" [14]. The infrastructure of IoT challenges the current data protection legislative framework for several reasons. Here are the problems highlighted by the Article 29 Working Party [15]:

- Lack of control and asymmetry: as the processing of the data involved in IoT environments relies on the coordinated intervention of several stakeholders, not only it will be difficult to establish the roles and responsibilities of data controller/processor, but it will also be hard to track the data flows that will be generated. This will entail a complete loss of control from the user as well as a self-exposure of all his/her data.
- Quality of the user's consent. One of the major problems of IoT is the awareness of the user of which objects are processing data from him/her. Classical mechanisms to obtain consent might not apply in this context, as it could be practically impossible to ask for consent each time.
- Inferences derived from data and repurposing of original processing. Modern techniques allow secondary, not pre-specified uses of the collected data very easily, and processing such data with a new aim or for a new use should be considered according to the European Data Protection legal framework.
- Intrusive extraction of behavior patterns and profiling. As this technology is going to be part of the private life of the users (because the wheelchair is used in the nursing home), the possibility to extract behavioral analysis of the collected data now is for real, something which clashes with the principal of data minimization.
- Limitation on the possibility to remain anonymous when using services. Because the idea behind IoT is the personalization of the offered services, it will

be very easy to identify the user of a particular technology. Furthermore, "large amount of data processed automatically [...] entails a risk of re-identification".

- Security risks: security versus efficiency. According to the Article 29 Working Party, manufacturers need to balance the implementation of confidentiality, integrity and availability measures at all levels of processing.

IoT combines the possibility to process personal data and also large quantities of sensor data, which can be used further on in data fusion. The main problem of data fusion is the use of data by third parties and, consequently, the loss of control over that data, both personal and non-personal and the unknown post behavioral analysis of this data [16]. The principle of transparency should play a major role in this data usage. Yet, the intrinsic labyrinthine structure of the data flow between devices, and back-end systems, providers and manufacturers, makes it practically impossible to track data. Tracking data is a key element for accounting reasons (e.g. black boxes) but the more the data collected, the more difficult it is to discover and track its flow [17]. In theory, the data minimization principle (derived from the principle of proportionality of the data processing) has a difficult task. In fact, on the one hand big data techniques are widely available today, on the other hand the intention of data collectors is to process all the available data in the world (e.g. Google's mission for instance is to organize the world's information and make it universally accessible and useful [18]).

All this information processed in data mining can turn into new surveillance options [19], a surveillance that could cause a big brother scenario. In fact, the N = All analysis aims at finding hidden connections that could be possibly useful for future developments [20]. The problem is that finding the correlation does not retrospectively justify obtaining the data in the first place [21], especially if there has been no consent for that. On the user's perspective, the use of several IoT connected devices could cause them anxiety [22], although there is no evidence of it yet.

The major problem in any case is similar to what happens in wearable technology, as the customers' perceptions of this technology, which tends to focus more on the benefits rather than on the risks [23]. This is caused by a disinformation on the actual risks: first, the providers are more interested in focusing on the benefits rather than on the risks; second, researchers tend to investigate the benefits of a certain technique or device rather than the bad consequences of its use; and third, costumers tend to compare the new device with other, more familiar devices although the latter might differ largely in terms of hardware architecture or functionality. In the end, "when one does not know that one does not know, one thinks one knows" [24].

Responsibility

Concerning the concept of agency, there has been a long discussion on whether machines should or not be granted agenthood. In 2011, Verbeek already considered technology as an active agent [25]; and so did Pagallo when he explained the "digital *peculium*" [26] This Roman legal institution was "the sum of money or property granted by the head of the household to a slave or son-in-power" for the master to avoid further responsibility for his slave's businesses. Pagallo suggests the possibility to apply the same principle in the digital era when robots perform legal transactions. This does not seem that far from reality after the National Highway Traffic Security Agency of the United States stated in 2016, for the first time in history, that driver of the Google car would be the artificial intelligent system.

The European Parliament expressed its worries concerning this topic in 2016. They argued that the more autonomous robots are, the less they can be considered tools in the hands of other actors [27]. This phenomenon was called "responsibility gap" and was identified by Andreas Matthias in 2004 [28]. The responsibility gap The responsibility gap theory suggests that, if robots learn as they operate, and the robots themselves can, on the course of operation, change the rules by which they act, then not the humans but the robots should be held responsible for their autonomous decisions [29] (Fig. 2).

There is no clarity at this moment concerning this possible gap. Although Johnson suggests that at the end it is a matter of the negotiations certain actors will have, the European Parliament is convinced that these capabilities have made them more similar to agents that interact with their environment and are able to change it exponentially. Because of that, the European Parliament suggests various things. First of all, they propose a general statement saying that roboticists should remain accountable for the social, environmental, and human health impacts that their robots may pose to current and future generations. Second, and concerning liability, they suggest to have (1) strict liability rules for the damaged caused by the robots (which would imply that only a causal link between the harm and the robot behavior should be proved), and (2) the responsibility of the teacher. However, and connecting this point with the last sub-section, as in the future the robot will be a thing of the internet of things, if the robot has learned from other devices or other robots, then it is not very clear whether the responsibility gap will be solved by the mere inclusion of the responsibility of the teacher.

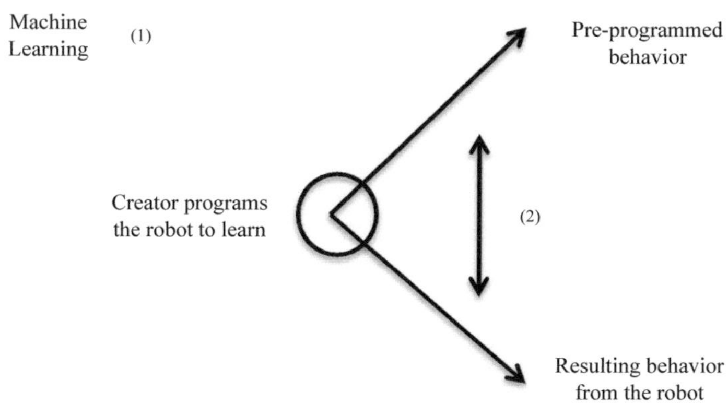

Fig. 2 Machine learning (1) and the responsibility gap (2)

In any case, the European parliament says that one of the solutions is to include an insurance schema behind robotic technology, without defining what types of robots should include it, and what would be the extent of the insurance.

3 Maria, Peter and the Exoskeletons

3.1 Consent in an Ubiquitous World

Consider the following use case:

> The hospital of Santa Barbara has bought several exoskeletons from the company Exoperfekt S.L. The company sells the device and also offers maintenance and updating services. Every 2 months, the exoskeletons are automatically updated. The Hospital is very happy with the service, as they improve substantially the performance of each device. Users are also very happy. Maria, a patient, feels as if the device knew already her movements.

This case relates to the use of personal data from companies that have already sold their devices to the users, e.g. the case of a smart TV that was processing personal data from the users to ameliorate their system [30]. During a research project, there is normally an ethical committee (Institutional Review Board, IRB) that approves and controls how the collection and processing of personal data is carried out. Once the company has put a device into the market, it is more difficult for an agency to control it (although the Data Protection Agencies are very active on this). The context where the robot is used, thus, matters [31].

In healthcare domain, the European Union gives special status and stronger protection to health data and considers it as sensitive data. There are some relevant considerations to make. First, the collection and processing of personal sensitive data needs to be balanced against other compelling interests (the protection of a person, the invasion of privacy); unequivocal informed consent of the user is needed; and the data collected and processed needs to be proportionate (for the intended task/the purpose which motivated the processing).

Some steps towards the creation of standards to anonymize data have been taken [32], although the anonymization of data does not involve per se the loss of the "personal" feature of data. In fact, although some companies advocate that only scattered information is processed (normally to escape from the data protection legislation) the Article 29 Working Party already warned that "the processing of that information only makes sense if it allows identification of specific individuals and treat them in a certain way", thus it should be considered as information relating to identifiable individuals [33]. As argued above, this anonymization would not even imply the fulfillment of the privacy-by-Design principle.

Physical assistant robots are designed to be personal data collectors as they work in a symbiotic manner with their user, despite being in non-medical contexts (as the ISO 13482:2014 pretends). In fact, they are fastened to the user to help a person perform actions according to the user's body characteristics and normal gait (which totally differs from the physical human-robot interaction with PCaR). The household exemption would not apply because all data is transferred to many different people (e.g. manufacturers, physicians, etc.) and not for household activities [34].

Some concerns concerning consent in non-social robots are: (a) awareness of the processing; (b) determining which information should be used for informed consent among special categories of users (elderly people, intellectual disabled people; children, etc.); (c) the exact extent to which the user may consent to the processing of data must be unambiguously defined:

(a) The principle of fairness requires that the data subject is informed and aware of the data collected. Failing to do so makes the processing unlawful and brings about consequences for the data controllers such as the duty to give compensation to the data subjects, or all the sanctions provided in the national legislations (or any measure in the GDPR). The more the devices will be fed by other structures (ambient intelligence, other sources), the more difficult this requirement will be to fulfill.
(b) Not only the data subjects need to be aware of the collected data, they also need to give their consent, especially if sensitive data are at stake (as they are regulated more stringently). Of note, informed consent had already some limitations, e.g. language, religious or false expectations [35], and such limitations increase when it comes to the smart devices [36] as the collection of information is not easy to be detected by everyone. The problem is to ensure a meaningful consent in this ubiquitous technology paradigm [37] where users cannot know how their information will be amalgamated or utilized in the future [38] and they need anyway to give their explicit consent [39]. Furthermore, although Art. 8.3 Data Protection Directive 95/46/EC (still applicable until the GDPR comes into force) states that the prohibition of collective sensitive information "shall not apply where the processing of data is required for the purposes of preventive medicine, medical diagnosis, the provision of care or treatment or the management of health-care services", these services need to be provided by health professional subjects under national laws, which is not the case when these devices are used for activities of the daily living.
(c) The purpose should be "specified, explicit and legitimate". There is an obligation for the data controller to extensively and explicitly describe why and for what purpose the data are being collected, especially if such data can have secondary uses. As the A29WP remarks, either for raw, extracted or displayed data, the controllers need to make sure that the used data is compatible with the original consent. If there is the intention to collect data for research, the controller not only needs to say so, he/she needs to have the consent of the user and set down all the appropriate safeguards to cope with that [40].

3.2 Cognitive Aspects and Ethics

Here us the last use:

> Peter on the contrary feels insecure with the exoskeleton. After some time, Peter also realizes the sessions with the therapist reduce. He starts feeling down. One day, tired of living, he decides to fall down the stairs with the exoskeleton. The exoskeleton prevents him from doing so and reports to the doctor this strange behavior.

As reported by Salem et al. certified safety and perceived safety are different [41]. Certified safety refers to the obtaining of standards and certificates that ensure the compliance of the device. Perceived safety, on the contrary, is the perception that the users have of the device. Subjective perceptions can sometimes constrain the performance of the device, especially in lower-limb PAR. As PAR work in a symbiotic manner with the user's movement, the users need to feel secure with the device during all gait cycle otherwise they might risk to activate the exoskeleton in an abnormal way [42]. The fear of falling, thus, should be taken into account in the design process of the device.

Although the Personal Care Robot Standard dose hint at the concepts of "mental stress" and "non-contact sensing", however it disregards other cognitive aspects related to this technology such as dependence, depression to decrease of human-human interaction, overreliance on the robot, frustration when robot performs different tasks because it has not understood human commands, etc. Article 3 EU CFR protects nevertheless both the physical and mental integrity of persons, and that is the European Parliament has pronounced itself: robots could cause psychological harm. All these aspects should be taken into account if roboticists want to place their robots into the market.

Sharkey and Sharkey noticed that one of the problems with assistive technology is the actual replacement of human therapists [43]. Although they referred to assistive technology that monitored elderly people, this also can happen when PAR are introduced in Healthcare facilities, especially if they are used for rehabilitation purposes. The actual use of this technology can reduce the supervision of a human, and this could undermine the dignity of the user. In the Care Robot section, the European Parliament also express this concern.

Some Japanese caregivers have reported something similar. In this case, they were the ones who complained about the insertion of this technology, because "autonomous wheelchair robots might decrease opportunities for rehabilitation". At the same time, they warned that "if seniors become dependent on such a robot and stop moving by themselves, their own physical activity will decrease'' [44].

Most of the times, nevertheless, a case-by-case study will have to be carried out in order to determine what is the actual negative impact of the use of a particular technology and how this is balanced with its benefits [31]. Personal care robots do not substitute any human intentionally, but try to promote a better human-human interaction, e.g. by allowing the person travel more easily to an intended destination, or to allow the person behave as a physically non-impaired person (using lower-limb exoskeletons).

What remains unclear is until what extent roboticists are the ones in charge to take into account all these aspects that are more, let's say, ethical. The recent BS 8611:2016 standard on the ethical design of robots might be one step towards promoting not only awareness on these topics but also ensure compliance with them. Beyond the discourse that industrial standards only serve the interests of the industry and whether society should leave the industry to determine what are the ethical aspects concerning robotic technology, it remains unclear what are the aspects that will have to be included in such compliance framework: should the robot preserve the human free will or his/her safety? How can the robot be sure that it understands the human commands? Could a robotic device as an accessory? As the robot capabilities will increase, the more they will have to face ethical dilemmas and the more aware of social norms they will have to be [45].

The draft of a law that could govern this type of technology could provide more clarity at this regard. For the moment, the European Parliament has only pushed for a directive to be effective in 10–15 years.

4 Conclusions

Non-social robots challenge the current legal order regardless of their compliance with current standards. In fact, the current industrial standards disregard several interdisciplinary aspects of robot technology that are crucial to offer a complete legal coverage to the citizens because they are solely concerned with the safety issues and the physical human-robot interaction. On the contrary, not only humans interact with robots in different manners (although physically, the interaction between a human and a PCaR and a person and a PAR is not the same; interaction can also be cognitive with them when mental communication is the only channel of communication), robots are perceived very differently regardless of their certification. Because of that, and because the perception of it can constraint the correct performance of the device (and by extension put at risk the safety of the user), cognitive aspects will have to be taken into consideration by roboticists. A case-by-case analysis will have to be carried out as cognitive aspects might have different meanings in different robots and in different contexts.

Concerning privacy, future robot technology needs to take into account data protection rules. This affects directly roboticists because the GDPR refers to the "privacy-by-default" which implies the embedment into the system of all security measures to protect the processing and collection of personal data. Although the regulation is not very clear at this respect, that does not exclude roboticists from compliance. Especially attention should be drawn to IoT environments, as there will be a lot of communications and sharing data between devices, most of the time not obvious. If the robot acts upon an ambient intelligent detector, then, clear rules between these objects concerning data protection should be established. In addition, other aspects such as the protection of the third uses of the collected data, informed consent, the legitimate purpose or the new data portability right need to be considered.

The fact that there will be different technology providers and the more and more the technology will be able to learn from the experience, attention will have to be drawn to the occurrence of harm and the subsequent allocation of responsibility. Although everyone tries to avoid the assumption of responsibility, new rules (the European Parliament recommendations) suggest that roboticists will remain accountable for the life-cycle of the robots: from their design to their implementation. Even for future impacts their technology could involve. And although this might sound dramatic to most of the researchers, it goes in line with the Responsible Research and Innovation framework of the European Union but also with the idea that, at the end of the day, one shall assume part of responsibility.

Other aspects such as the protection of the mental integrity of the person are going to gain more and more importance with the growing use of Brain-Computer Interfaces. Very soon there will be the need to answer very interesting questions such as "what if your brain reveals important personal information of the user?". In the World Economic Forum in 2016 this question led to a debate where several aspects regarding the intersection of neuroscience and the Law were discussed: from the way neuroscience techniques could be applied to improve the current legal system (to avoid the current existing bias in the decision-making process), to what would happen if a person could use his/her brain to prove his/her alibi [46].

In the end, it is important to start thinking about other sides of robotics and create technology that is safer because, beside traditional safety aspects, other aspects such as privacy, data protection, autonomy and dignity are carefully taken into account. In this way, robots and robotic devices will promote better human-human interaction, which is the final and most important goal of all.

References

1. ISO 13482:2014: Robots and Robotics Devices—Safety Requirements for Personal Care Robots
2. Graaf, M.M.A., et al.: What makes robots social? A user's perspective on characteristics for social human-robot interaction. In: Social Robotics, pp. 184–193. Springer International Publishing (2015)
3. Sorell, T., Heather, D.: Robot carers, ethics, and older people. Ethics Inf. Technol. **16**(3), 183–195 (2014)
4. Tucker, et al.: Control strategies for active lower extremity prosthetics and orthotics: a review. J. Neuroeng. Rehabil. **12**, 1 (2015)
5. Fosch-Villaronga, E.: ISO 13482:2014 and its confusing categories. In: Wenger et al. (eds.) New Trends in Medical and Service Robots. Machine Science, vol. 39 (2016)
6. Kim, B.K., Tanaka, H., Sumi, Y.: A low cost robotic wheelchair system using a pan-tilt camera and a visual marker. Appl. Mech. and Mater. **789–790**, 652–657 (2015)
7. Article 7 European Charter of Fundamental Rights. http://www.europarl.europa.eu/charter/pdf/text_en.pdf

8. European Regulation 2016/679 on the protection of natural persons with regard to the processing of personal data and on the free movement of such data, and repealing Directive 95/46/EC (General Data Protection Regulation)
9. Yang, J., et al.: A language for automatically enforcing privacy policies. In: ACM SIGPLAN Notices, vol. 47, no. 1, pp. 85–96. ACM (2012)
10. Cavoukian, A.: 7 Foundational Principles of Privacy by Design (2011)
11. See the BBC (Sept 2015) Millions of Fingerprints Stolen in the US Government. http://www.bbc.com/news/technology-34346802
12. Dr. Hawking Connected Wheelchair Project. http://www.intel.la/content/www/xl/es/internet-of-things/videos/dr-hawkings-connected-wheelchair-video.html
13. Markoff, J.: Google car exposes regulatory divide on computers as drivers. NY Times. http://www.nytimes.com/2016/02/11/technology/nhtsa-blurs-the-line-between-human-and-computer-drivers.html?_r=0 (2016)
14. Rose, K., et al.: The internet of things: an overview. In: The Internet Society (ISOC) (2015)
15. Article 29 Working Party (2014) Opinion 8/2014 on the on Recent Developments on the Internet of Things: http://ec.europa.eu/justice/data-protection/article-29/documentation/opinion-recommendation/files/2014/wp223_en.pdf
16. Howard, P.N.: Pax Technica: How the Internet of Things May Set Us Free or Lock Us Up. Yale University Press (2015)
17. Medaglia, C.M., Serbanati, A.: An overview of privacy and security issues in the internet of things. In: The Internet of Things, pp. 389–395. Springer, New York (2010)
18. Information. https://www.google.com/about/company/
19. Holler, J., et al.: From Machine-to-Machine to the Internet of Things: Introduction to a New Age of Intelligence. Academic Press (2014)
20. Mayer-Schönberger, V., Cukier, K.: Big data. In: A Revolution that will Transform How We Live, Work and Think. John Murray (2013)
21. Information Commisisoner's Office UK Big Data and Data Protection. https://ico.org.uk/media/for-organisations/documents/1541/big-data-and-data-protection.pdf (2014)
22. Becker, M., et al.: Cyberpsychol. Behav. Soc. Netw. **16**(2) 132–135 (2013). http://www.liebertpub.com. doi:10.1089/cyber.2012.0291
23. Heetae, Y., et al.: User acceptance on wearable devices: an extended perspective of perceived value. Telem. Inform. **33**, 256–269 (2016)
24. Erevelles, S., et al.: Big data consumer analytics and the transformation of marketing. J. Bus. Res. **69**, 897–904 (2016)
25. Verbeek, P.P.: Moralizing Technology: Understanding and Designing the Morality of Things. University of Chicago Press (2011)
26. Pagallo, U.: The Laws of Robots, vol. 200. Springer, Heidelberg (2013)
27. European Parliament: Draft Report with recommendations to the Commission on Civil Law Rules on Robotics (2015/2103(INL)) (2016)
28. Matthias, A.: The responsibility gap: ascribing responsibility for the actions of learning automata. Ethics Inf. Technol. **6**(3), 175–183 (2004)
29. Johnson, D.G.: Technology with no human responsibility? J. Bus. Ethics **127**(4), 707 (2015)
30. BBC (2015) Not in front of the telly: Warning over 'listening' TV. http://www.bbc.com/news/technology-31296188
31. Fosch-Villaronga, E.: Creation of a care robot impact assessment. In: XVII International Conference on Social Robotics (2015)
32. Similar to Hamblen M.: UL creating a standard for wearable privacy and security. In: Computerworld. http://www.computerworld.com/article/2991331/security/ul-creating-standard-for-wearable-privacy-and-security.html (2015)
33. Opinion 04/2007 on the Concept of Personal Data. Article 29 Work in Party. http://ec.europa.eu/justice/policies/privacy/docs/wpdocs/2007/wp136_en.pdf
34. Article 3(2) of the current Data Protection Directive (95/46/EC) states that the Directive shall not apply to the processing of personal data done by a natural person in the course of a purely

personal or household activity. Vid.: http://ec.europa.eu/justice/data-protection/article-29/documentation/other-document/files/2013/20130227_statement_dp_annex2_en.pdf
35. Nijhawan, L.P., et al.: Informed consent: issues and challenges. J. Adv. Pharm. Technol. Res. **4**(3), 134–144 (2013)
36. Big Data and Smart Devices and Their Impact on Privacy DG for Internal Policies. Policy Department. Citizen's Rights and Constitutional Affairs. http://www.europarl.europa.eu/RegData/etudes/STUD/2015/536455/IPOL_STU(2015)536455_EN.pdf (2015)
37. Office of the Privacy Commissioner of Canada (OPC) Guidance Documents, Seizing Opportunity: Good Privacy Practices for Developing Mobile Apps. https://www.priv.gc.ca/information/pub/gd_app_201210_e.pdf (2012)
38. Office of the Privacy Commissioner of Canada (OPC) Guidance Documents: Wearable Computing. Challenges and Opportunities for Privacy Protection. http://www.priv.gc.ca/information/research-recherche/2014/wc_201401_e.pdf (2014)
39. Article (8.2.a) Directive 95/46/CE on the protection of individuals with regard to the processing of personal data and on the free movement of such data
40. Art. (6.1.b) of the EU Data Protection Directive: further processing of data for historical, statistical or scientific purposes shall not be considered as incompatible provided that Member States provide appropriate safeguards
41. Salem, M., et al.: Towards safe and trustworthy social robots: ethical challenges and practical issues. In: Tapus, A., et al. (eds.) ICSR, LNAI 9388, pp. 584–593 (2015)
42. F. Zhang et al.: Preliminary study of the effect of the user intention recognition errors on volitional control of powered limbs prostheses. In: 34th International Conference of the IEEE Engineering in Medicine and Biology Society (2012)
43. Sharkey, A., Sharkey, N.: Granny and the robots: ethical issues in robot care for the elderly. Ethics Inf. Technol. **14**(1), 27–40 (2012)
44. Shiomi, M., et al.: Effectiveness of social behaviors for autonomous wheelchair robot to support elderly people in Japan. PLoS One **10**(5), 1–15 (2015)
45. Steinert, S.: The five robots—a taxonomy for roboethics. Int. J. Soc. Robot. **6**(2), 249–260 (2014)
46. World Economic Forum What if Your Brain Confesses Debate. www.weforum.org/events/world-economic-forum-annual-meeting-2016/sessions/what-if-your-brain-confesses (2016)

Test Bench for Space Remote Docking System

A. Pisla, C. Vaida and F. Covaciu

Abstract The paper presents the main components of the preliminary research in developing an IOS (Instructor Operator Station) as a testing system for components, algorithms and human reactions in related space applications i.e. spacecraft docking. The mechanical, actuating and control solution for the IOS test bench is considered. The contributions are the result of a joint activity between teams from the DSSL (Dynamic Systems Simulation Laboratory) and CESTER.

Keywords Instructor operation station · Docking · Platform for spacecraft control

1 Introduction

Nowadays the number of space travel applications is continuously increasing. The **ISS** (International Space Station) is the largest structure placed by man in space as an artificial satellite of Earth. ISS has over 400 tones and was served by a multitude of spacecraft models: the Russian TMA (Transport Modified Anthropometric) Soyuz and the cargo spacecraft Progress; the ESA ATV (Automated Transfer Vehicle); the NASA Space Shuttle; the Japanese HTV (HII Transfer Vehicle) Kounotori; and lately the Dragon developed by SpaceX and the NASA's Cygnus (Fig. 1).

A. Pisla (✉) · F. Covaciu
Department of Engineering Design and Robotics, Technical University of Cluj-Napoca, Cluj-Napoca, Romania
e-mail: adip@mail.utcluj.ro

F. Covaciu
e-mail: florin.covaciu@mep.utcluj.ro

C. Vaida
CESTER, Research Center for Industrial Robots Simulation and Testing, Technical University of Cluj-Napoca, Cluj-Napoca, Romania
e-mail: calin.vaida@mep.utcluj.ro

M. Husty and M. Hofbaur (eds.), *New Trends in Medical and Service Robots*, Mechanisms and Machine Science 48, DOI 10.1007/978-3-319-59972-4_18

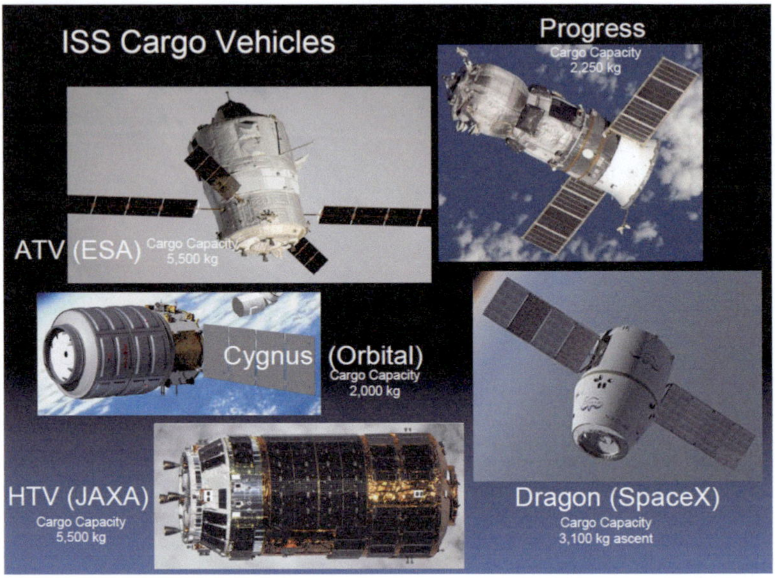

Fig. 1 Chaser vehicles (Credit: [2])

The **US Space Shuttle** programme ended in 2011, since then, the Soyuz rockets became the only provider to transport the ISS astronauts and the **Dragon** made by SpaceX remained the only provider of bulk services (cargo-return-to-Earth).

The Space Exploration Technologies Corporation, or SpaceX, was founded in 2002 and is the only private company that operates on ISS under commercial agreement with NASA, for 12 robotic supply flights and aim to fly astronauts by 2017.

The docking system refers to the coupling of two free-flying space vehicles. Before and after Moon landing, in order to couple two flying objects in space missions used the **docking** and the **berthing** methods. **The berthing systems** imply an inactive vehicle that is placed to the mating interface via a robotic arm. Berthing systems seem to be quicker, safer and less laborious than the manual docking and therefore selected as future solution for emergency case crew evacuation, but manual docking remains open in case that the robotic arm is damaged or there is no one to operate it.

NASA considers the development of the un-crewed berthing system for non-cooperative space vehicles, concerning the approach, orbital and attitude changes. With the missions development the docking systems also evolved, from the early non-androgynous design (that is forming a gender-mating solution where each spacecraft has a unique design and the roles cannot be reversed), to the androgynous docking and berthing using an identical interface for both space vehicles.

Four different docking solutions were developed in the space operation: the US Gemini and Apollo Docking System, the Russian Original and the Modern Docking System, the US Russian APAS-75, the Russian APAS-89 and US APAS-95. The later development solutions are for berthing: the Common Berthing Mechanism used by Dragon and Cygnus; and for the docking and berthing is the IDA (International Docking Adapter) and the NASA's with the Docking System for future US vehicles and the IBDM (International Berthing and Docking Mechanism).

Future research is made by ESA in cooperation with SNC (Sierra Nevada Corporation) to use IBDM for the SNC's Dream Chaser, a small reusable spacecraft, and a possible competitor for Dragon II (both being capable to transport 7 people).

A significant development in various technologies is required for an autonomous chaser vehicle capable of rendezvous and docking maneuvers. The proximity operations and the docking on LEO (Low Earth Orbit) situation which applies currently to the ISS are extremely delicate and precise, requiring accurate relative position and velocity state estimation.

Within the DSSL, Technical University in Cluj-Napoca, the development of an IOS (Instructor Operation Station) as a new testing device for simulation and training, designed as a dual (virtual and physical) solution has started. The IOS is conceived as a computer based system that enables the manual or the automatic scenarios generation under an instructor supervision and intervention. The conceived HMI (Human Machine Interface) for the IOS is a versatile designed solution with several specific features: the switching between manual and automatic control, emergency case intervention, mapping and visualization facilities, etc.

2 The Docking Procedures in Space

For the actual docking systems, the docking maneuvers are made in the area of LEO where the chaser body-fixed frame must coincide with target body-fixed frame at the docking moment. The correct docking procedures are mainly based on the attitude dynamics in order to determine the appropriate strategy that facilitates the chaser approach to the docking system.

The LQR (Linear Quadratic Regulator) approach presents an optimal control design that provides linearized closed-loop error dynamics for tracking. The chaser-target rendezvous mission is divided into the following phases: launch, phasing, far/close rendezvous and the docking.

Within the docking simulation are used the V-R bar operations, considered necessary to have minimum accelerations to control the spacecraft. The simulation results obtained in our model have comparable characteristics with existing models.

For now only the attitude rendezvous is achieved, proximity and docking operations requiring highly precise maneuvers. The close range rendezvous operations are usually divided in a preparatory phase to the final approach corridor and the physical docking. Curve (1), Fig. 2 is considering the phasing to the approach

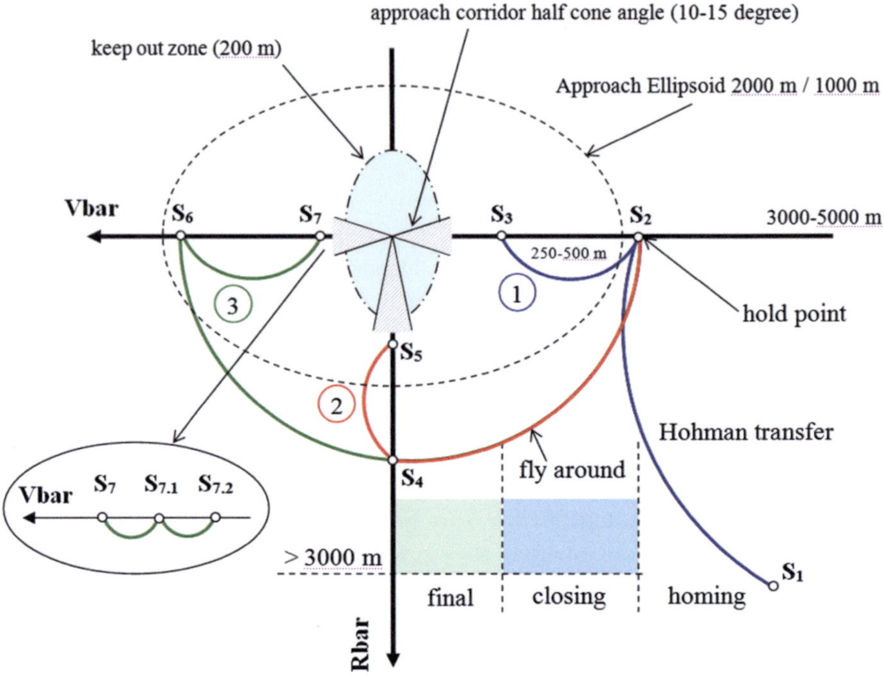

Fig. 2 Proximity operations strategies (Credit STRAERO)

ellipsoid and the intended far away rendezvous. Curves (2) and (3) represent the R-bar and V-bar far rendezvous toward the keep out zone. The close rendezvous is made in the approach corridor to the adequate distance for docking/berthing.

3 The Mobile Mechanical Platform

The IOS physical simulator consists in a mobile mechanical platform that together with the actuating and control algorithms forms the SMS (Spacecraft Mechanical Simulator). The mechanical structure of the SMS is designed in two versions: the full size 1:1 scale one capable to manipulate 2000 kg payload remaining here with the SMS name and the 1:12 scaled one capable to manipulate in the initial version 2 kg payload, entitled MMP (Mechanical Motion Platform). The initial research is made on MMP and any confirmed phase will be remodeled for the SMS.

The NX design of the mechanical structure is depicted with the actual coordinating system and the defined geometrical parameters for the mathematical model (Fig. 3).

The working space generation is based on the IKP and the DKP models, having a given start position for direct kinematics model. The main program is

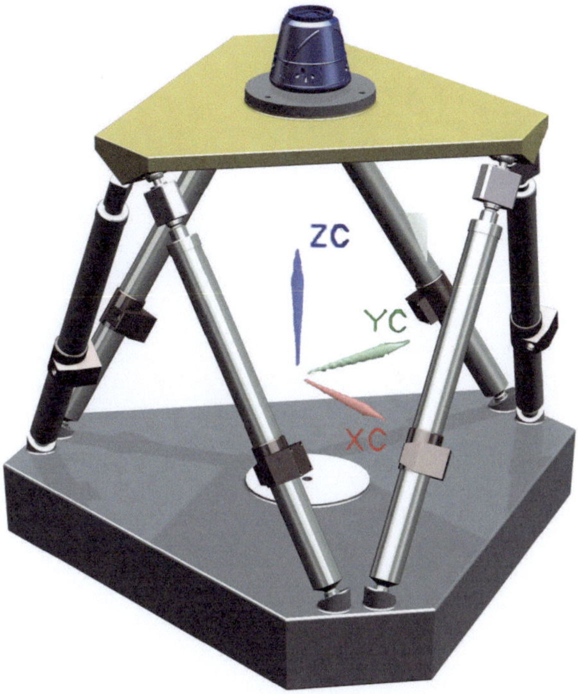

Fig. 3 Mechanical motion platform

parameterized in order to offer the specific geometric parameters, as input data, for the motion generation and the overall simulation. The parameterization is related to the PB (Base Platform) and the PM (Mobile Platform), in between being placed the linear actuating motors connected to the platforms with spherical joints.

In the model, the linear actuators are placed on circles with specific radius for each platform: dM = 40 mm—distance between spherical joints on PB; R = 271 mm—placement radius on PB on which the joints are positioned; lmin = 418 mm—minimum length of the qi arm corresponding to qi = 0; qmax = 120 mm—maximum stroke of the each active joint; dm = 40 mm—distance between spherical joints on PM; r = 200 mm—placement radius on the PM.

For both kinematic models, homogenous coordinating system was used also to express the rotation of the coupled joint from the PM in respect with the base PB.

For simulating the rendezvous, the RDT (Real Docking Trajectory) must be scaled to the robotic platform working space, in the first instance, for MMP. In the actual study the SDT (Scaled Docking Trajectory) must fit in the determined MMP working space considered for the Dragon mockup placed in the middle of the mobile platform as is represented in Fig. 4.

In MATLAB, a program was developed having the SDT as input trajectory. The program generates the motion trajectory as discrete points with orientation and the general coordinates qi, i = 1 ÷ 6, using the IKP.

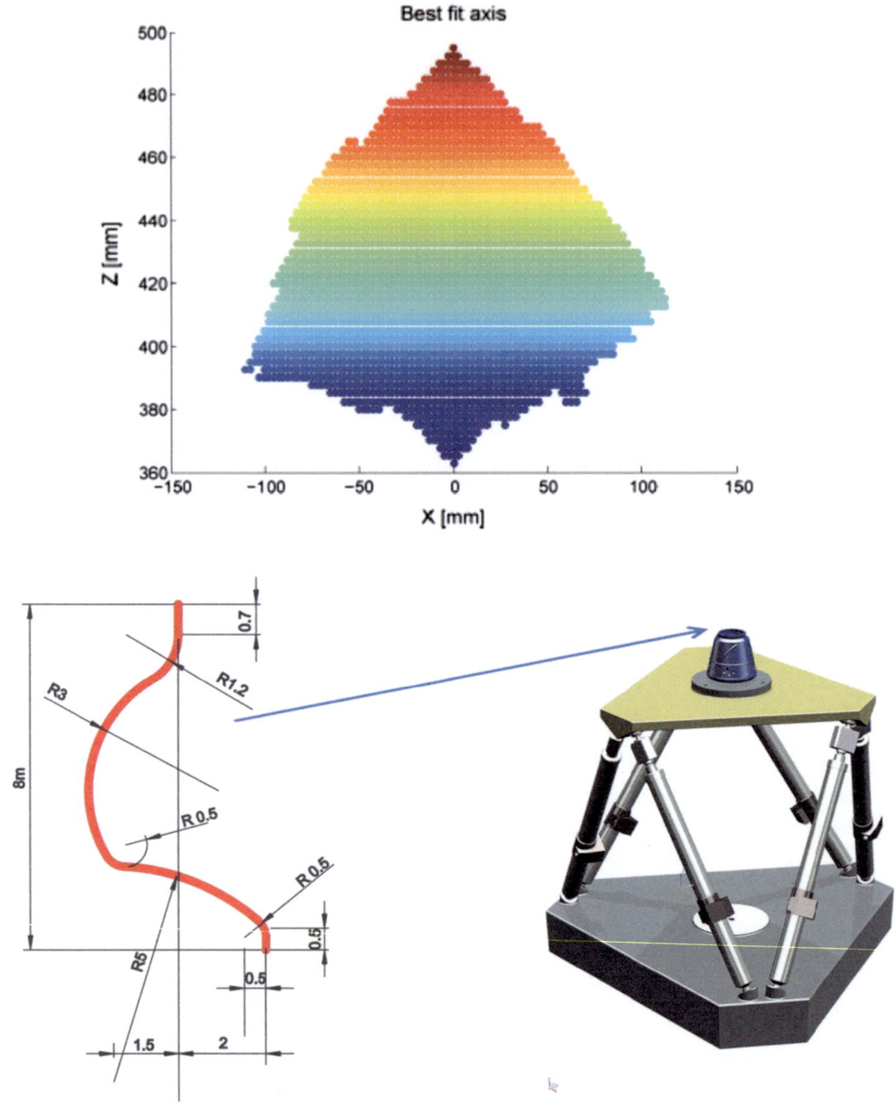

Fig. 4 MMP working space and the simulation trajectory for the Dragon mockup

The running time, on a standard computing desktop, for the given motions was between 200 and 300 μs. The motion generalized program enables the SDT description in an analytical form. For the positions and motion validation the calculated vectors which characterize the variation at the level of the each active joint were used as input data in the motion simulation module of Siemens NX and the resulting trajectory was compared with STD.

4 Mobile Mechanical Platform Control Unit

The software bundle used for IOS development is formed by four programming environments: the Siemens PLM NX for the CAD modeling and simulation and the CAM manufacturing process; the MATLAB-Simulink for the mathematical modeling and simulation; Visual Studio for the communication and the User Interface (HMI); and the Automation Studio for actuating and control of the mobile platform.

The system computing time and the mobile platform are not critical for the real time control and therefore the actual solution uses the Windows 7 Premium on 32 bits, as operating system, fully compatible with all the other programming environments.

The MMPCU (Mechanical Motion Platform Control Unit) is divided in two: the HMI graphical Interface and the PCU (Platform Control Unit).

4.1 HMI Graphical Interface

The first version of the HMI is depicted in Fig. 5. On the left side, M1 ÷ M6, are the progressive bars that represent the linear actuating strokes showing the actual position of each linear actuator. For each linear actuator the programmed velocity and the current axial force (V, F) are represented.

Below the progressive bars is represented the position and the orientation (the attitude) of the TCP (Terminal Center Point), namely in the six text boxes (X, Y, Z, α, β, φ), followed by the Tool ("Viteza TCP") for the TCP velocity and acceleration estimation. The evolution in time of several parameters such as: feed or acceleration of a selected linear actuator or the TCP velocity and acceleration etc.; may be displayed in the grid graphic area.

The standard predefined positions for this robotic structure are: DOWN, SADDLE and UP. Accordingly the X, Y, Z coordinates are displayed and the orientation

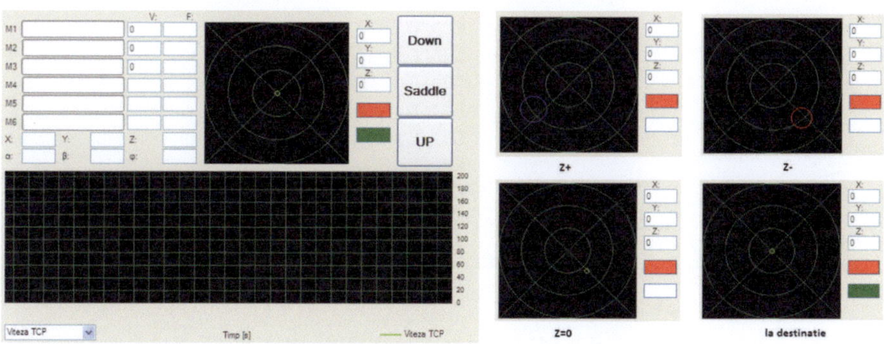

Fig. 5 The human machine interface display

angles are considered zero. The interactive motion indicators are (the upper) green = in motion, red = STOP, (the lower) green = target reached, white = a different position is reached.

On the radar screen display the TCP actual spatial position is graphically represented using a circle of variable radius. The radius is zero (a white point) when the TCP is on target and increases proportional with the distance to the target. The circle is colored blue if the TCP is above the target and turns red if the TCP exceeds the target.

The keyboard control is programmed to use the arrows for the translations and the numerical pad for rotations. The input terminals are: the PC keyboard (safe input for validation); the Joystick (standard solution for berthing and docking); and the Path scenarios stored on PC. For the interface programming are used standard and automation libraries, as shown below.

```
//-----------------------------Libraries-----------------------------------------------------------------//
    using System;
    using System.Collections.Generic;
    using System.ComponentModel;
    using System.Data;
    using System.Drawing;
    using System.Text;
    using System.Windows.Forms;
    using BR.AN.PviServices; //Libraries to connect the OPC Server
//------------------------------------------------------------------------------------------------------//
```

- drawing variables and functions, for the graphical interface design;
- OPC Server connection and setting variables, to initiate the communication between the motion control functions, sensors, motors and the variables change;
- plotting variable and functions, for the motion parameters.

```
//--------------------------------OPC--Variable------------------------------------------//
                Name                                          Type
    poz1                                    INT
    br_a                                    DINT
    br_b                                    DINT
    br_g                                    DINT
    br_x                                    DINT
    br_y                                    DINT
    br_z                                    DINT
    brDown                                  BOOL
    brSadle                                 BOOL
//---------------------------------------------------------------------------------------//
```

In the actual stage, for the MMP control are defined 126 Global Variables and another 126 Local variables for the actuating PCU.

4.2 HMI Graphical Interface

For the MMP was developed a special PCU based on B&R standard components, but customized for the type of actuation existing on the mobile platform and the imposed real time. The PCU uses an X20 CP1483 B&R controller. For the control program implementation an open standard interface OPC is used. The OPC server (**O**LE (Object Linking and Embedding) for **P**rocess **C**ontrol) for the PLC (Programmable Logic Controller) allows Windows programs to communicate with industrial hardware devices, implemented in Server/client pairs. Any program that needs to connect the hardware (motor, HMI, etc.), getting data or sending commands, converting the hardware communication protocol used by a PLC into the OPC protocol, acts as an OPC client software.

In order to connect the X20 CP1483 controller with the six motors of the robotic platform a new type of acquisition board and the required PCB (Printed Circuit Board) was designed and optimized for the application, Fig. 6.

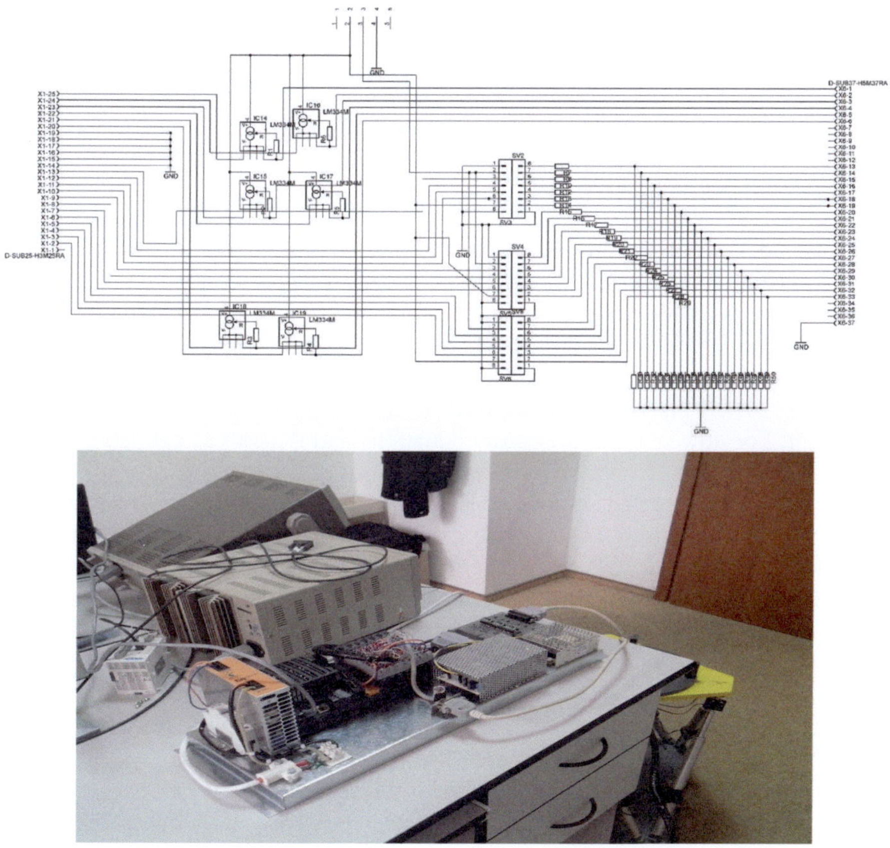

Fig. 6 The designed and optimized PCB

On the acquisition board the controllers are placed for the six motors and the circuits that connect the sensors, located on the motors, with the PLC modules. The command input data, from the User interface, are transferred to the actuating controller of the mobile platform.

Interfaced with the motion control program, the PLC is used for the direct control of all six actuating elements, fulfilling the following tasks:

- Read the actual position from the analog positioning sensors, value that must be linearized and scaled first for all six axes;
- Read the speed value from the tachogenerators, also analogical inputs;
- Send digital control signals for the drivers placed on the acquisition board, two for each motor (rotation sense using logical type signals on-off and the PWM signal for speed and position control. The motors motion algorithms uses a PI positioning algorithm in a negative reaction positioning feed-back loop and the motors correlation version;
- The feed-back loop integration in order to satisfy all above mentioned requirements;
- The implementation of the IKP, in the (motors) actuating components positioning to place the TCP in the desired position and orientation.

5 Modeling and Simulation Results

From the docking procedures in space were selected the docking V-R bar operations. These are considering the minimum accelerations to control the spacecraft, namely the close rendezvous made in the approach corridor for docking. To initiate the simulation process and due to the reduced scale of the mechanical motion platform, the SDT is approximated with linear and circular interpolation curves.

The MATALB path generator module accepts different forms for the trajectory data input. For now only the trajectory equations and the curves defined by points are accepted.

The result of the scaled docking trajectory processing (SDT), generates a list of points with orientation (LPO), whose coordinates must be located in the MMP defined working space resulted from the imposed orientation (the space shuttle attitude).

The generation of the LPO depends not only on the curve shape and the robotic dimensions, but also on the imposed velocity and acceleration that determines the resolution of the SDT approximation based on the minimal time increment (MTI) defined for the entire motion. The definition of the MTI is made with an in house developed algorithm, in this simulation case MTI = 50 μs.

From the LPO are calculated: the spatial distance between two successive points, the change in velocity and the resulted accelerations for each linear or angular motion.

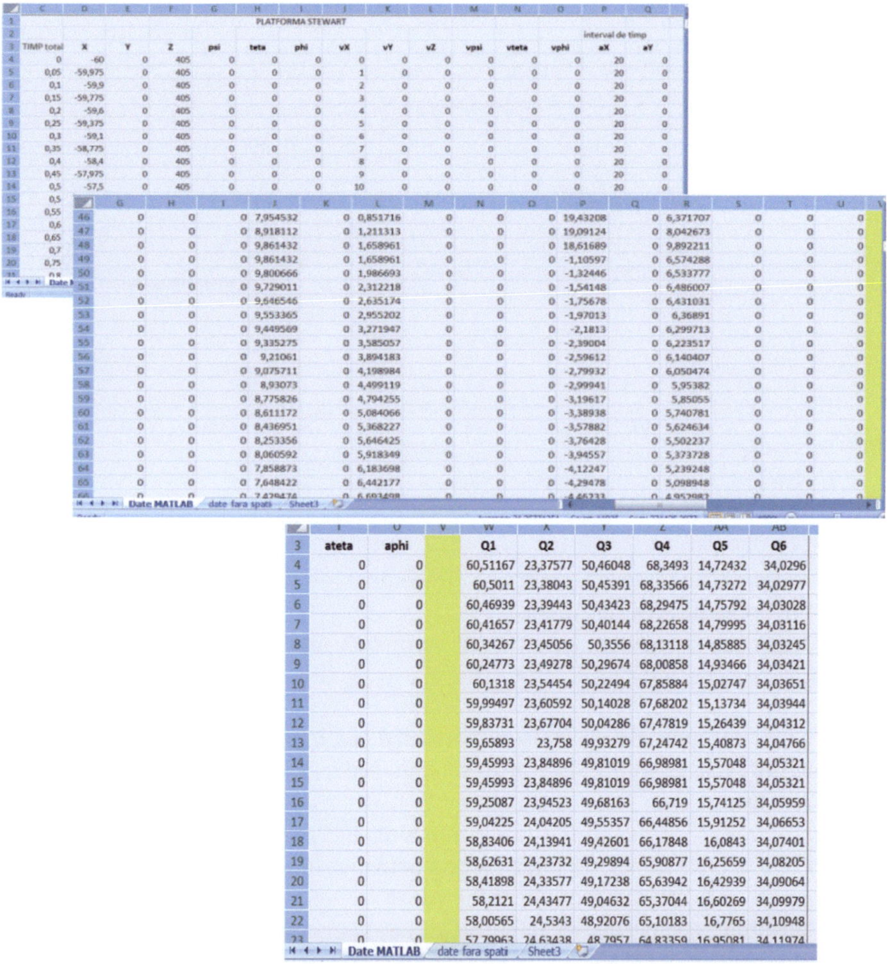

PLATFORMA STEWART

TIMP total	X	Y	Z	psi	teta	phi	vX	vY	vZ	vpsi	vteta	vphi	aX (interval de timp)	aY
0	-60	0	405	0	0	0	0	0	0	0	0	0	20	0
0,05	-59,975	0	405	0	0	0	1	0	0	0	0	0	20	0
0,1	-59,9	0	405	0	0	0	2	0	0	0	0	0	20	0
0,15	-59,775	0	405	0	0	0	3	0	0	0	0	0	20	0
0,2	-59,6	0	405	0	0	0	4	0	0	0	0	0	20	0
0,25	-59,375	0	405	0	0	0	5	0	0	0	0	0	20	0
0,3	-59,1	0	405	0	0	0	6	0	0	0	0	0	20	0
0,35	-58,775	0	405	0	0	0	7	0	0	0	0	0	20	0
0,4	-58,4	0	405	0	0	0	8	0	0	0	0	0	20	0
0,45	-57,975	0	405	0	0	0	9	0	0	0	0	0	20	0
0,5	-57,5	0	405	0	0	0	10	0	0	0	0	0	20	0

0	0	0	7,954532	0	0,851716	0	0	0	19,43208	0	6,371707	0	0	0
0	0	0	8,918112	0	1,211313	0	0	0	19,09124	0	8,042673	0	0	0
0	0	0	9,861432	0	1,658961	0	0	0	18,61689	0	9,892211	0	0	0
0	0	0	9,861432	0	1,658961	0	0	0	-1,10597	0	6,574288	0	0	0
0	0	0	9,800666	0	1,986693	0	0	0	-1,32446	0	6,533777	0	0	0
0	0	0	9,729011	0	2,312218	0	0	0	-1,54148	0	6,486007	0	0	0
0	0	0	9,646546	0	2,635174	0	0	0	-1,75678	0	6,431031	0	0	0
0	0	0	9,553365	0	2,955202	0	0	0	-1,97013	0	6,36891	0	0	0
0	0	0	9,449569	0	3,271947	0	0	0	-2,1813	0	6,299713	0	0	0
0	0	0	9,335275	0	3,585057	0	0	0	-2,39004	0	6,223517	0	0	0
0	0	0	9,21061	0	3,894183	0	0	0	-2,59612	0	6,140407	0	0	0
0	0	0	9,075711	0	4,198984	0	0	0	-2,79932	0	6,050474	0	0	0
0	0	0	8,93073	0	4,499119	0	0	0	-2,99941	0	5,95382	0	0	0
0	0	0	8,775826	0	4,794255	0	0	0	-3,19617	0	5,85055	0	0	0
0	0	0	8,611172	0	5,084066	0	0	0	-3,38938	0	5,740781	0	0	0
0	0	0	8,436951	0	5,368227	0	0	0	-3,57882	0	5,624634	0	0	0
0	0	0	8,253356	0	5,646425	0	0	0	-3,76428	0	5,502237	0	0	0
0	0	0	8,060592	0	5,918349	0	0	0	-3,94557	0	5,373728	0	0	0
0	0	0	7,858873	0	6,183698	0	0	0	-4,12247	0	5,239248	0	0	0
0	0	0	7,648422	0	6,442177	0	0	0	-4,29478	0	5,098948	0	0	0

ateta	aphi		Q1	Q2	Q3	Q4	Q5	Q6
0	0		60,51167	23,37577	50,46048	68,3493	14,72432	34,0296
0	0		60,5011	23,38043	50,45391	68,33566	14,73272	34,02977
0	0		60,46939	23,39443	50,43423	68,29475	14,75792	34,03028
0	0		60,41657	23,41779	50,40144	68,22658	14,79995	34,03116
0	0		60,34267	23,45056	50,3556	68,13118	14,85885	34,03245
0	0		60,24773	23,49278	50,29674	68,00858	14,93466	34,03421
0	0		60,1318	23,54454	50,22494	67,85884	15,02747	34,03651
0	0		59,99497	23,60592	50,14028	67,68202	15,13734	34,03944
0	0		59,83731	23,67704	50,04286	67,47819	15,26439	34,04312
0	0		59,65893	23,758	49,93279	67,24742	15,40873	34,04766
0	0		59,45993	23,84896	49,81019	66,98981	15,57048	34,05321
0	0		59,45993	23,84896	49,81019	66,98981	15,57048	34,05321
0	0		59,25087	23,94523	49,68163	66,719	15,74125	34,05959
0	0		59,04225	24,04205	49,55357	66,44856	15,91252	34,06653
0	0		58,83406	24,13941	49,42601	66,17848	16,0843	34,07401
0	0		58,62631	24,23732	49,29894	65,90877	16,25659	34,08205
0	0		58,41898	24,33577	49,17238	65,63942	16,42939	34,09064
0	0		58,2121	24,43477	49,04632	65,37044	16,60269	34,09979
0	0		58,00565	24,5343	48,92076	65,10183	16,7765	34,10948

Date MATLAB / date fara spati / Sheet3

Fig. 7 LPO, LOQ, LPO diagrams

The obtained data are used to determine the generalized coordinates for the MMP, in a list form named LOQ (List of generalized coordinates). From the LPO is generated the simulated curve and the LOQ is transferred to the PCU.

The simulation inputs are: SDT, motion velocity and the motion acceleration.

The simulation outputs are: MTI, LPO, LOQ, LPO-diagrams, LOQ-diagrams.

The LOQ is used in the MMP control, where the MMP motion is recorded and the traced curves (LOQ-diagrams) are used also for the comparison the SDT.

The final result is the deviation of the imposed docking trajectory in the modeling and simulation system and in the mechanical platform motion. In Fig. 7 are presented the LPO and the LOQ.

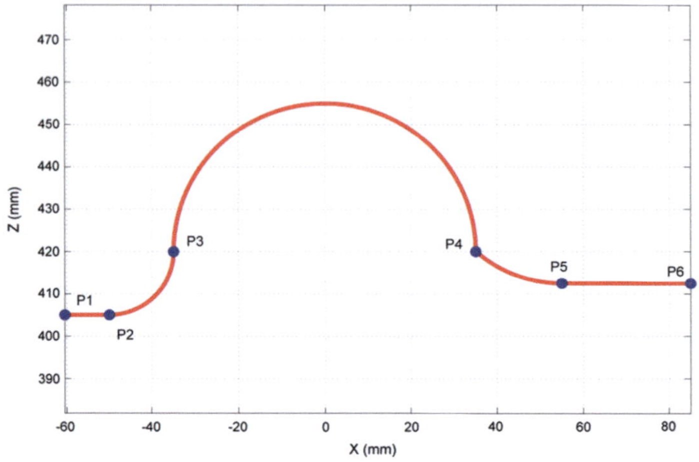

Fig. 8 The generation of the docking curve interpolation

The shape of the imposed trajectory for the docking is calculated and scaled to fit inside the workspace of the robot.

The trajectory is a scaled down real approach and the IOS training platform integrates, besides the MMP and HMI the replicate conditions for the Dragon shuttle.

In Fig. 8, an optimal trajectory is presented, with six control points where the pilot should actuate the shuttle thrusters in order to align the target onto the trajectory.

For this trajectory, using the fast computing IKP, are determined the position, velocity and accelerations variations at the active joints level in order to obtain the input data to simulate the motion of the MMP.

The position, speed and acceleration variations, at the level of the target coordinates (the scaled Dragon shuttle) are presented in Fig. 9, emphasizing the location of each control point where the thrusters have to be engaged.

The resulted displacements for each actuated joint (the generalized coordinates) are depicted in Fig. 10, but as long as they are to be analyzed together and in parallel, the superposed diagram being presented in Fig. 11.

The resulted output data (from the trajectory generation using the IKP), are the input data in the defined virtual model of the MMP, designed with Siemens NX software. In NX the advanced motion simulation features are used to obtain the simulation based on the sequence of numeric values resulted from the MATLAB model generated data.

Similar inputs are used also for the MMP control (Path scenarios). The real motion is monitored with position and force sensors. The position sensors will record each actuated joint position to be compared with the input data. The resulting simulation, which used absolutely no data from the IKP, illustrates the same

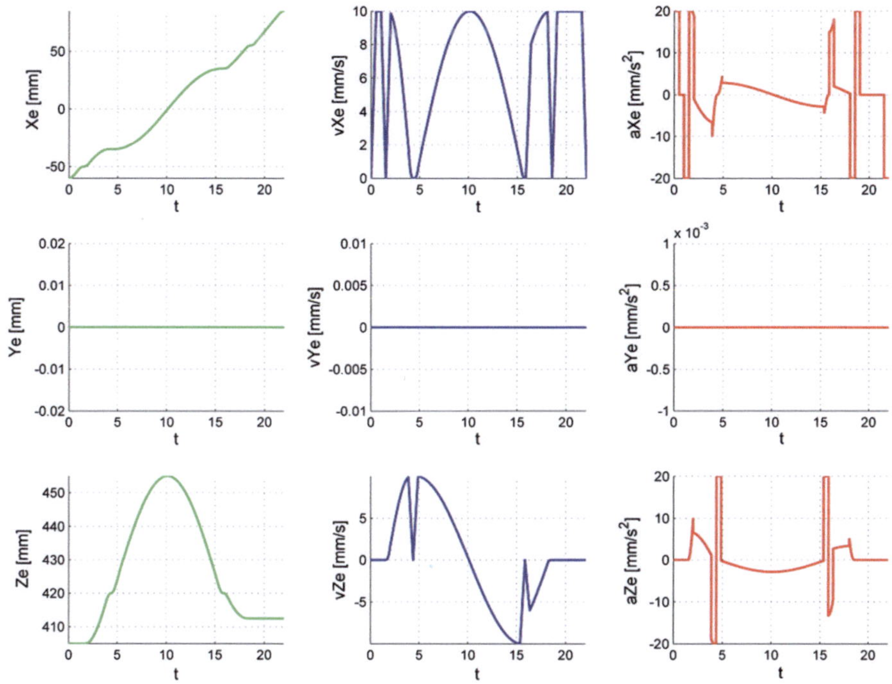

Fig. 9 Positions, speeds and accelerations for the scaled Dragon shuttle tip

(identical) behavior of the platform, which represents also a validation of the developed mathematical model, Fig. 12.

The force sensors offer the components for the Propulsion vector. Together with position sensors, these enables the safe use of the mathematical equations inside the control unit of the robot (PCU) and helps to create the training platform software for the docking procedure simulation. In Fig. 13 are depicted the identified forces in each actuating system.

Except spinning reduction all the other motions of the scaled space shuttle can be simulated to identify the scaled "trust force", that must be induced in each Dragon thrusters. SpaceX's Dragon spacecraft uses Draco thrusters to maneuver in the vacuum space and upon reentry into the Earth's atmosphere.

There are 18 Draco thrusters on each Dragon, distributed across four pods, two housing four thrusters each and two housing five thrusters each.

From the MMP force distribution diagram, Fig. 14, are extracted the propulsion vector for the spacecraft positioning, and the acceleration and breaking vectors for positioning.

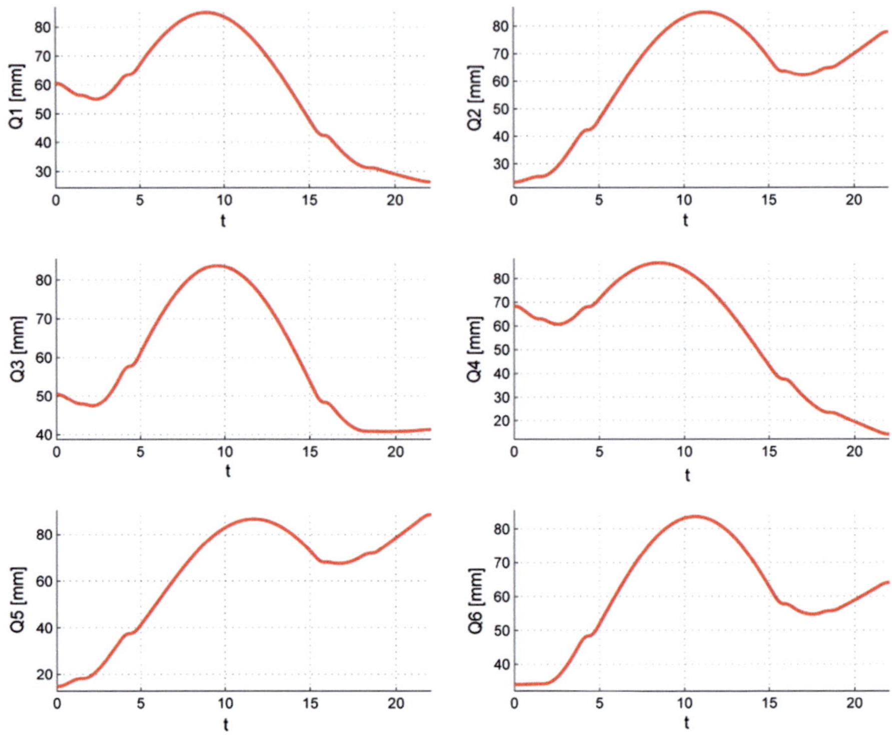

Fig. 10 The generalized coordinates for each actuating system

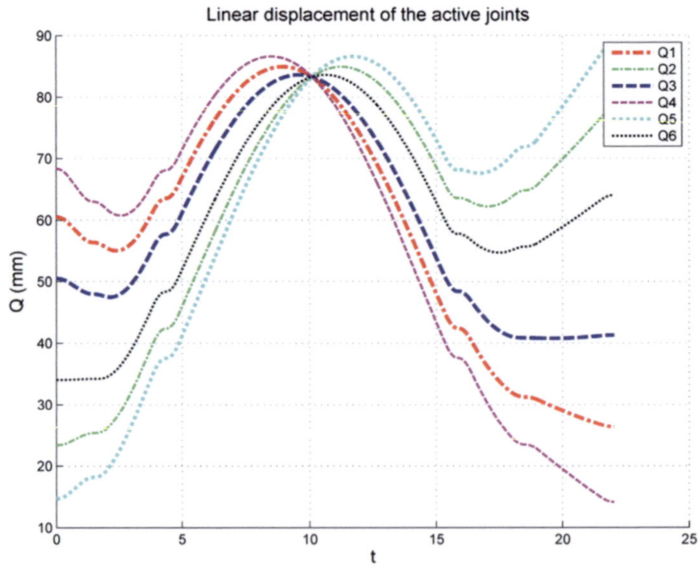

Fig. 11 The superposed positions of the six actuating systems

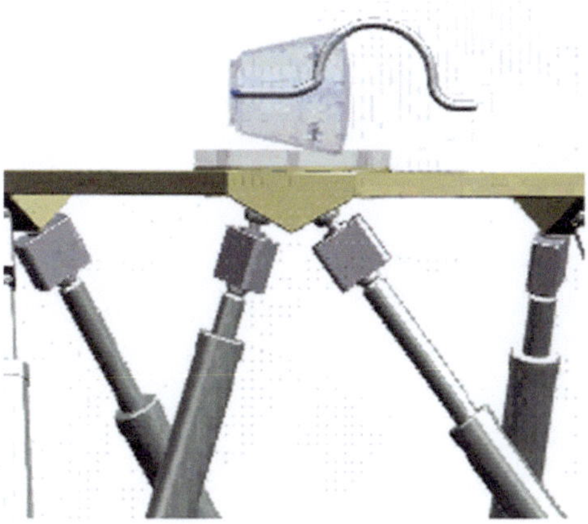

Fig. 12 The traced trajectory during the simulation process

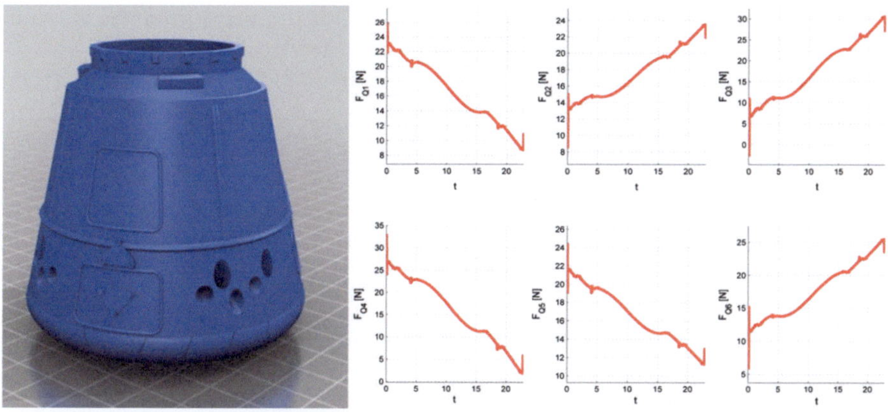

Fig. 13 The superposed positions for the six actuating systems

6 Conclusions

In the paper is presented the first stage of the research with results in updating a scaled mechanical structure 1:12, relative to the full sized one.

The mechanical solution was modeled using Siemens PLM software platform. In simulation were used trajectories derived from the real docking procedures.

Using maxon DC motors (similar with the ones provided for aerospace applications and the Mars rovers) a new actuating control unit was developed with B&R components. B&R company is providing also solutions for aerospace industry.

The MATLAB implementation of the mathematical model enables simulations having as result the trajectories for the MMP (Mechanical Motion Platform)

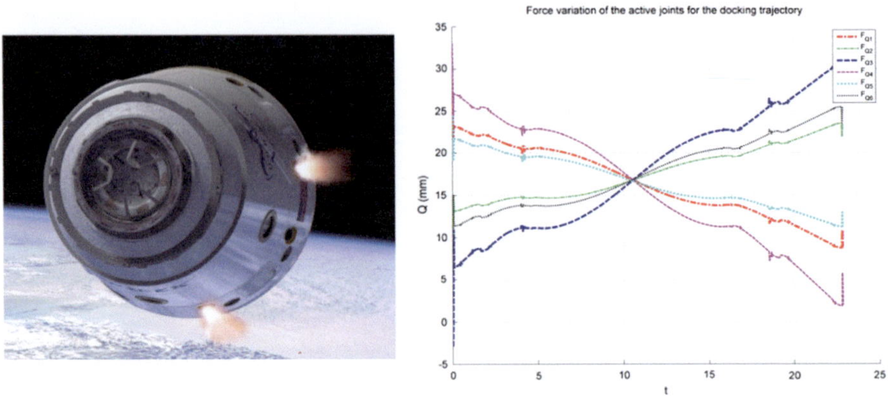

Fig. 14 The MMP force distribution diagram

generating the list of positions, velocities and acceleration for all six actuation elements. The values in the list are compared with the ones from the imposed trajectory and with the ones measured during the MMP motion.

From the dynamical point of view in the Siemens PLM software platform the payload is the one considered for the SpaceX Dragon spacecraft scaled to maximum 2 kg payload on the MMP robotic application.

Relative to the full scaled structure, the SMS, this is a 1:1000 weight scaling factor applied in order to identify the axial forces on the all six actuation elements, with the aim to obtain a composed vector (direction and spinning) that will be transformed in force-time diagram for the existing 18 Draco thrusters on the Dragon spacecraft.

In the end may be considered the achievement of a scaled version for the IOS (Instructor Operation Station) designed to simulate space maneuvers and testing new devices and control algorithms, as a dual (virtual-physical) solution.

Acknowledgements This work was supported by a grant of the Romanian National Authority for Scientific Research, Program for research-Space Technology and Advanced Research—STAR, project number 95.

References

1. Husty, M.: An algorithm for solving the direct kinematic of stewart-gough-type platforms. McGill Center for Intelligent Machines, McGill University, Montreal, Quebec, Canada June (1994)
2. Jones, L., Peck, M.: Control strategies utilizing the physics of flux-pinned interfaces for spacecraft. In: AIAA Guidance, Navigation, and Control Conference. Portland, OR (2011)
3. McKee, J.W., Lyndon, B.: APOLLO experience report-crew-support activities for experiments performed during manned space flight, Johnson Space Center, Houston, Texas 77058. National Aeronautics and Space Administration (NASA), Washington, D.C. September (1974)

4. Sellmaier, F., Boge, T., Spurmann, J., Gully, S., Rupp, T., Huber, F.: On-orbit servicing missions: challenges and solutions for spacecraft operations (2010)
5. Zebenay, M., Lampariello, R., Boge, T., Choukroun, D.: A new contact dynamics model tool for hardware-in-the-loop docking simulation. In: International Symposium on Artificial Intelligence, Robotics and Automation in Space (i-SAIRAS) (2012)
6. Pisla, A., Vaida, C.: Testing capacity for space technology suppliers. In: New Trends in Medical and Service Robots, Challenges and Solutions, pp. 369–384 (2014)

Rob'Autism: How to Change Autistic Social Skills in 20 Weeks

S. Sakka, R. Gaboriau, J. Picard, E. Redois, G. Parchantour, L. Sarfaty, S. Navarro and A. Barreau

Abstract Rob'Autism proposes an approach to improve social skills of people with autistic spectrum disorders. The program focuses on linking voice to gestures, and checks the emotional effects of this linkage. Rob'Autism is divided into 20 sessions of 1 h each, alternating preparatory sessions and robotics sessions. During the preparatory sessions, the subjects register their voices reading a story. During the robotics sessions, the subjects program the robot gestures according to the registered voices. In this program, the robots are used as an extension, and not as a companion as traditionally performed in other research programs. Consequently, the subjects immediately use it for their communication with others, showing consequent improvements of their communication skills, inside and outside the sessions, in a very short time.

S. Sakka (✉)
Research Institute for Communications and Cybernetics of Nantes, Nantes, France
e-mail: Sophie.Sakka@irccyn.ec-nantes.fr

S. Sakka
Non Profit Organization Robots!, Nantes, France

R. Gaboriau · J. Picard · E. Redois · G. Parchantour · L. Sarfaty
Medical University Center of Nantes, CPGEA, Nantes, France
e-mail: Gaboriau@chu-nantes.fr

J. Picard
e-mail: Picard@chu-nantes.fr

E. Redois
e-mail: Redois@chu-nantes.fr

G. Parchantour
e-mail: Parchantour@chu-nantes.fr

L. Sarfaty
e-mail: Sarfaty@chu-nantes.fr

S. Navarro
Non Profit Organization STEREOLUX, Nantes, France
e-mail: sonia.navarro@stereolux.org

A. Barreau
Ecole Centrale de Nantes, Nantes, France
e-mail: direction.recherche@ec-nantes.fr

M. Husty and M. Hofbaur (eds.), *New Trends in Medical and Service Robots*, Mechanisms and Machine Science 48, DOI 10.1007/978-3-319-59972-4_19

The program has also proven to length in time, as 6 months after its end, its effects on the subjects can still be observed. This article review the preliminary results of Rob'Autism, validated with 6 young test subjects with autism, aged 11–15.

Keywords Rob'Autism · Autistic spectrum disorder · Voice · Gesture · Robot · Programming

1 Introduction

The use of robots to improve skills for subjects with autistic spectrum disorder started in the late 90's with Dautenhahn's work [4, 14]. Since then, the AURORA European project led by Dautenhahn [5] and grouping worldwide researchers (Robins et al. [10], Billard et al. [2], Dickerson et al. [6], Werry and Dautenhahn [15], etc.) allowed many developments and various protocols on different robotic platforms (human like or not). Many other projects appeared since 2010 thanks to the appearance of the affordable platform NAO (Aldebaran Robotics).

Dautenhahn suggested the use of a robot as a companion for autistic young subjects, introducing the concept of *Robots as social actors*: the robot should be equipped with a specific software that makes it look as an autonomous person, in the sense that the robot comes with its own personality, and could exchange with the subjects on topics proposed by the therapist approach. For example, the robot would show the child different images, and ask him/her to point out an apple, or a boat, and so on. Then the child must show the selected image to the robot, which validates the selection or ask to choose again. In this framework, solicitations come from the robot and are performed as would a non-autistic adult do. The concept is based on the fact that autistic subject have a natural attraction to robots. Immediate search for interaction can be observed, curiosity and desired communication with the machine that was difficult to perform with human persons.

All other worldwide researchers tracked the same approach using the robot as a companion. Then the approaches explored different situations and exercises, aiming at improving one specific skill at each contact such as social interaction or communication, imagination, spontaneousness, free talking, proximity acceptance, focus and concentration, care for objects, imitation. More and more researchers are working with robots for autism, especially since the appearance of the robot NAO on the market (2009) for an available cost [1, 3, 12, 13].

The appearance of the robot was particularly studied by Feil-Safer et al. [7] and Robins et al. [9]. All authors showed that a humanoid shape was more efficient on children progresses than other (animals or mascots) shapes. It was mentioned that robots do not replace human beings, but may increase their capabilities [8, 11]. Still, the social companion approach has not been questioned yet, even though this approach is equivalent to replacing human being with a robot.

The Rob'Autism project proposes another approach using the humanoid robot NAO (Aldebaran Robotics): it is not used as a robot companion, but as a machine that does not do anything without the programing of the subjects. As a consequence, the robot is directly approached as an extension that allows safe communication. This paper will describe the context of the project, its sequences and the observations made in its preliminary stage.

2 Context of Rob'Autism Project

2.1 The Project

Rob'Autism is a multidisciplinary project linking medical, arts and sciences fields. It was born in 2014, and can continue thanks to the collaboration of four partners: 2 academic institutions: CHU-Nantes (CPGEA Samothrace: day hospital for autistic young ones) and *Ecole Centrale de Nantes* (school of engineering), and 2 non-profit organizations: Stereolux (science and culture) and *Robots!* (Robotics and arts). Rob'Autism consists in a therapeutic support for autistic people, which lasts 20 weeks and is based on interactions between subjects and robots. Rob'Autism is organized in 20 sessions of 1 h each, once in a week. The sessions alternate 10 non-robotics and 10 robotics work groups.

2.2 Subjects and Material

Six young teenagers aged from 11 to 15 years old participated in this experiment, 5 boys and 1 girl. All subjects'parents gave written informed consent before entering the study. Ethic approval was granted by the ethic committee of the Hospital Center of Nantes. These test subjects suffer from autistic spectrum disorders. The 6 subjects have some ability to read and write, and they are familiar with the use of a computer. They have known each other and the medical staff members for four years, and had participated to another work group using a software dedicated to voice exercises. The location of the work group for the robotics sessions was chosen the same as their previous working sessions, so the working environment was also familiar to the subjects.

The program uses 3 humanoid robots NAO from Aldebaran Robotics. The robots are programmed by the subjects using the software interface *Choregraphe*, which is the classical programming interface sold with the robots (i.e., no specific software was used for the programming).

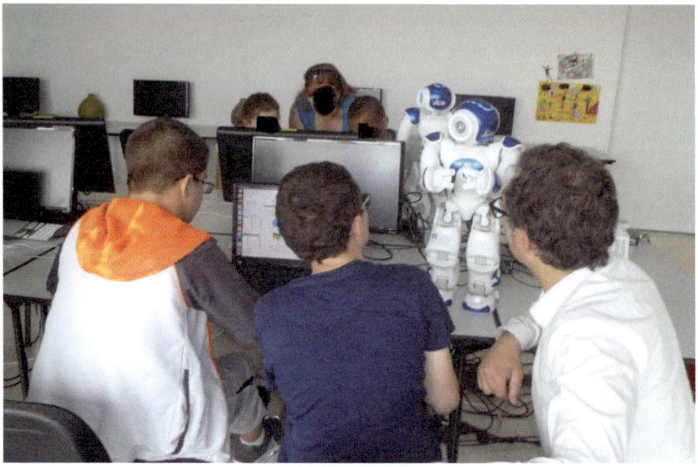

Fig. 1 Two out of three working groups during Rob'Autism working session. Each group contains two subjects and one nurse

2.3 *Organization*

The robotics sessions make the subjects program the robots and are organized as follows: two children per robot, using the same computer (See Fig. 1). The three groups face each other: the working tables are in the center of the room in such disposition that each group can see the two other ones. Each group is assisted by one nurse trained in robot programming, and a robotics specialist is also present in the room to help with specific programming requests (see below for the sessions content). When the children enter the room, they find the robots and computers always at the same place. The computers are switched on, but not the robots (except for the first session).

For the non-robotics sessions, a sound specialist leads the working progress of the 6 children, assisted by three nurses and a speech therapist. The room is located at the CPGEA center, with no tables but cushions on the floor.

3 Sequences

We present in this section the sequences of the project, describing the sessions and their context, the program preliminary- and post-work.

3.1 *Before the 20 Weeks Rob'Autism Program*

The medical staff was trained to program the robots during 12 h (one and a half day) before the start of the program to get the ability to share the robot experience with the subjects and help them with simple programming questions. This knowledge is absolutely necessary as the medical staff can keep the children focused on the session objectives by helping them when necessary. Still, as the medical staff is not specialized in robot programming, the presence of a robot specialist is required during the 10 robotics sessions.

3.2 Non-robotics Sessions

The non-robotics sessions aim at preparing the robotics sessions. The project focuses on linking voice to gestures. So the program was set to make the robot tell a story, using the voices of the subjects. The chosen story is *Voices in the park*, by Anthony Brown: four characters share a story in a park, and the four tell the story with their own interpretation. During the non-robotics session, the children were asked to read the story, and their voices were saved to be replayed by the robots. The global organization was the following one:

- Session 1: Draw a Robot
- Session 3: First reading of the story/Discuss security (fragility) of the robot/talk about first contact made in session 2
- Session 5: Registering voice 1/acting voice 1 (with gestures)
- Session 7: Registering voice 2/acting voice 2 (with gestures)
- Session 9: Registering voice 3/acting voice 3 (with gestures)
- Session 11: Registering voice 4/acting voice 4 (with gestures)
- Session 13: listening to voices 1 and 2/discussing tone, gestures and emotions. Modifying some passages (registering)
- Session 15: listening to voices 3 and 4/discussing tone, gestures and emotions. Modifying some passages (registering)
- Session 17: Associating emotions to eyes colors/prepare decor for the show (1)
- Session 19: Draw a robot/prepare decor for the show (2).

Once the voices are saved in mp3 files, they are divided into several shorter sound files in preparation to the robotics sessions. Each short sound file will be treated by a group to program the corresponding gestures and emotions of the robots.

The first and last non-robotics sessions are dedicated to subjects interpretation of how they imagine a robot. They were asked to draw a robot, explaining the content of their drawings. These drawings are used to link imagination to experience and feelings. The drawings of two subjects are illustrated in Fig. 3, they will be discussed in the results section.

3.3 Robotics Sessions

The robotics sessions consisted in programming the motion of the robot according to the registered voices telling the story. As the subjects had acted the story in the non-robotics sessions, they already had an idea of desired movements. The sessions were organized as follows.

- Session 2: First contact: short explanations (security) and make the robot talk (program ready, subjects only have to tape the text to be pronounced by the robot)
- Session 4: Make the robot talk (use the behavior library to get the *say* box)
- Session 6: Make the robot talk then move (use the library for pre-registered motions: *sit*, *get up*, *wave*, aso.), move then talk, move and talk at the same time
- Session 8: Switch on robot/Make motions using *timeline*. Explain configurations versus motions.
- Session 10: Play the recorded sounds, program desired motions (voice 1)/Switch off robot
- Session 12: Play the recorded sounds, program desired motions (voice 1)
- Session 14: Play the recorded sounds, program desired motions (voice 2)
- Session 16: Play the recorded sounds, program desired motions (voice 3)
- Session 18: Play the recorded sounds, program desired motions (voice 4), change eyes LEDs colors
- Session 20: Program emotions using eyes LEDs colors.

Even though the children could concentrate the complete hour from session 14, they were limited to 45 mn of work. The remaining 15 mn were used to play with the voice synthesizer and make the robots talk. Robot programming using Choregraphe consists in choosing a desired function in a library on the left of the window. The user must drag and drop the chosen function in the robot interface, which is a white initially empty area in the center of the window. The function appears as a box in the window, with its name on it. The box must be connected to the robot input, then clicking on the send button, sent to robot control. The difficult part is the choice of the desired function in the library, which is in English (the subjects only speak French, and show difficulties to read even if they can approximately manage). So the first time they had to use a given function, they would arrive at the session with the function already in the robot interface, connected and ready to use. The following session, they would be asked (with verbal help) to find it in the library, drag and drop it in the robot interface, connect it and send it to robot control.

The robot was switched on for the first three robotics session, during which the subjects were learning how to take care of the robot and insure its security. For all the robotics sessions, one subject was programming, then asked for security assistance, the second subject would stand next to the robot during the whole robot motion (Fig. 2). Once the motion is finished, could the security assistance stop.

3.4 After the 20 Weeks Rob'Autisme Program

A public representation of the robotic show programmed by the children was organized, grouping 12 strangers as spectators. The spectators were officials supports of the project. The sessions organizers (robotics and sound specialists, the medical

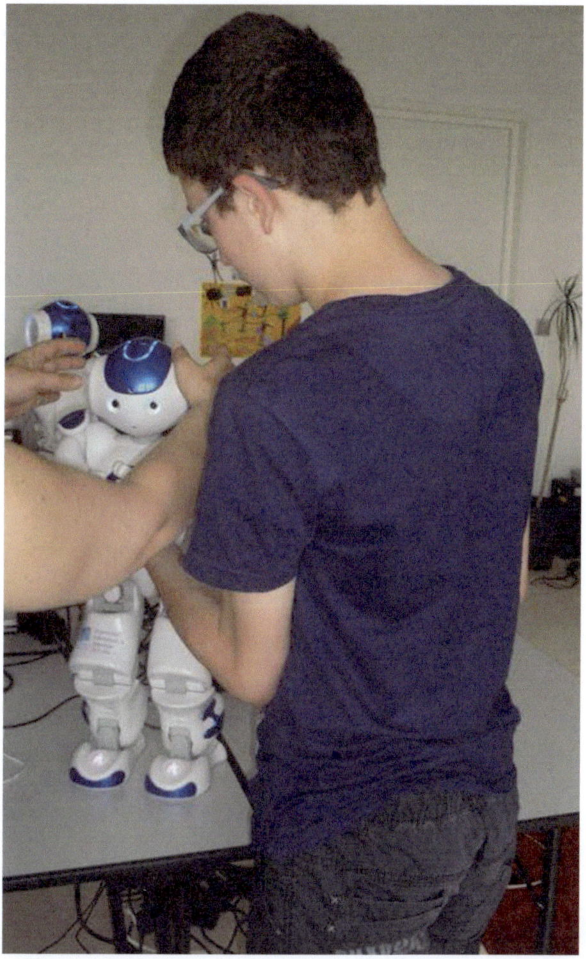

Fig. 2 Assuring security of the robot while his colleague programs motion

staff) were also present in the room. The show took place in the same room as the robotic sessions, at STEREOLUX. The room was re-organized as follows: the working tables were removed from the center of the room, a scene was set along one of the wall and chairs were placed in the center of the room, facing the scene. This setting was performed before the arrival of the subjects. A lunch grouping the work group (subjects, medical staff, robot and sound specialists, Stereolux organizer) was organized, then all went to the room to welcome the spectators. The children sat in front of the scene, directly on the ground. The spectators were sitting in their back, on the chairs. The program was explained to the public, then the show was performed. Once finished, questions and remarks of the public were answered during a 20 min discussion. Finally, strangers could get up and go out of the room.

4 Results

Consistent improvements in focus, communication and social skills were observed. We will summarize here the most important ones. Three general observations should be pointed, concerning (1) the impressive velocity of the changes in subjects behaviors and attention; (2) the memory of the subjects from robotics session to robotics session: they remembered everything learned at the last robotics session even if it was two weeks back (sometimes more because of holidays) and (3) the changes outside the sessions, that could be observed from the third robotics session.

The first programming contact with the robot consisted in making it talk. The subject had to enter the text from the keyboard. The global following points could be observed.

- *Concentration time*: The nurses had great difficulties to make the subjects focus continuously during more than 12 min when the program started. Breaks were organized to make them relax (explanations, interactions). At robotics session 14, the subjects were able to work the complete session on programming the robot movements. But it was observed that they were getting tired, and started to go away from the robot. To avoid tiredness and keep them close to the robot, the working time was limited to 45 min. The 15 min left were dedicated to playing with the voice synthesizer, making the robot talk in funny ways or in forbidden ways.
- *Sharing with others*: The first talks of the robots were trials. The subjects made the robot talk for themselves, following nurses "instructions". Each time a subject finished taping a sentence, silence and attention of the others were required, and everybody would listen to the robot talk. With this approach, the subjects very quickly switched to programming to show to the others, and a kind of contest started, which aim was to find the more silly thing to make the robot say. The same organization was performed when programming the robot movements: once a movement is finished by one subject, everybody stops and looks at the robot performance. Doing so, the subject could enjoy the pride to share their respective work with others, to work with the objective of showing / sharing.
- *Acquiring robot programming abilities*: Choregraphe software is very simple to understand. Still, some great difficulties occur for the studied population: the software is in English (subjects are French), the function library contains a lot of functions, so finding a specific function (in English) is a difficult task. Moreover, saving the work was far from a programming reflex when the subjects started the sessions. At each robotics session, the programmer's how-to was re-said, re-explained until the knowledge was acquired by the subjects. Programming a desired movement was the most difficult part of the training, as the notion of body configuration (static) and body trajectory (dynamic) is particularly difficult to integrate. Added to this, the necessity to remember to save the configurations: the robot will understand what to do, not once it is shown how to do it, but once what to do is saved in its file. Most basics robot programming knowledge was acquired by the 6 subjects

at the end of the program. The subjects also remembered this knowledge 6 months after the end of the program.

- *Voluntary communication*: The changes in voluntary communication started at the end of the first robotics session. They were the most spectacular changes, that came from two facts: the understanding that the robot is theirs and can talk for them and the showing to (sharing with) the other groups. The puppet master effect (see below) led to spectacular results: first the subjects used the robot to talk for them, using forbidden vocabulary. The sentences are short and mainly limited to series of slang words. Then the robots say complete sentences borrowed to movies or personal life scenes, or they say slang with different intonations (playing with the level and speed of the voice synthesizer). Then, the robot expresses things directly connected to the subject state of mind. Finally the subjects directly express themselves, as typing becomes to slow to say things. The puppet master effect is described in more details in Sect. 4.3.
- *Verbal communication*: The subjects using the robots build a strong relation with the object, allowing the robots to say things the subjects would have never express. Once again, they benefit the puppet master effect, as when the robot talks, people look at it and accept anything said by it. It gives the subjects an example of positive reaction to what is said by the robot, then they feel safer saying it themselves. Verbal communication was very low at the program start. One of the subjects even did not talk at all. Focusing on the robot programming, the subjects' desire to use the robot was the strongest: verbal communication started with shy, short and rare questions about the programming. Then it became more and more often, up to the level of discussion (any subject). It took five robotics sessions before voluntary verbal communication with eye contact. The subject who was suffering the most with language skills took longer, but volunteered for the voices to be given to the robot.
- *Taking care of objects*: Security of the robot was explained from the very first session (non robotics). The robot NAO is a fragile platform, and during the sessions one subject was programming while the other one would insure robot security: standing next to it, ready to catch it if the robot falls. An interesting fact was observed at the sixteenth session: one of the robots fell down because of a motor breakdown: the motor generated a sudden motion of the knee, which had a consequence of robot jumping then falling from the table. A spare robot was immediately given to replace the damaged one, so the session could continue. The six subjects showed very concerned by the fall, but instead of caring for the objects, turned naturally to the robotics specialist and expressed their being sorry for the fall of the robot. This clearly illustrates their understanding of the machine the robot is, and what the robot helps them with. They have accepted the machine as a helping tool for communication. They have accepted to care for the machine, but doing so they have shown respect, not to the machine, but to the machine specialist (human being). This also has illustrated how important it is *not to lie* about the robot nature (funny machine vs. companion), as using the robot as a machine enhance the link to the human beings behind the robot. At the end of the program, the subjects would very carefully put back the robot in its box. They were very

proud of this responsibility (the subjects asked to do it). Once the robot is in the box, they look back up to the robot specialist, hoping they have done well.

- *Writing and reading* (foreign language): the subjects writing abilities were slow at the beginning of the program, with many orthographic and grammatical errors. They quickly got autonomous self-correction, thanks to the voice synthesizer, as it would say whatever was taped without any interpretation of the meaning. They would tape, listen to the result, modify (sometimes ask the nurse for help), listen again. Only when the saying was correct, would they accept to make the other listen to their performance. The three first robotics sessions needed a lot of concentration for correctness of the writing, then the focus eased as the orthographic and grammar abilities increased. Once they became comfortable with this point, the subject started playing with the voice synthesizer, experimenting nonexistent words and generating sounds. Choregraphe software uses a functions library, the functions are described with an English word and a representative drawing. The English language was completely unknown to most subjects. The fact that the functions were described with English words did not seem to annoy their use, as the subjects easily recognized the drawings associated to the functions.
- *Organization, focus and efficiency*: To program the movements of the robot using the function *timeline*, it was needed to first imagine which movements are desired, then decompose the motion into fixed configurations that have to be saved in the software. Then the software generates trajectories from one registered configuration to the next one. There are two possibilities to register a configuration: (1) from the software interface, act on the motors of the virtual robot and put them one by one at the desired values; (2) release the tension in the motors of the real robot, put it in the desired configuration and put the tension back. This second situation is much easier to use, and was the one chosen for the application. Still, imagining the needed configurations and registering them required a strong focus from the subjects, even for simple motions. The first time they used the function (session 8), they managed 15 min of focus (time to make a gesture with the arms). The next time (session 10) they managed a 35 min of focus, as they were using the registered voice 1 and were building the motion with it.

4.1 Robot Image

The subjects' resulting drawings before (left) and after (right) Rob'Autism program are illustrated in Fig. 3. Most had first represented a robot as a threat, equipped with heavy weapons, before the program starts. The first contact with the robots was disappointing for them, as it looked not scary at all, even looked fragile and did not move as in their imagination (like a super hero). At the end of session 2, their disappointment had disappeared, replaced with amusement and interest. After the program has finished, the robot emotions are drawn first. Some are still equipped with weapons, but they have become protective robots and emotionally capable. These could be

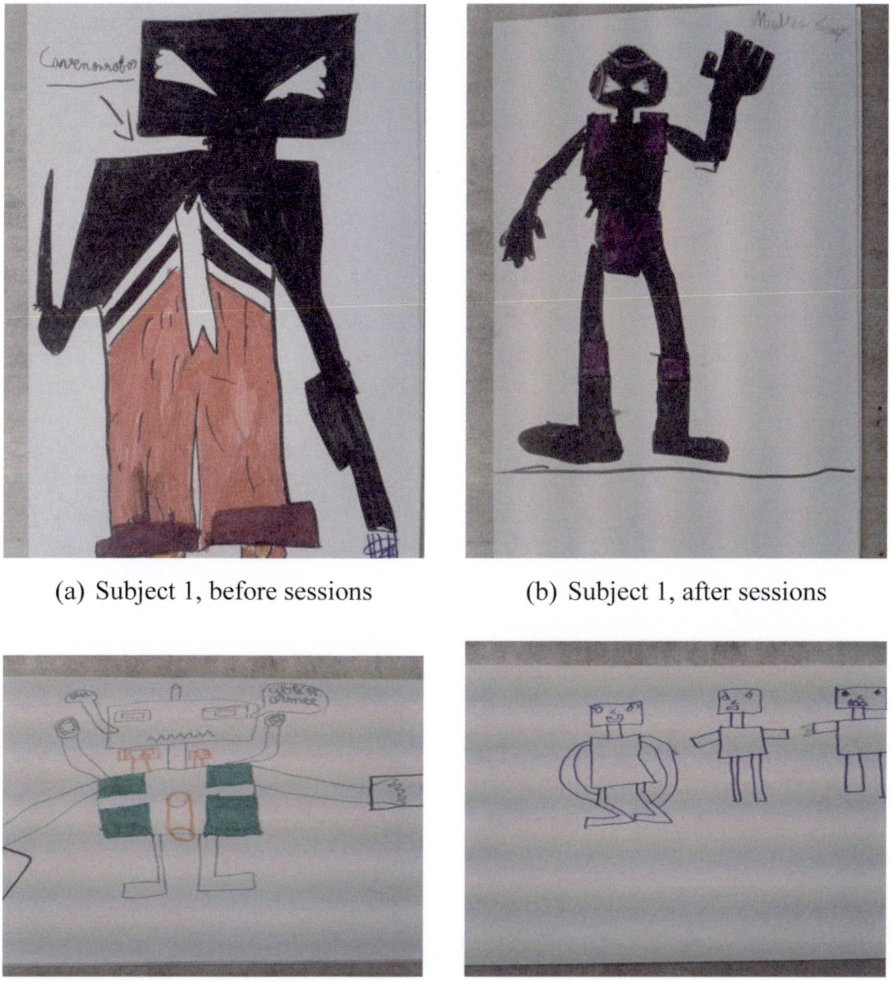

(a) Subject 1, before sessions

(b) Subject 1, after sessions

(c) Subject 6, before sessions

(d) Subject 6, after sessions

Fig. 3 Robot representation for two subjects, before and after Rob'Autism program

interpreted as the robot as social companion, as enhanced by so many authors. But a discussion with one of the children should be mentioned here:

- The robot is smiling because he is happy?
- No, the robot is smiling because *I* am happy.
- So this is you smiling?
- Yes.
- Why are you happy?
- (direct eye contact, with smile) Maybe the robot will tell you later.

This discussion had summarized most of the concept that was developed in Rob'Autism project: the use of a robot as a tool for communication, and not as a companion. There is no ambiguity for the subjects about the mechanical nature of the robot, which remains an object, such as a toy. But the subjects have used it to express emotions and say things.

4.2 The Public Show

The public show was organized with a limited number of strangers (12), sitting in the back of the children. The children were present in the room to welcome the arrival of the strangers. The show (introduction, performance, discussion) lasted around 90 min, during which the children sat quietly, listening to the introduction, watching the show and listening to the discussions afterward, answering questions when asked. They were solicited to interfere in the discussion, with the following questions: *Who was the first voice of the robot?*. The children did not move, and after a short time two of them pointed their colleague, who smiled looking down at his feet. The second question asked who was the second voice. After a few seconds, 5 children pointed "the second voice" saying his name and laughing. The pointed one said nothing but smiled, watching the ground. It was obvious that he was waiting to be pointed. Same scenario for the third and fourth voices. During the whole moment, the children never looked back at the public, remained sit.

When the public went out of the room, the children were at the door shaking hands and saying goodbye. Some people who attended the show asked afterward if the children really were autistic, which illustrates the amazing change in their behaviors with this program, as there was no doubt on this point when they first entered the room at the beginning of Rob'Autism.

There was no guaranty on the children behaviors with this public show. A few months before, it would have been impossible to perform it. The change concerns the desire of the children to share with the society what they had created. They were proud of their work, and proud to show it. The proud feeling was stronger that day than the stress of meeting strangers, the stress was naturally forgotten. After the departure of the strangers, all stayed in the room and enjoyed a drink with the team (medical staff, robotic and sound specialists). The children could follow organized discussion even among themselves, with normal tone of voices. Then they cheered a goodbye to the robot and sound specialists, taking them in their arm and wishing good holiday time with happiness smiles.

To conclude with this public robotic show: A program started in this year with the same children (Rob'Autism level 2), 6 months after the 2015 robotic show. At the second robotics session, one of the children stood up and asked in the name of his friends (watching him but remaining seated) to organize another show at the end of the program. Even though the children were surprised with the 2015 show, they clearly enjoyed it whole. The request, and the way they made it, illustrate the progress in communication skills they have made, and their will for improvement. The children have become actors of their project, not just attendees of the sessions.

4.3 Puppet Masters

Rob'Autism puts the robots as screens protecting the programmers from a direct interference with other human beings. The programmer is like a puppet master, acting in the shadow while doing great things. The use of robots for autistic children is classically made differently: the robot arrives with its own abilities, as a companion, and requires from the subjects like an adult could be requiring. Oppositely, in Rob'Autism, the robot is presented as an extension. The puppet master technique amplifies the robot abilities to make the autistic subject communicate. As the subject remains hidden, he/she is free of saying and doing anything. The public will look at the robot, and the responsibility of what was said or done is left to the robot: the programmer is not involved. This is a very comfortable way to start interfering with the world when ones do not have natural abilities for interaction. This point, actually, is the post important one in this project, and its effects should be evaluated and compared to the classical approach.

5 Conclusion

This paper explains the 20 weeks Rob'Autism protocol aimed at improving autistic people communication capabilities. The 20 sessions were described, as well as preparation and conclusion of the program. Several key points were addressed to perform the program, which uses three robots for six subjects: (1) the necessity to train the medical staff to program the robot, and the obligations to have a robot specialist in the room; (2) The importance for the programming subjects to see the other programmers' contributions and show their own; (3) The importance to alternate robotics and non-robotics sessions; (4) The importance to organize a final *public* show. This work was a preliminary study, questioning the efficiency of robot companion approach and proposing an extension approach based on the puppet master technique. Observed results showed fast changes in communication behavior, to the point that even though the autistic characteristic was obvious for all the subjects with a quick look at them when they started the program, but not so obvious at the end of the program, after only 20 h of training (only 10 h with the robots). The effects were observed during the sessions, but also very quickly outside the sessions. Finally, the progresses were still effective 6 months after the end of the program.

The next step should answer other questions on the program effects: are the changes permanent, or is it necessary to restart regularly a robot training session? Do the subject continue to improve with the same velocity their communication skills if using the robot longer, or do their skill stabilize? Also a larger population should be studied to check the generalizations of the results and the limits of this approach.

Acknowledgements Rob'Autism project was made possible thanks to the contribution of CHU-Nantes, Ecole Centrale de Nantes, and the two non-profit organizations Stereolux and *Robots!*. We also would like to thank MAIF and EPSI for the financial support they have provided.

References

1. Bekele, E.T., Lahiri, U., Swanson, A.R., Crittendon, J.A., Warren, Z.E., Sarkar, N.: A step towards developing adaptive robot-mediated intervention architecture (aria) for children with autism. IEEE Trans. Neural Syst. Rehabil. Eng. **21**(2) (2013)
2. Billard, A., Robins, B., Nadel, J., Dautenhahn, K.: Building robota, a mini-humanoid robot for the rehabilitation of children with autism. RESNA Assist. Technol. J. (2006)
3. Cabibihan, J.-J., Javed, H., Ang Jr, M., Aljunied, S.M.: Why robots? a survey on the roles and benefits of social robots in the therapy of children with autism. Int. J. Soc. Robot. **5**(4) (2013)
4. Dautenhahn, K.: I could be you: the phenomenological dimension of social understanding. J. Cybern. Syst. (1997)
5. Dautenhahn, K.: Robots as social actors: Aurora and the case of autism. In: Third International Cognitive Technology Conference (1999)
6. Dickerson, P., Robins, B., Dautenhahn, K.: Where the action is: a conversation analytic perspective on interaction between a humanoid robot, a co-present adult and a child with an asd. Interact. Stud. **14**(2) (2013)
7. Feil-Seifer, D., Black, M., Mataric, M.J., Narayanan, S.: Designing interactive technologies for supporting research in autism spectrum disorders. USC Interaction Lab Technical Report CRES-09-001 (2009)
8. Feil-Seifer, D., Mataric, M.J.: Using robots to augment (not replace) people in therapeutic settings. In: Robotics Science and Systems Workshop on Human-Robot Interaction: Perspectives and Contributions to Robotics from the Human Sciences (2011)
9. Robins, B., Dautenhahn, K., Dubowski, J.: Does appearance matter in the interaction of children with autism with a humanoid robot? Interac. Stud. **7**(3) (2006)
10. Robins, B., Dickerson, P., Stribling, P., Dautenhahn, K.: A case study in robot-human interaction. Interaction studies, Robot-mediated joint attention in children with autism (2004)
11. Scassellati, B.: How social robots will help us to diagnose, treat, and understand autism. In: International Symposium of Robotics Research (2005)
12. Shamsuddin S., Yussof H., Ismail L., Hanapiah F.A., Mohamed S., Piah, H.A., Zahari N.I.: Initial response of autistic children in human-robot interaction therapy with humanoid robot nao. In: International Colloquium on Signal Processing and its Applications (2012)
13. Tapus, A., Peca, A., Aly, A., Pop, C., Jisa, L., Pintea, S., Rusu, A.S., Daniel, O.D.: Children with autism social engagement in interaction with nao, an imitative robot: a series of single case experiments. Interact. Stud. **13**(2) (2012)
14. Werry, I., Dautenhahn, K.: Applying mobile robot technology to the rehabilitation of autistic children. In: International Symposium on Intelligent Robotic Systems (1999)
15. Werry, I., Dautenhahn, K.: Modeling biology: structures, behaviors, evolution – vienna series in theoretical biology. In: Human-Robot Interaction as a Model for Autism Therapy: An Experimental Study with Children with Autism, pp. 283–299 (2007)

Force Balance Conditions of Complex Parallel Mechanisms with Mass Equivalent Modeling

V. van der Wijk

Abstract A shaking force balanced mechanism is a mechanism that does not exert dynamic reaction forces to its base and to its surrounding for any motion. For mobile mechanisms such as exoskeletons, humanoid robots, drones, and anthropomorphic hands force balance is an important property for, among others, their dynamic behavior, stability, safety, control, and low energy consumption. For the design of force balanced mechanisms with multiple closed loops it can be a significant challenge to obtain the balance conditions, especially when the mechanism consists of closed loops that depend on other closed loops. In this paper it is shown how with mass equivalent modeling the force balance conditions can be derived of a complex multi-degree-of-freedom parallel mechanism with multiple closed loops of which one or more depend on other closed loops. It is shown how such a mechanism can be divided in mass equivalent linkages such as mass equivalent dyads and mass equivalent triads for which each can be analyzed individually with principal vectors and linear momentum equations.

Keywords Force balance · Mass equivalent modeling · Parallel mechanism · Center of mass

1 Introduction

A shaking force balanced mechanism is a mechanism that does not exert dynamic reaction forces to its base and to its surrounding for any motion. The sum of the linear momenta of all moving elements of a force balanced mechanism is constant for all motion which most of the times implies that the center of mass (CoM) of the mechanism is in a stationary point in the base. Also the motion of a force balanced mechanism is not affected by any translational motion of the base, i.e. the base and the mechanism are dynamically decoupled for translational motion of the base.

V. van der Wijk (✉)
Faculty of Natural and Mathematical Sciences, Department of Informatics, Centre for Robotics Research, King's College London, Strand, London, UK
e-mail: Volkert.vanderWijk@kcl.ac.uk

M. Husty and M. Hofbaur (eds.), *New Trends in Medical and Service Robots*, Mechanisms and Machine Science 48, DOI 10.1007/978-3-319-59972-4_20

For mobile mechanisms such as exoskeletons, humanoid robots, drones, and anthropomorphic hands force balance is an important property for their dynamic behavior [6], stability and control [2], safety, and ergonomics [5]. Since force balanced mechanisms are also statically balanced—gravity does not affect their motion, they lead to energy friendly actuation [3] and also to an increase of safety of large moving structures such as bridges [6]. For fast moving robotic manipulators force balance reduces the base vibrations such that cycle times can be shorter [10].

For the design of force balanced mechanisms with multiple closed loops it can be a significant challenge to obtain the general force balance conditions, especially when the mechanism consists of closed loops that depend on other closed loops. Common methods to derive the balance conditions require the explicit formulation of the closed-loop relations which then need to be included in the other equations where the linear dependent relations among the links need to be eliminated [1]. If at all possible, this leads to considerable efforts.

With mass equivalent modeling the loop closure relations can be considered implicitly. This has already shown to have potential to derive the force balance conditions of simple parallel mechanisms by balancing each arm individually [4, 11, 12] and also for complex parallel mechanisms by the design of inherently balanced closed-chain linkage architectures [6, 7] and by the design of mass equivalent dyad and triad linkages [8, 9]. The essence of this approach for complex linkages is that one or multiple links together are modeled with real and virtual equivalent masses, which subsequently are projected on the remaining open-chain linkage and included for analysis.

The goal of this paper is to show how with mass equivalent modeling the force balance conditions can be derived of a complex multi-degree-of-freedom (multi-DoF) parallel mechanism with multiple closed loops of which one or more depend on other closed loops. It is shown how such a mechanism can be divided in mass equivalent linkages such as mass equivalent dyads and mass equivalent triads for which each can be analyzed individually. First a two-DoF force balanced planar parallel mechanism with three closed loops is presented. This linkage is divided in one mass equivalent dyad and two mass equivalent triads. Then the balance conditions of the mass equivalent dyad are explained and subsequently the balance conditions and design parameters of the mass equivalent triads are obtained.

2 Two-DoF Force Balanced Planar Parallel Mechanism with Three Closed Loops

Figure 1a presents a planar parallel linkage which has two-DoF motion and three closed loops of which one depends on the other two. This new mechanism consists of the two four-bar linkages $A_0A_1A_2A_3$ and $A_4A_5A_6A_7$, with common base link $A_0A_3A_7A_4$, and a dyad $B_1C_1B_2$ of which B_1 and B_2 are revolute pairs with the coupler links of each four-bar linkage. Where each four-bar linkage has a single independent closed loop, the dyad gives a third dependent closed loop following a path through

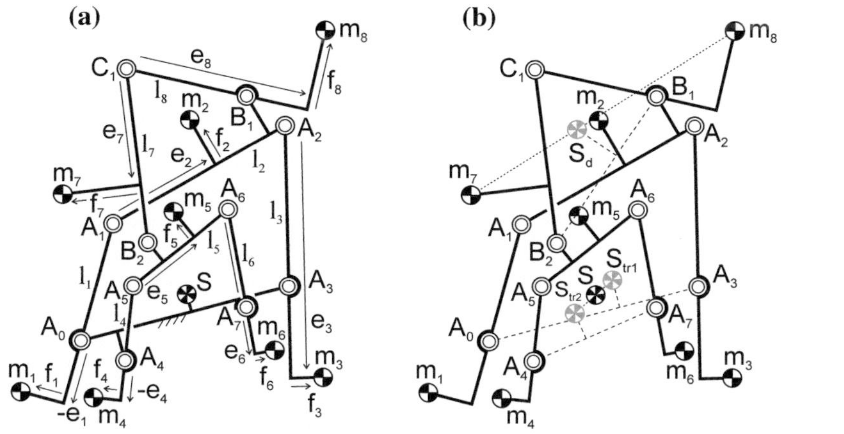

Fig. 1 **a** Force balanced parallel mechanism composed of two 4R four-bar linkages with common base and a dyad pivoted with each coupler link (*drawn to scale*); **b** The dyad and the two triads representing the 4R four-bar linkages are shown with their mass equivalent elements from which the force balance conditions are derived

each four-bar linkage. From the perspective of a driven parallel manipulator, both four-bar linkages can be moved individually with two actuators at the base whereby the motion of the dyad with joint C_1 as the end-effector is determined. Such a mechanism could be useful, for instance, as a manipulator on a service and inspection drone to move around rapidly without dynamically affecting (destabilizing) the hovering and manoeuvring drone itself.

Each link i of the mechanism has a mass m_i with its CoM defined by parameters e_i and f_i relative to the line through the joints of the link as illustrated in Fig. 1a. This means that each of the eight links can have a general design, i.e. mass symmetry is not required.

For specific relations among the link masses and the link CoMs the common CoM of all links together is in a stationary point S in the base link for all motion of the mechanism. These relations are named the *(shaking) force balance conditions* which in fact are design criteria for the links. The mechanism in Fig. 1a is shown with one of the many force balance solutions and is drawn to scale for a realistic impression.

With common methods such as the linear independent vector method [1] it is specifically challenging to handle the closed loop by the dyad because of its dependency on the closed loops of each four-bar linkage. However with mass equivalent modeling this can be considered in a systematic and insightful manner.

To derive the general force balance conditions the mechanism can be divided in three parts which each then is analyzed by means of a mass equivalent model. These three parts are the dyad $B_1C_1B_2$ with links masses m_7 and m_8, and each of the two four-bar linkages. In the next section the dyad is investigated for mass equivalence and the four-bar linkages are investigated for mass equivalence in the subsequent section.

3 Mass Equivalent Dyad

For force balance of the mechanism in Fig. 1a the dyad $B_1C_1B_2$ needs to have constant mass properties with respect to joints B_1 and B_2 for all motion such that these mass properties can be included in the force balance of the two four-bar linkages. This is since the motion of the dyad is nonlinearly related with the motion of the other links by which the design of the other links cannot contribute fully to the balance of the dyad links in another way. It can also be said that the dyad needs to be force balanced with respect to the 'imaginary dyad base link' B_1B_2. This imaginary link is shown in Fig. 1b where S_d is the common CoM of m_7 and m_8. Due to the motion of the mechanism the size of this imaginary link varies. As long as the triangle $B_1B_2S_d$ remains similar of shape for all motion while being scaled and rotated, the mass properties of the dyad relative to B_1 and B_2 are constant. The triangle $B_1B_2S_d$ with a mass $m_7 + m_8$ in S_d then is regarded a mass equivalent model of the dyad [8]. Also, from another viewpoint, for force balance the dyad needs to be mass equivalent to the model of the triangular element $B_1B_2S_d$ with mass $m_7 + m_8$ in S_d.

The conditions for which the triangular element $B_1B_2S_d$ and the dyad are mass equivalent have been derived as [8]

$$m_7e_7 = m_d^a l_7, \quad m_7f_7 = m_d^c l_7, \quad m_8e_8 = m_d^b l_8, \quad m_8f_8 = m_d^c l_8 \tag{1}$$

Here $m_d^a = (m_7 + m_8)(1 - \lambda_{d1})$ and $m_d^b = (m_7 + m_8)\lambda_{d1}$ are real equivalent masses with $m_d^a + m_d^b = m_7 + m_8$ and $m_d^c = (m_7 + m_8)\lambda_{d2}$ is a virtual equivalent mass. λ_{d1} and λ_{d2} are the similarity parameters, i.e. the properties that define the shape of the triangle $B_1B_2S_d$ by describing the location of S_d relative to line B_1B_2.

These conditions are the first four force balance conditions of the mechanism. For instance when l_7, l_8, m_7, m_8, e_7, and f_7 are given then e_8 and f_8 can be derived for force balance of the linkage in Fig. 1. Generally this means that the CoM of one of the dyad links is located beyond the joint with the coupler link as illustrated for m_8 that is located beyond joint B_1. In practice this implies the need of a countermass on link B_1C_1.

4 Mass Equivalent Triads

For force balance the two four-bar linkages need to have constant mass properties with respect to the base link $A_0A_3A_7A_4$, i.e. they need to be force balanced with respect to the base, for all motion. Since each four-bar linkage consists of three moving links, they can be regarded as triads $A_0A_1A_2A_3$ and $A_4A_5A_6A_7$ which, similar to the dyad, need to have constant mass properties with respect to their joints A_0, A_3, A_4, and A_7. This means that also the triads need to be mass equivalent to single-element models [9]. This is illustrated in Fig. 1b where triangle $A_0A_3S_{tr1}$ represents the equivalent mass model of triad $A_0A_1A_2A_3$ and triangle $A_4A_7S_{tr2}$ represents the equivalent mass model of triad $A_4A_5A_6A_7$.

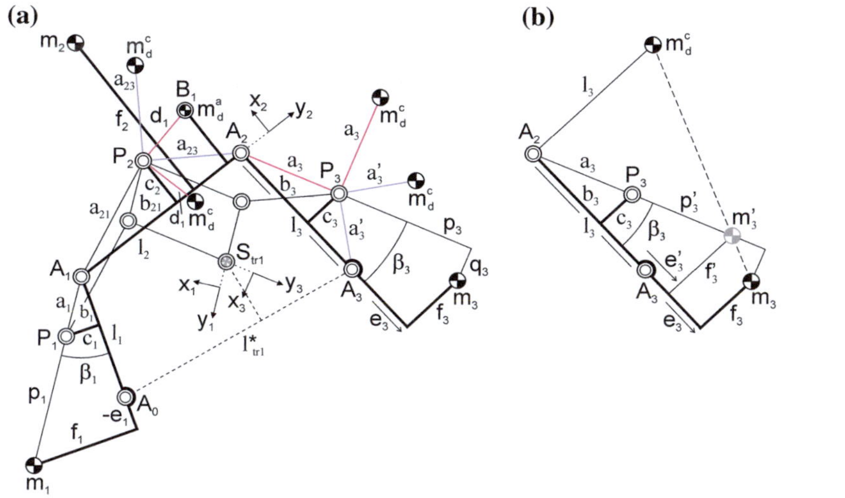

Fig. 2 **a** Triad 1 as a 3-DoF principal vector linkage with mass projection of the equivalent dyad with m_d^a in B_1 and m_d^c about P_2 and P_3; **b** For analysis of DoF 3 the masses in link A_2A_3 can be combined as m_3'

Since the dyad is located on top of the two triads, the mass of the dyad needs to be included in the triads as well. This means that the mass model $A_0A_3S_{tr1}$ includes the mass of triad $A_0A_1A_2A_3$ and part of the dyad mass with their common CoM in S_{tr1} and that the mass model $A_4A_7S_{tr2}$ includes the mass of triad $A_4A_5A_6A_7$ and the other part of the dyad mass with their common CoM in S_{tr2}. Both mass models lay in the base link with the common CoM of S_{tr1} and S_{tr2} located in S, which is the common CoM of the complete mechanism.

The force balance conditions of the triads can be derived with the methodology presented in [6, 8, 9] by analyzing each DoF of the triad independently with principal vectors. First these principal vectors are investigated, then the balance conditions are obtained with linear momentum equations for each relative DoF individually followed by the calculations of the mass parameters of the triad from the mass equivalent model.

Figure 2a shows the triad $A_0A_1A_2A_3$ as a 3-DoF principal vector linkage with a principal point P_1, P_2, and P_3 in each of the three principal elements—the triad links. These principal points define together with the principal joints A_1 and A_2 the three illustrated parallelograms which trace the common CoM in S_{tr1} for all motion. The lengths of the sides of the parallelograms a_1, a_{21}, a_{23}, and a_3 are the principal dimensions which are constants. This means that the parallelograms can be seen as rigid-body linkages with revolute pairs moving along with the triad. The location of the principal point in each principal element is defined with parameters b_i and c_i relative to the lines through the joints of the links.

In addition to the masses m_1, m_2, and m_3 of the triad, in Fig. 2a also the equivalent masses m_d^a and m_d^c of the dyad are projected. The real equivalent mass m_d^a is projected in B_1 and the virtual equivalent mass m_d^c is projected twice about P_2 and twice about P_3. About P_2 m_d^c is located at a distance $d_1 = \|B_1P_2\|$ from P_2 perpendicular to line B_1P_2 as illustrated and m_d^c is located at a distance $a_{23} = \|A_2P_2\|$ from P_2 perpendicular to line A_2P_2 as illustrated. About P_3 m_d^c is located at a distance $a_3 = \|A_2P_3\|$ from P_3 perpendicular to line A_2P_3 as illustrated and m_d^c is located at a distance $a_3' = \|A_3P_3\|$ from P_3 perpendicular to line A_3P_3 as illustrated.

The fundamentals of the mass projections are explained in detail in [6, 7]. The virtual equivalent mass m_d^c determines the positions of the link CoMs of the dyad perpendicular to the lines through the links' joints. To include this property in the triads they have to be projected about each principal point along a closed loop. The closed loop chosen here runs along $B_1P_2A_2P_3A_3 - A_7P_6A_6P_5B_2$, i.e. via triad 1, the base, and triad 2 with principal points P_5 and P_6 as shown in Fig. 4.

With the method of rotations about the principal joints (RAPJ) [6, 8] DoF 1 and DoF 3 can be analyzed. DoF 1 is the rotational motion of principal element A_0A_1 about principal joint A_1 with the other two principal elements immobile. This means that only mass m_1 is moving and for force balance its linear momentum should equal the linear momentum of the total mass of the triad moving along in joint S_{tr1}. The linear momentum of this motion can be written with respect to the aligned reference frame x_1y_1 as

$$\frac{\overline{L}_1}{\dot{\theta}_1} = \begin{bmatrix} m_{tr1}a_1 \\ 0 \end{bmatrix} = \begin{bmatrix} m_1(a_1 + p_1) \\ 0 \end{bmatrix} \tag{2}$$

with $m_{tr1} = m_1 + m_2 + m_3 + m_d^a$ the total mass of the triad model. The resulting force balance condition of this DoF is directly found as

$$m_1p_1 = (m_2 + m_3 + m_d^a)a_1 \tag{3}$$

DoF 3 is the rotational motion of principal element A_2A_3 about principal joint A_2 with the other two principal elements immobile and is analyzed similarly as DoF 1. It is useful to first combine all masses in principal element A_2A_3 as shown in Fig. 2b where the location of the total mass $m_3' = m_3 + m_d^c$ is defined by e_3' and f_3' which are calculated as

$$e_3' = \frac{m_3e_3}{m_3'}, \quad f_3' = \frac{m_3f_3 + m_d^cl_3}{m_3'} \tag{4}$$

Then for the motion of DoF 3 only mass m_3' is moving and for force balance its linear momentum equals the linear momentum of the total mass of the triad moving along in joint S_{tr1}. The linear momentum of this motion can be written with respect to the aligned reference frame x_3y_3 as

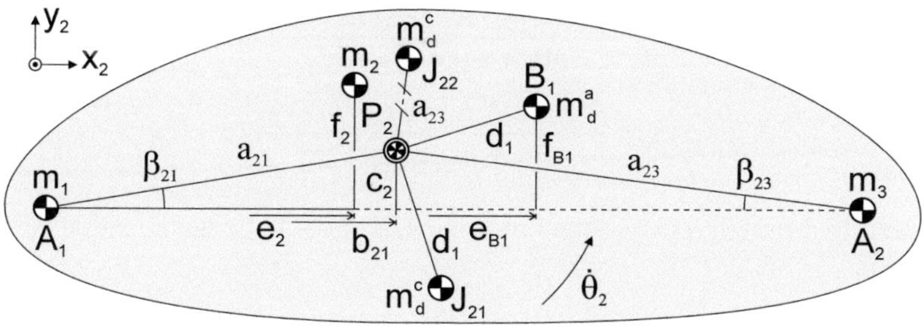

Fig. 3 Equivalent Linear Momentum System of DoF 2 of triad 1 of which P_2 is the center of mass for force balance

$$\frac{\overline{L}_3}{\dot{\theta}_3} = \begin{bmatrix} m_{tr1}a_3 \\ 0 \end{bmatrix} = \begin{bmatrix} m_3'(a_3 + p_3') \\ 0 \end{bmatrix} \tag{5}$$

with p_3' the distance between m_3' and P_3 as illustrated. The resulting force balance condition for this DoF is found as

$$(m_3 + m_d^c)p_3' = (m_1 + m_2 + m_d^a - m_d^c)a_3 \tag{6}$$

For DoF 2 the method of rotations about the principal points (RAPP) needs to be used [6, 9]. DoF 2 is the rotational motion of element A_1A_2 about principal point P_2 with elements A_0A_1 and A_2A_3 solely in translational motion. The linear momentum of this motion must equal zero for force balance since the total mass in joint S_{tr1} is stationary. To assist formulating the linear momentum equations, the mass motion can be modeled with the Equivalent Linear Momentum System shown in Fig. 3, which is a mass model with the same linear momentum for rotational motion about P_2. From this model the linear momentum of the motion of DoF 2 can be written with respect to the aligned reference frame x_2y_2 as

$$\begin{aligned} \frac{\overline{L}_2}{\dot{\theta}_2} = \begin{bmatrix} 0 \\ 0 \end{bmatrix} = m_1 \begin{bmatrix} c_2 \\ -b_{21} \end{bmatrix} + m_2 \begin{bmatrix} c_2 - f_2 \\ -(b_{21} - e_2) \end{bmatrix} + m_d^a \begin{bmatrix} c_2 - f_{B1} \\ -(b_{21} - e_{B1}) \end{bmatrix} - \\ m_d^c \begin{bmatrix} b_{21} - e_{B1} \\ c_2 - f_{B1} \end{bmatrix} + m_3 \begin{bmatrix} c_2 \\ -(b_{21} - l_2) \end{bmatrix} + m_d^c \begin{bmatrix} b_{21} - l_2 \\ c_2 \end{bmatrix} \end{aligned} \tag{7}$$

The resulting force balance conditions for this DoF are directly obtained as

$$\begin{aligned} m_1c_2 + m_2(c_2 - f_2) + m_d^a(c_2 - f_{B1}) - m_d^c(l_2 - e_{B1}) + m_3c_2 = 0 \\ m_1b_{21} + m_2(b_{21} - e_2) + m_d^a(b_{21} - e_{B1}) - m_d^c f_{B1} + m_3(b_{21} - l_2) = 0 \end{aligned} \tag{8}$$

To calculate the design parameters of the links, when parameters e_2 and f_2 are chosen the parameters b_{21} and c_2 of P_2 are obtained from Eqs. (8) as

$$b_{21} = \frac{m_2 e_2 + m_d^a e_{B1} + m_d^c f_{B1} + m_3 l_2}{m_1 + m_2 + m_3 + m_d^a} \quad (9)$$
$$c_2 = \frac{m_2 f_2 + m_d^a f_{B1} + m_d^c (l_2 - e_{B1})}{m_1 + m_2 + m_3 + m_d^a}$$

Subsequently the design parameters of links A_0A_1 and A_2A_3 can be calculated from the relations

$$\frac{p_1 + a_1}{a_1} = \frac{e_1}{b_1} = \frac{f_1}{c_1}, \quad \frac{p_3' + a_3}{a_3} = \frac{e_3'}{b_3} = \frac{f_3'}{c_3} \quad (10)$$

with which the link CoM parameters can be derived to depend on b_i and c_i as

$$e_1 = (\frac{p_1}{a_1} + 1)b_1 = (\frac{m_2 + m_3 + m_d^a}{m_1} + 1)b_1$$
$$f_1 = (\frac{p_1}{a_1} + 1)c_1 = (\frac{m_2 + m_3 + m_d^a}{m_1} + 1)c_1 \quad (11)$$
$$e_3' = (\frac{p_3'}{a_3} + 1)b_3 = (\frac{m_1 + m_2 + m_d^a - m_d^c}{m_3 + m_d^c} + 1)b_3$$
$$f_3' = (\frac{p_3'}{a_3} + 1)c_3 = (\frac{m_1 + m_2 + m_d^a - m_d^c}{m_3 + m_d^c} + 1)c_3$$

The relations for a triad to be mass equivalent with the element $A_0A_3S_{tr1}$ are [9]

$$m_{tr_i}^a (l_1 - b_1) = m_{tr_i}^b b_1, \qquad m_{tr_i}^c l_1 = (m_{tr_i}^a + m_{tr_i}^b) c_1$$
$$m_{tr_i}^a b_{21} = m_{tr_i}^b (l_2 - b_{21}), \qquad m_{tr_i}^c l_2 = (m_{tr_i}^a + m_{tr_i}^b) c_2 \quad (12)$$
$$m_{tr_i}^a b_3 = m_{tr_i}^b (l_3 - b_3), \qquad m_{tr_i}^c l_3 = (m_{tr_i}^a + m_{tr_i}^b) c_3$$

with the equivalent triad masses $m_{tr_1}^a$, $m_{tr_1}^b$, and $m_{tr_1}^c$. With b_{21} and c_2 known, they are obtained from these relations as

$$m_{tr_1}^a = m_1 + m_2 + m_3 + m_d^a - m_{tr_1}^b \quad (13)$$
$$m_{tr_1}^b = \frac{m_1 + m_2 + m_3 + m_d^a}{l_2} b_{21}, \quad m_{tr_1}^c = \frac{m_1 + m_2 + m_3 + m_d^a}{l_2} c_2$$

and subsequently c_1, c_3, b_1, and b_3 can be calculated as

$$b_1 = \frac{m^a_{tr_1}}{m_1 + m_2 + m_3 + m^a_d} l_1, \quad c_1 = \frac{m^c_{tr_1}}{m_1 + m_2 + m_3 + m^a_d} l_1$$
$$b_3 = \frac{m^b_{tr_1}}{m_1 + m_2 + m_3 + m^a_d} l_3, \quad c_3 = \frac{m^c_{tr_1}}{m_1 + m_2 + m_3 + m^a_d} l_3 \tag{14}$$

Herewith all parameters are known for force balance. In addition, the similarity parameters of triad 1 defining the shape of element $A_0A_3S_{tr1}$ can be found as

$$\lambda_{tr11} = \frac{m^b_{tr_1}}{m_1 + m_2 + m_3 + m^a_d}, \quad \lambda_{tr12} = \frac{m^c_{tr_1}}{m_1 + m_2 + m_3 + m^a_d} \tag{15}$$

and the principal dimensions a_1, a_{21}, a_{23}, and a_3 can be calculated as

$$\begin{aligned}
a_1 &= \sqrt{b_1^2 + c_1^2} = l_1\sqrt{(1-\lambda_{tr11})^2 + \lambda_{tr12}^2} \\
a_{21} &= \sqrt{b_{21}^2 + c_2^2} = l_2\sqrt{\lambda_{tr11}^2 + \lambda_{tr12}^2} \\
a_{23} &= \sqrt{(l_2 - b_{21})^2 + c_2^2} = l_2\sqrt{(1-\lambda_{tr11})^2 + \lambda_{tr12}^2} \\
a_3 &= \sqrt{b_3^2 + c_3^2} = l_3\sqrt{\lambda_{tr11}^2 + \lambda_{tr12}^2}
\end{aligned} \tag{16}$$

For triad 2 the force balance conditions and the design parameters are derived similarly to triad 1. Figure 4a shows the triad $A_4A_5A_6A_7$ as a 3-DoF principal vector linkage with a principal point P_4, P_5, and P_6 in each of the three principal elements. These principal points define together with the principal joints A_5 and A_6 the three illustrated parallelograms which trace the common CoM in S_{tr2} for all motion. The lengths of the sides of the parallelograms are the principal dimensions a_4, a_{54}, a_{56}, and a_6.

In Fig. 4a also the equivalent masses m^b_d and m^c_d of the dyad are projected with the real equivalent mass m^b_d in B_2 and the virtual equivalent mass m^c_d projected twice about P_5 and twice about P_6. About P_5 m^c_d is located at a distance $d_2 = ||B_2P_5||$ from P_5 perpendicular to line B_2P_5 as illustrated and m^c_d is located at a distance $a_{56} = ||A_6P_5||$ from P_5 perpendicular to line A_6P_5 as illustrated. About P_6 m^c_d is located at a distance $a_6 = ||A_6P_6||$ from P_6 perpendicular to line A_6P_6 as illustrated and m^c_d is located at a distance $a'_6 = ||A_7P_6||$ from P_6 perpendicular to line A_7P_6 as illustrated.

Following the same procedure as for triad 1, the linear momentum of DoF 1 of triad 2, which is the rotational motion of A_4A_5 about A_5 with the other triad links immobile, can be written relative to the aligned reference frame x_4y_4 as

$$\frac{\bar{L}_4}{\dot{\theta}_4} = \begin{bmatrix} m_{tr2}a_4 \\ 0 \end{bmatrix} = \begin{bmatrix} m_4(a_4 + p_4) \\ 0 \end{bmatrix} \tag{17}$$

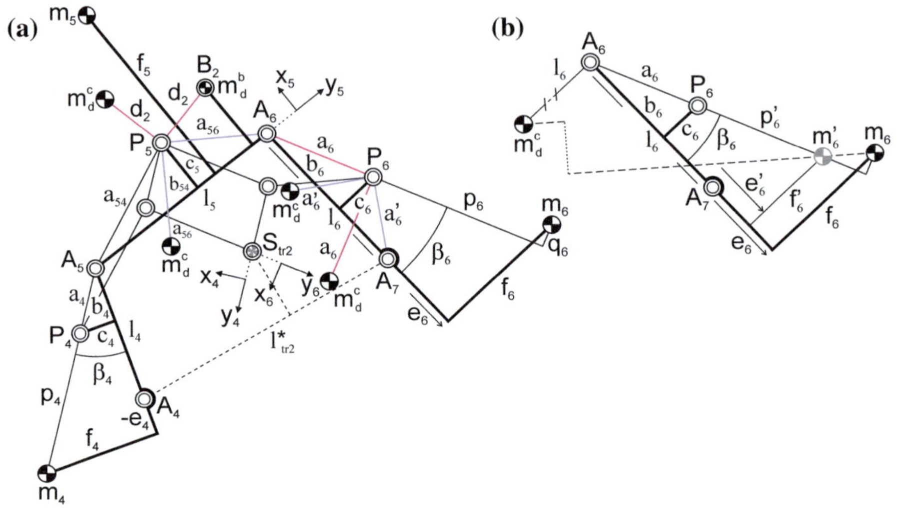

Fig. 4 **a** Triad 2 as a 3-DoF principal vector linkage with mass projection of the equivalent dyad with m_d^b in B_2 and m_d^c about P_5 and P_6; **b** For analysis of DoF 3 the masses in link A_6A_7 can be combined as m_6'

with $m_{tr2} = m_4 + m_5 + m_6 + m_d^b$ the total mass of the triad model with CoM in joint S_{tr2}. The masses in principal element A_6A_7 can be combined in total mass $m_6' = m_6 + m_d^c$ with CoM defined by e_6' and f_6' which are calculated as

$$e_6' = \frac{m_6 e_6}{m_6'}, \quad f_6' = \frac{m_6 f_6 - m_d^c l_6}{m_6'} \tag{18}$$

Then the linear momentum of DoF 3 of triad 2, which is the rotational motion of principal element A_6A_7 about principal joint A_6 with the other two principal elements immobile, can be written relative to the aligned reference frame x_6y_6 as

$$\frac{\bar{L}_6}{\dot{\theta}_6} = \begin{bmatrix} m_{tr2}a_6 \\ 0 \end{bmatrix} = \begin{bmatrix} m_6'(a_6 + p_6') \\ 0 \end{bmatrix} \tag{19}$$

For DoF 2, the rotational motion of element A_5A_6 about principal point P_5 with elements A_4A_5 and A_6A_7 solely in translational motion, Fig. 5 shows the Equivalent Linear Momentum System. For force balance P_5 is the CoM of this mass model. From this model the linear momentum can be written with respect to the aligned reference frame x_5y_5 as

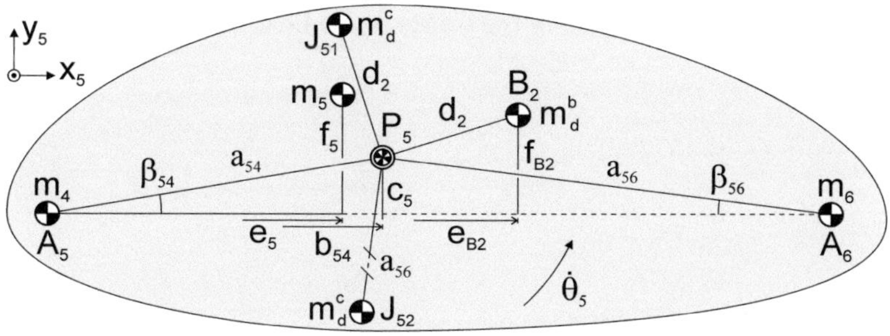

Fig. 5 Equivalent Linear Momentum System of DoF 2 of triad 2 of which P_5 is the center of mass for force balance

$$
\frac{\overline{L}_5}{\dot{\theta}_5} = \begin{bmatrix} 0 \\ 0 \end{bmatrix} = m_4 \begin{bmatrix} c_5 \\ -b_{54} \end{bmatrix} + m_5 \begin{bmatrix} c_5 - f_5 \\ -(b_{54} - e_5) \end{bmatrix} + m_d^b \begin{bmatrix} c_5 - f_{B2} \\ -(b_{54} - e_{B2}) \end{bmatrix} + m_d^c \begin{bmatrix} b_{54} - e_{B2} \\ c_5 - f_{B2} \end{bmatrix} + m_6 \begin{bmatrix} c_5 \\ -(b_{54} - l_5) \end{bmatrix} - m_d^c \begin{bmatrix} b_{54} - l_5 \\ c_5 \end{bmatrix} \tag{20}
$$

From Eqs. (17), (19) and (20) the force balance conditions for triad 2 are obtained as

$$
\begin{aligned}
m_4 p_4 &= (m_5 + m_6 + m_d^b) a_4 \\
(m_6 + m_d^c) p_6' &= (m_4 + m_5 + m_d^b - m_d^c) a_6 \\
0 &= m_4 c_5 + m_5 (c_5 - f_5) + m_d^b (c_5 - f_{B2}) + m_d^c (l_5 - e_{B2}) + m_6 c_5 \\
0 &= m_4 b_{54} + m_5 (b_{54} - e_5) + m_d^b (b_{54} - e_{B2}) + m_d^c f_{B2} + m_6 (b_{54} - l_5)
\end{aligned} \tag{21}
$$

Similarly as for triad 1, the parameters of the principal points P_4, P_5, and P_6 can be calculated as

$$
\begin{aligned}
b_4 &= \frac{m_{tr_2}^a}{m_4 + m_5 + m_6 + m_d^b} l_4, & c_4 &= \frac{m_{tr_2}^c}{m_4 + m_5 + m_6 + m_d^b} l_4 \\
b_{54} &= \frac{m_5 e_5 + m_d^b e_{B2} - m_d^c f_{B2} + m_6 l_5}{m_4 + m_5 + m_6 + m_d^b}, & c_5 &= \frac{m_5 f_5 + m_d^b f_{B2} - m_d^c (l_5 - e_{B2})}{m_4 + m_5 + m_6 + m_d^b} \\
b_6 &= \frac{m_{tr_2}^b}{m_4 + m_5 + m_6 + m_d^b} l_6, & c_6 &= \frac{m_{tr_2}^c}{m_4 + m_5 + m_6 + m_d^b} l_6
\end{aligned} \tag{22}
$$

with

$$
\begin{aligned}
m_{tr_2}^a &= m_4 + m_5 + m_6 + m_d^b - m_{tr_2}^b \\
m_{tr_2}^b &= \frac{m_4 + m_5 + m_6 + m_d^b}{l_5} b_{54}, \quad m_{tr_2}^c = \frac{m_4 + m_5 + m_6 + m_d^b}{l_5} c_5
\end{aligned} \tag{23}
$$

and subsequently the parameters of the CoMs of the links can be calculated with

$$\begin{aligned} e_4 &= \frac{m_4 + m_5 + m_6 + m_d^b}{m_4} b_4, & f_4 &= \frac{m_4 + m_5 + m_6 + m_d^b}{m_4} c_4 \\ e_6' &= \frac{m_4 + m_5 + m_6 + m_d^b}{m_6 + m_d^c} b_6, & f_6' &= \frac{m_4 + m_5 + m_6 + m_d^b}{m_6 + m_d^c} c_6 \\ e_6 &= \frac{m_6 + m_d^c}{m_6} e_6', & f_6 &= \frac{(m_6 + m_d^c) f_6' + m_d^c l_6}{m_6} \end{aligned} \tag{24}$$

Herewith all parameters are known for force balance of triad 2. The similarity parameters of triad 2 which define the shape of element $A_4A_7S_{tr2}$ can be found as

$$\lambda_{tr21} = \frac{m_{tr_2}^b}{m_4 + m_5 + m_6 + m_d^b}, \quad \lambda_{tr22} = \frac{m_{tr_2}^c}{m_4 + m_5 + m_6 + m_d^b} \tag{25}$$

and the principal dimensions a_4, a_{54}, a_{56}, and a_6 can be calculated as

$$\begin{aligned} a_4 &= \sqrt{b_4^2 + c_4^2} = l_4 \sqrt{(1 - \lambda_{tr21})^2 + \lambda_{tr22}^2} \\ a_{54} &= \sqrt{b_{54}^2 + c_5^2} = l_5 \sqrt{\lambda_{tr21}^2 + \lambda_{tr22}^2} \\ a_{56} &= \sqrt{(l_5 - b_{54})^2 + c_5^2} = l_5 \sqrt{(1 - \lambda_{tr21})^2 + \lambda_{tr22}^2} \\ a_6 &= \sqrt{b_6^2 + c_6^2} = l_6 \sqrt{\lambda_{tr21}^2 + \lambda_{tr22}^2} \end{aligned} \tag{26}$$

5 Discussion and Conclusion

In this paper it was shown how with mass equivalent modeling the force balance conditions can be derived of a complex multi-degree-of-freedom parallel mechanism with multiple closed loops of which one depends on the other closed loops. By dividing the mechanism in three parts it was investigated as a combination of a mass equivalent dyad on top of two mass equivalent triads. With the method of principal vectors and the linear momentum equations of each relative degree-of-freedom the force balance conditions were derived and the design parameters were calculated for each of three parts individually.

The approach of mass equivalent modeling can also be used for the *synthesis* of complex force balanced mechanisms by composing the new mechanism of combined mass equivalent linkages. There is a wide variety of possibilities to do this, already when solely using mass equivalent dyads and triads. The advantage with mass equivalent modeling is that the closed-loop relations do not need to be formulated but are considered implicitly. Also it is possible to apply this method for spatial mechanisms. For instance by applying two mass equivalent triads as balanced four-bar linkages with common base as in this paper but placing them in different planes under a relative angle instead of having them in the same plane, with a spatially moving mass equivalent dyad on top.

Acknowledgements This publication was financially supported by the Niels Stensen Fellowship

References

1. Berkof, R.S., Lowen, G.G.: A new method for completely force balancing simple linkages. Eng. Ind. 21–26 (1969)
2. Brown, G.W.: Suspension system for supporting and conveying equipment, such as a camera, patent US-4710819 (1987)
3. Chung, W.K., Cho, H.S.: On the dynamic characteristics of a balanced PUMA-760 robot. Ind. Electron. **35**(2), 222–230 (1988)
4. Gosselin, C.M., Vollmer, F., Côté, G., Wu, Y.: Synthesis and design of reactionless three-degree-of-freedom parallel mechanisms. IEEE Trans. Robot. Autom. **20**(2), 191–199 (2004)
5. Ishida, K., Matsuda, T.: Performance characteristics and working comfortableness of forest workers of a new non-vibrating chain saw utilizing perfectly balanced rotation-reciprocation device. In: Proceedings of the Fifth World Congress of Theory of Machines and Mechanisms, pp. 951–954. ASME (1979)
6. van der Wijk, V.: Methodology for analysis and synthesis of inherently force and moment-balanced mechanisms—theory and applications (dissertation). University of Twente (2014). (free download: doi:10.3990/1.9789036536301)
7. van der Wijk, V.: Closed-chain principal vector linkages. In: Flores, P., Viadero, F. (eds.), New Trends in Mechanism and Machine Science, vol. 24, pp. 829–837. Springer (2015)
8. van der Wijk, V.: Mass equivalent dyads. In: Bai, S., Ceccarrelli, M. (eds.), Recent Advances in Mechanism Design for Robotics, vol. MMS 33, pp. 35–45. Springer (2015)
9. van der Wijk, V.: Mass equivalent triads. In: Proceedings of the 14th IFToMM World Congress in Mechanism and Machine Science, p. OS13.131/10.6567 (2015)
10. van der Wijk, V., Krut, S., Pierrot, F., Herder, J.L.: Design and experimental evaluation of a dynamically balanced redundant planar 4-RRR parallel manipulator. Int. J. Robot. Res. **32**(6), 744–759 (2013)
11. Wu, Y., Gosselin, C.M.: Design of reactionless 3-DOF and 6-DOF parallel manipulators using parallelepiped mechanisms. IEEE Trans. Robot. **21**(5), 821–833 (2005)
12. Wu, Y., Gosselin, C.M.: On the dynamic balancing of multi-dof parallel mechanisms with multiple legs. Mech. Des. **129**, 234–238 (2007)

Numerical Simulations and Experimental Human Gait Analysis Using Wearable Sensors

D. Tarnita, I. Geonea, A. Petcu and D.N. Tarnita

Abstract The paper presents a comparison between an experimental study of flexion-extension movement in human legs joints and numerical simulations on a virtual mannequin computed in ADAMS virtual environment. Using Biometrics system which is a data acquisition system based on electrogoniometers, data were collected for the right and left ankle, knee and hip during experimental gait overground on force platforms. The mean flexion-extension cycles for legs joints were obtained. The obtained experimental data series were be introduced as input data in the joints of the virtual mannequin and a walking simulation was performed in ADAMS environment software. The variation of ground forces during walking are obtained by experimental data and by virtual simulation.

Keywords Human gait · Kinematics · Ground reaction forces · Electrogoniometers · Force platforms · Virtual mannequin · ADAMS simulation

1 Introduction

In last years, several humanoids robots are able to walk and perform human-like movements, several humanoid friendly robots that assist human activities in human daily environments such as in homes, offices, and hospitals, have been developed

---

D. Tarnita (✉) · I. Geonea · A. Petcu
University of Craiova, Craiova, Romania
e-mail: tarnita.daniela@gmail.com

I. Geonea
e-mail: igeonea@yahoo.com

A. Petcu
e-mail: petcu.alin.i@gmail.com

D.N. Tarnita
University of Medicine and Pharmacy, Craiova, Romania
e-mail: dan_tarnita@yahoo.com

M. Husty and M. Hofbaur (eds.), *New Trends in Medical and Service Robots*,
Mechanisms and Machine Science 48, DOI 10.1007/978-3-319-59972-4_21

[1–5]. In papers [4, 5] the authors present a human-oriented approach to the study of the biped gait for a humanoid robot. Starting from the analysis of the human lower-limbs, they pointed the main features of the human legs for a correct walking motion useful in the mechanical design of a humanoid robot. Humanoid robots will be developed in next future because of anthropomorphism applicability of locomotion.

Objective gait analysis techniques are based on the use of different devices to capture and measure information related to the various gait parameters [6].

The main four clinical applications of wearable sensors and acquisition data systems are: (a) identifying movement disorders, (b) assessing surgical outcomes, (c) improving walking stability, and (d) reducing joint loading [7]. Recent technological advances have produced sensors that are smaller, lighter, and more robust than previous versions [7]. Wearable sensing systems make it possible to analyze data outside the laboratory and capture information about the human gait during the person's everyday activities. Different types of sensors are used to capture the various signals that characterize the human gait [8, 9].

Goniometers can be used to study the angles for ankles, knees, hips and other human joints [10–15]. The main advantages of the wearable sensing systems are presented in [6]: Transparent analysis and monitoring of gait during daily activities and on the long term; Allows the possibility of deployment in any place, not needing controlled environments; Wireless systems enhance usability; In clinical gait analysis, promotes autonomy and active role of patients.

The force platform is now an indispensable tool in a state-of-the-art motion analysis laboratory which is used together with kinematic and EMG measurements in order to obtain maximum clinical implementation and interpretation of force plate measurements [16]. Force platforms are used in gait analysis to measure the gait by pressure or force sensors and moment transducers when the subject walks on them. Ground reaction force sensors (GRF) which measure the force exerted by the subject's feet on the floor when he walks are determined using force platforms. GRF measurement was used earlier in the various gait analysis studies, i.e. identification of muscle forces in human lower limbs during sagittal plane movements in the monitoring of the patients physiotherapy process [17, 18].

The first objective of this study is to measure the variation of flexion-extension angles of the human legs joints while the subject performs normal walking on a set of force platforms. The obtained experimental data series will be introduced as input data in the joints of a virtual mannequin and a virtual walking simulation will be performed in ADAMS environment software. The variation of ground forces will be obtained by experimental data and by virtual simulation and will be compared. The second objective supposes the determination, by numerical simulation, of the reactions forces developed in the lower limbs joints in order to perform an analysis with the finite element method and obtain the stresses and deformations maps for the normal joints, for the osteoarthritic joints and for prosthetic joints.

2 Experimental Study

The experimental method which allows obtaining the kinematic parameters diagrams for the human knee joint uses a Biometrics Ltd data acquisition system based on electrogonimeters and on force platforms. Biometrics Ltd is a world leader in the design, manufacture and distribution of technologically advanced sensors, instruments and software for the demanding needs in biomedical and engineering research [19]. DataLog MWX8 is the latest in data acquisition technology for portable data collection and ambulatory monitoring on 8 channels simultaneously in human gait, human performance, medical research, robotics [19]. A lot of research studies used for human gait analysis various wearable sensors such as, electogoniometers, and the Biometrics data acquisition system [20, 21].

Using Biometrics system and the appropriate sensors (electrogoniometers and force platforms), in our study the experimental measurements were performed for five trials of ten consecutive walking cycles of a male subject. The subject was pain-free and had no evidence or known history of motor and skeletal disorders or record of surgery to the lower limbs. The experimental data were acquired for the right and left ankle joints, right and left knee joints and right and left hip joints, for overground walking cycles on six force platforms. In Table 1 the values for anthropometric data of male subject are presented.

In the performed experiments six force platforms, 3 for right leg and 3 for left leg, type FP4, from Biometrics system were used. These were arranged on a flat surface so the distance between them is equal to the steps of the subject. Taking into account the anthropometric data of the subject, the distance between the first and second force platform representing a step has been selected for a value equal to 580 mm and the distance between the left and right force platforms was chosen 280 mm. For data acquisition a 8-channel DataLOG at a frequency of 500 Hz (MWX 8 Biometrics Ltd) was used, each platform being assigned to a channel numbered from 1 to 6 in order of settlement on the floor surface. DataLOG was connected with each platform using a H2000 cable, and transfer data from the computer DataLOG was conducted in real time via Bluetooth.

For measuring angles variation during the gait, for the six joints of both lower limbs, six flexible electrogoniometers were used. For the ankle joint for both left and right legs were used two twin axis goniometers SG100. Attachment to the ankle

Table 1 Values of anthropometric data

Age (years)	Weight (kg)	Height (cm)	Leg length (cm)	Hip–knee length (cm)	Knee–ankle length (cm)
35	68	168	81	42	39

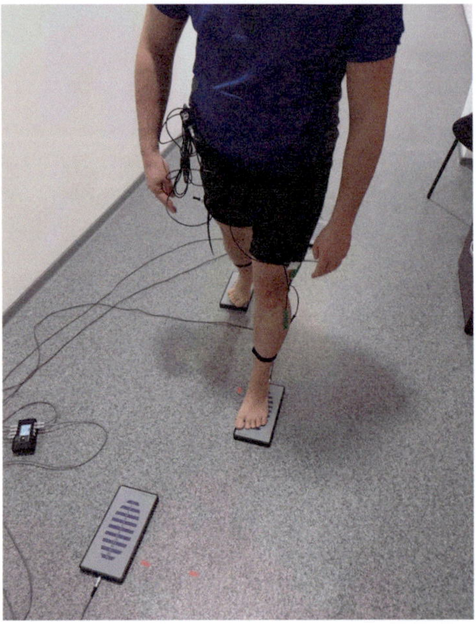

Fig. 1 Subject with mounted Biometrics data acquisition system

joint was performed in two steps. First the distal endblock of the SG110 was attached on the back of the heel. After flexion of ankle, the proximal endblock was attached to the posterior of the leg so that the axis of the leg and endblock coincide. For knee and hip joints of both legs, four twin axis goniometers SG 150 were used. For knee joint, starting with the subject standing in the neutral position with the foot on a flat surface, the distal endblock was mounted laterally on the leg so the axes of the leg and endblock coincide, when viewed in the sagittal plane, with the leg fully extended in the position of reference extend the goniometer to maximum length and attach the proximal endblock to the thigh so the axes of the thigh and endblock coincide. For hip joint, with the limb in position of reference, the goniometer was extend to maximum length and the distal endblock was attached to the thigh so the axes of the thigh and endblock coincide. All measurements were performed with a frequency of 500 Hz.

The experimental trials were approved by the University of Craiova human ethics research committee and they were performed in the biomechanics laboratory at INCESA Research Centre, University of Craiova. Before starting the experiments there were collected anthropometric data from the human subject. In Fig. 1 the data acquisition system mounted on the subject is shown. In Fig. 2 different Biometrics flexible electrogoniometers and the DataLog device are presented.

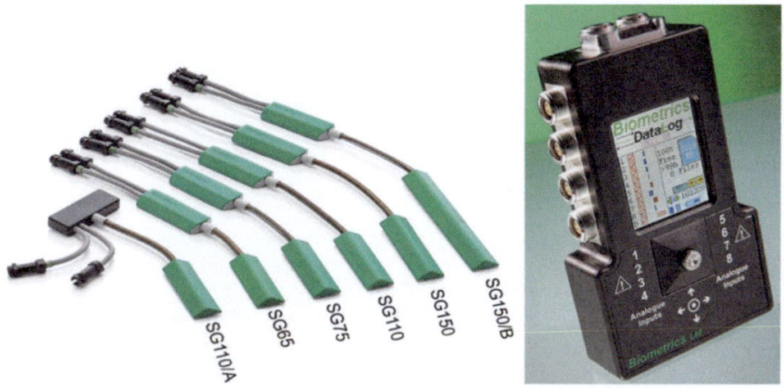

Fig. 2 Biometrics flexible goniometers and Data Log data acquisition system [19]

3 Numerical Simulations

3.1 Multibody Model of a Mannequin Walking

Multi-Body Systems environment uses virtual prototyping techniques which allows modeling mechanical systems, simulating their motion under real conditions and their optimization [22, 23]. Multibody methods are used for human gait analysis when the investigation is focused on mechanical aspects, such establish of joints reaction forces [24]. For that purpose, the inverse dynamics approach is used, based, as inputs data, on the human leg joints angular variations to establish the joints reaction forces and torques.

In this research a virtual mannequin in the assumption of ground walking is modeled as a multibody model. The virtual model of the mannequin, which follows the anthropometric data of human subject, taken from Table 1 is developed in Solid Works virtual environment. A detail of designed mannequin presenting 14 rigid parts is presented in Fig. 3.

Mannequin walking is a special kind of the multibody system with the occurrence of impacts, friction and slipping. All these aspects observed during the foot-ground contact have to be introduced into the model to make it real. In this research, both the slips and impacts are taken into consideration. The model was developed in ADAMS environment [25].

Mannequin legs are modeled realistically consisting of 3 parts: thigh, shank and foot. Each revolute joint, representing the hip, knee and ankle, is additionally constrained by a motion generator, as presented in Fig. 3.

Motion laws of the human leg joints, established experimentally, are introduced in ADAMS using a spline function and the Akima fitting method [26] (Fig. 4). The impact and friction effects are considered in the ground reaction forces modeling. It is used the impact model contact in ADAMS, and the friction is specified according Coulomb model. A number of test simulations are performed in order to choose proper values of estimated stiffness **k** of the foot in shoe and proper values of

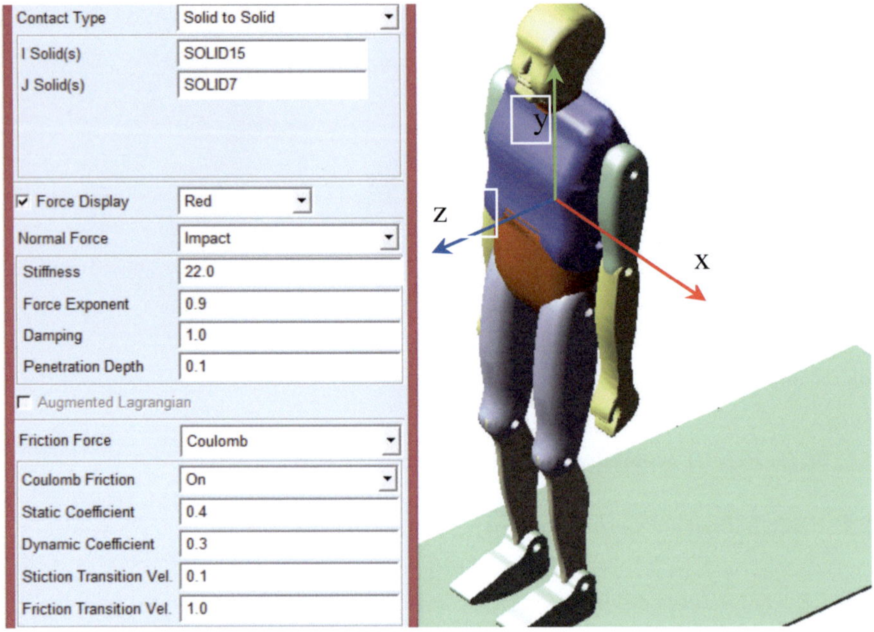

Fig. 3 Virtual model of a mannequin in ADAMS and ground-foot contact parameters

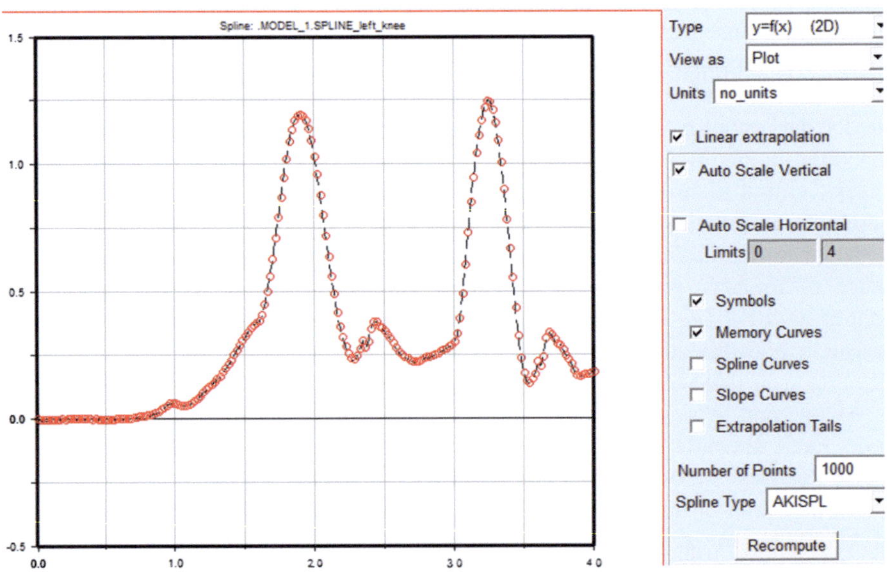

Fig. 4 Left knee angular motion obtained in ADAMS by using spline function

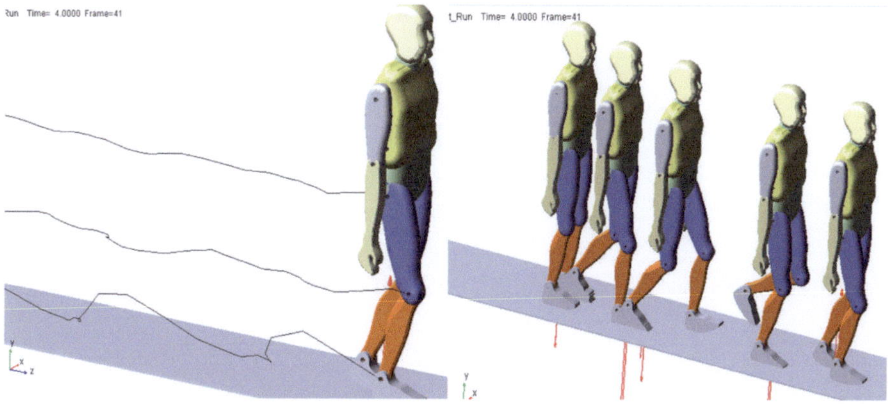

Fig. 5 Mannequin leg joints trajectory and superimposed walking frames, computed in ADAMS

damping parameters ***d*** and ***C***. Contact parameters according to this model are presented in Fig. 3. For this simulation approach the ground reaction forces are computed in ADAMS (they do not play the role of input data). Comparison of the measured ground reaction forces with the calculated ones are used to validate the model. The calculated and the measured results are similar, however there are some differences. These differences are caused mostly by the fact that foot is modeled as rigid.

To obtain better results the model of foot and the model of contact should be made more complex [27].

Dynamic simulation in ADAMS is performed using the WSTIFF solver and SI2 integrator [28]. The gait patterns of the markers attached to the ankle, knee and hip, obtained from ADAMS dynamic simulation, are shown in Fig. 5. Also superimposed frames from mannequin walk animation are shown.

4 Results

The angular variations of the six human joints flexion-extension during the gait performed on the treadmill were obtained from the report generated by the acquisition system as data files. For a good accuracy of the collected data, the transient data were removed, so the first two and the last two cycles were removed.

The results of measurements were exported in .txt as datasets and then imported into SIMIMOTION software. The diagrams of Ground Reactions Forces corresponding to the trial 1, obtained for the six force platforms are shown in Fig. 6 and the corresponding diagrams of the ankle, knee and hip flexion-extension angles collected using the acquisition data system for both legs (right and left) are shown in Fig. 7. The graphs were divided into gait cycles starting with the point of

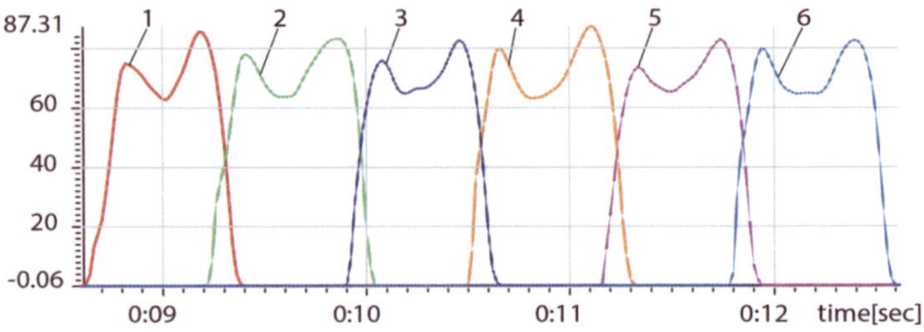

Fig. 6 The experimental Ground Reactions Forces variations on the six force platforms

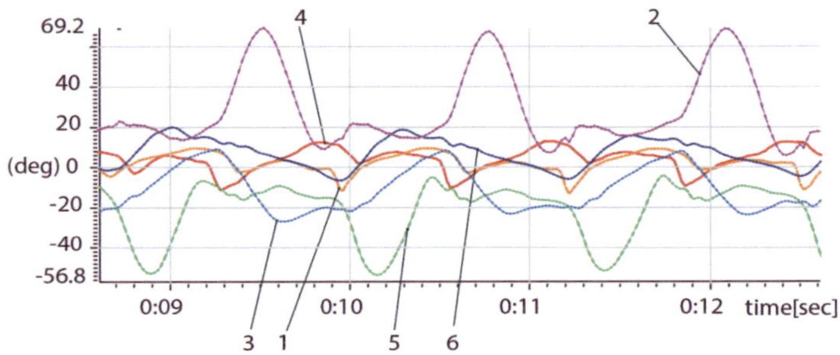

Fig. 7 The experimental diagrams obtained for six joints (right and left ankle, knee and hip)

beginning of the first force platform and ending with the end of the six force platform.

After splitting the initial cycles, the normalized flexion-extension cycles for each of six human joint and for each of six force platforms were obtained.

To obtain the average cycles of each movement cycle joints, in SIMIMOTION were introduced the gait cycles for the six joints of both legs. The mean cycle of experimental Ground Reaction Forces obtained from the six platforms during five walking trials, for right leg and for left leg are presented in Fig. 8. The mean angular flexion-extension experimental cycles for the six joints obtained from the collected data of the five walking trials are also presented in Fig. 8c–h.

From Figs. 6 and 8a, b we can see that the maximum value experimentally recorded is found in the second extreme point and it is 810 N (P1), is 1.22 BW (body weight) where BW = 660 N. In the first extreme point is recorded the value 780 N (P2), is 1.18 BW, and the minimum is 780 N (P3), is 0.92 BW. The results are similar to those obtained in the papers [29, 30] where the maximum values are comprised in the interval [1.15 BW; 1.25 BW] and the minimum values are comprised in the interval [0.82 BW; 0.95 BW]. The maximum value corresponds to an abscissa value equal to the percentage 50%, when for a normalized gait cycle correspond 100% percentages on abscissa.

Comparing the results from the papers [29, 30] we notice that the percentage values are similar, because 50% of the full cycle is equivalent to ≈80% of the active cycle

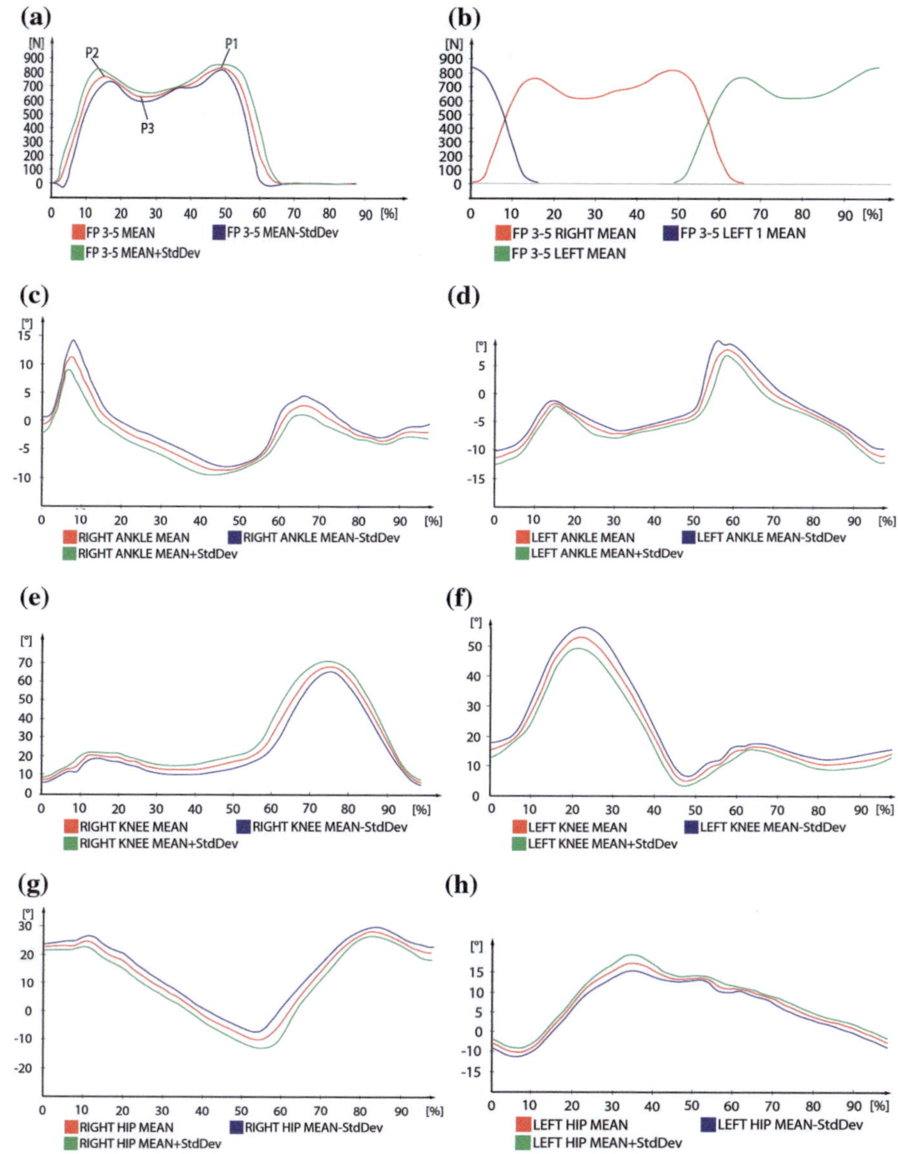

Fig. 8 Medium experimental cycles obtained from collected data computed in SIMIMOTION: **a** Mean Ground Reaction Forces for right leg cycle; **b** Mean Ground Reaction Forces for right leg and left leg cycles, corresponding to a complete right leg cycle; Flexion-extension cycles during a walking cycle for lower limbs joints: **c** right ankle; **d** left ankle; **e** right knee; **f** left knee; **g** right hip; **h** left hip

(the period of contact of the foot with the force platform), as it is presented in the cited papers. From the Fig. 8c–h, it results a good repeatability of cycle gait corresponding to the five trials, obvious fact by parallel curves: Mean, Mean + StdDev, Mean − StdDev and by the fact that the standard deviation is <10%, excepting the areas corresponding to the maximum values of normalized cycles.

Referring to Fig. 9a–c, we can conclude that the subject is executing larger movements with the right foot in comparison with the left foot. By comparison the maximum values of flexion angles are: for the right ankle the value is 13° versus left ankle which is 7°; for the right knee the maximum value is 68° while for the left knee is 52°; for the right hip the value is 21° versus the hip left value which is 17°. The results obtained in the present study are comparable to those obtained in the papers [2, 29, 30] both in terms of asymmetry and maximum values. The second set of results are the ones obtained by numerical simulations of mannequin walking, performed in ADAMS environment. Ground contact forces variations in time obtained by virtual simulation, for right and left leg are presented in Fig. 10.

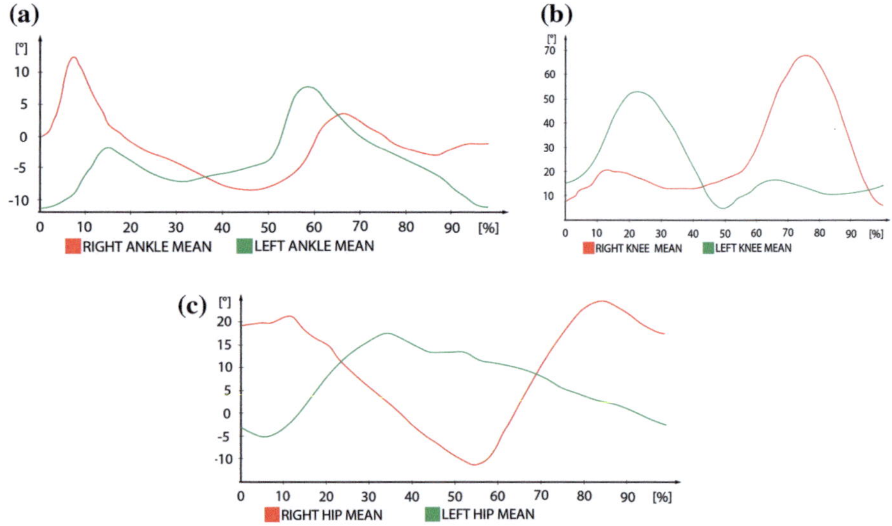

Fig. 9 Experimental flexion-extension medium cycles for: **a** right and left ankles; **b** right and left knees; **c** right and left hips

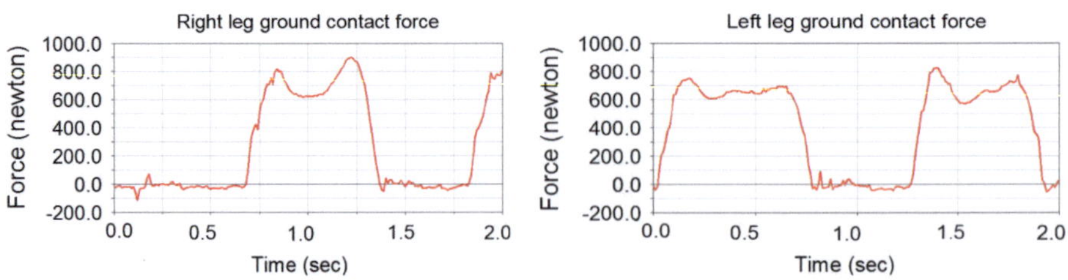

Fig. 10 Ground contact forces for right and left leg, computed in ADAMS simulation

Comparing the values of the ground reaction forces obtained by experimental tests on the force platforms and by numerical simulations in ADAMS we observe that they are similar, the maximum values of about 900 N being occurred when the heel touches the floor and when the toes push off. The maximum values of the ground reaction force computed in ADAMS for the right leg is 900 N and for the left leg is about 840 N. The values obtained from ADAMS simulation for the ground reaction forces are comparable with the experimentally measured ground reaction forces, presented in Fig. 6. The differences could appear because of the contact conditions during mannequin walking. The horizontal displacements (on z-axis which represents the movement direction) and vertical displacements (on y-axis) of right hip attached marker, resulted from ADAMS simulation are presented in Fig. 11. Similar diagrams were obtained for the other five joints.

Another simulation results consist in legs joints reaction forces and joints torques. Vertical reaction forces developed in the virtual knee joint, for right and left leg, are presented in Fig. 12. Similar diagrams were obtained for the other joints.

The joints torques is computed in ADAMS simulation. In Fig. 13 are shown the variations in time of torques magnitudes for both (right and left) mannequin knee joints. Similar diagrams of torques magnitude were obtained for the other joints.

The obtained values of the joint torques from ADAMS simulation are comparable with those results obtained by other researchers [27].

The reaction forces developed in every lower limb joint are very useful for understanding normal and pathological musculoskeletal motion and for the study of

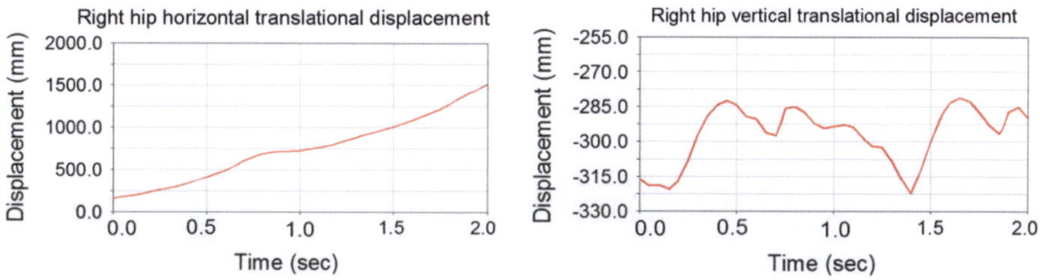

Fig. 11 Right hip translational displacements, upon horizontal direction (on z-axis) and vertical direction (on y-axis) computed in ADAMS

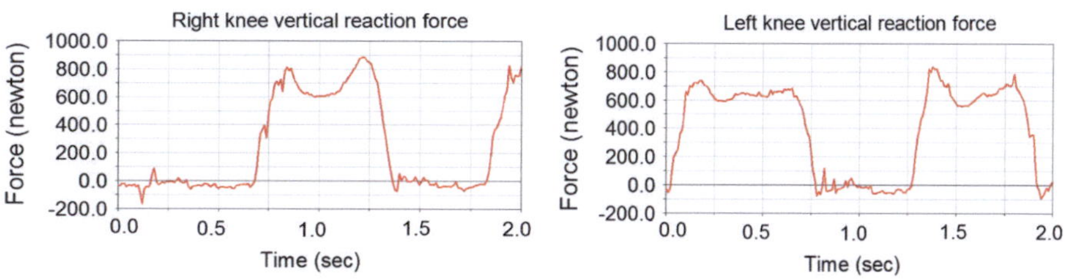

Fig. 12 Right and left knee vertical reaction forces (on y-axis), computed in ADAMS simulation

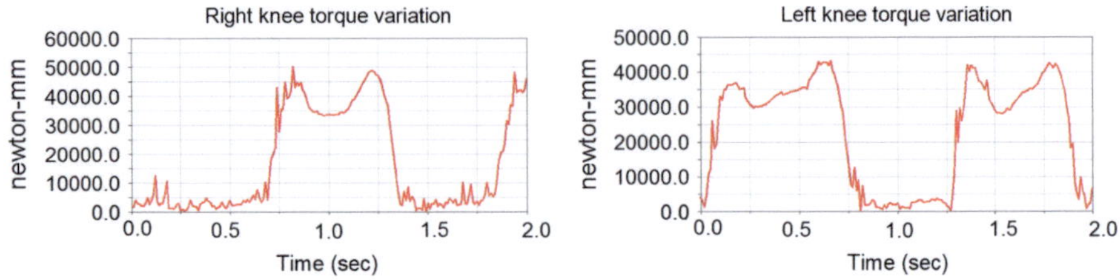

Fig. 13 Right and left knee joints torques magnitude computed in ADAMS

the stresses and displacements developed in normal joints, in affected and prosthetic or orthotic joints, using the Finite Element Method [31–33, 36, 37]. Considering the reaction forces obtained in knee joint by numerical simulation, the stress and deformation maps developed in the knee prosthetic joint could be obtained, as in Fig. 14 [31]. The reaction force could be used to determine the stress and displacements maps for an osteoarthritic knee and for an orthotic device designed for rehabilitation of the knee mouvements are shown in Fig. 15 [32, 33]. The ground reaction forces are useful to study the behavior of the medical devices based on advanced composite materials [34, 35] or to simulate and analyze the osteosynthesis process of lower limbs fractures [36].

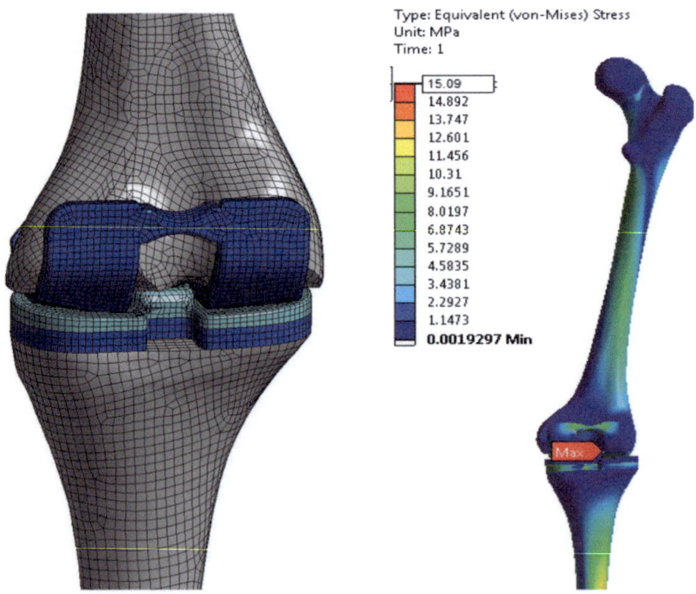

Fig. 14 The prosthetic knee assembly joint; stress map in the prosthetic knee joint for a compression force of 800 N [31]

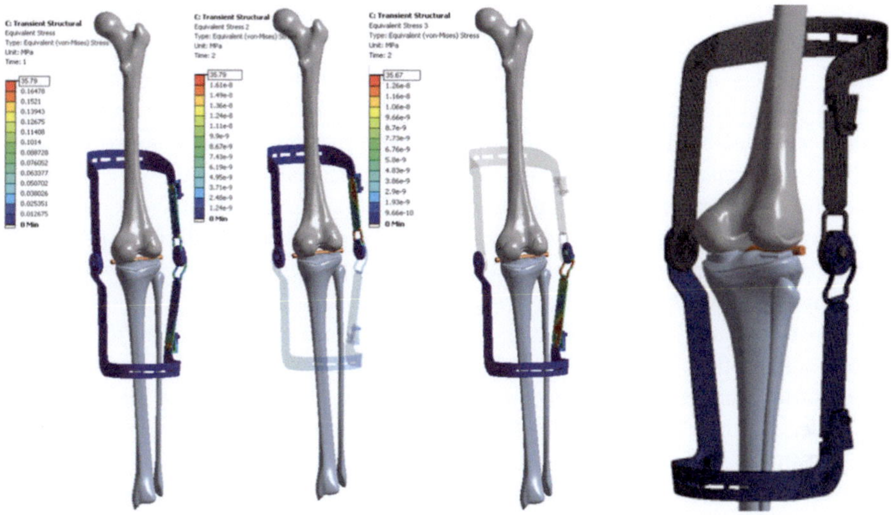

Fig. 15 Von Mises stress for the assembly knee-orthotic device; the orthotic device [33]

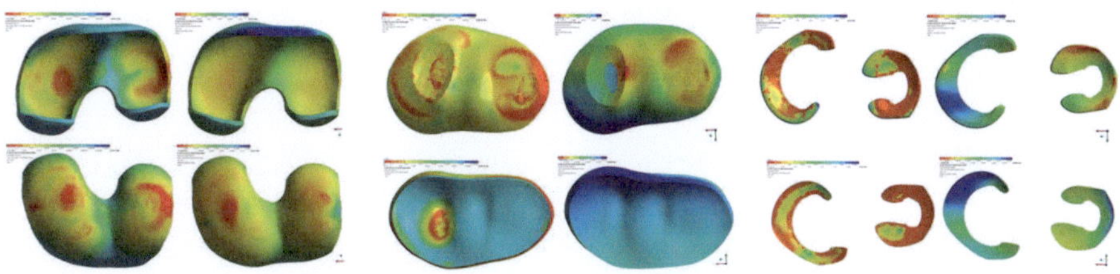

Fig. 16 Von Mises stress on the femoral cartilage, on the tibial cartilage and on the menisci for healthy knee [37]

The reaction force developed in knee joint could be, also, used to investigate the role of the articular cartilage in the developing of the osteoarthritis, to analyze and simulate the biomechanical behavior of the knee joint cartilages (Fig. 16) [37].

For future work, the obtained results, the numerical simulation and experimental results could be used to design and develop human-inspired robotic structures used in medical, assistive or rehabilitation fields [38, 39].

5 Conclusions

A study based on the tools of gait analysis of human knee movement is presented. The purpose of this study was to investigate the human flexion-extension movements of the human lower limb joints and the ground reaction forces developed during walking on the platform forces. The study presents a comparison based on the experimental data collected during walking cycles for both legs joints of a healthy subject and on the numerical simulations in ADAMS environment. Biometrics acquisition system was considered to collect the data files from the six human joints of both legs and from the six force platforms. The kinematic data of the flexion extension angles for human ankle, knee and hip joints were obtained. Based on the average human anthropometric data and using SolidWorks software, the virtual model of a mannequin was developed and then transferred to ADAMS simulation environment in order to obtain the reaction forces in the six joints of both lower limbs. The results of ADAMS simulation obtained for the ground reaction forces are similar with the experimental measurements. The joint torque values and profiles of the simulated gait are similar with the results presented in other works. The reaction forces developed in every lower limb joint are very useful for understanding normal and pathological musculoskeletal motion and for the study of the stresses and displacements developed in normal joints, in affected and prosthetic or orthotic joints, using the Finite Element Method. In a similar manner, the experimental and numerical analysis can be applied to the joints and the bones of the upper limb. For future work, the numerical simulation and experimental results could be used to design and develop human-inspired robotic structures used in medical, assistive or rehabilitation fields.

References

1. Tlalolini, D., Christine, C., Yannick, A.: Human-like walking: optimal motion of a bipedal robot with toe-rotation motion. Trans. Mechatron. Inst. Electr. Electron. Eng. **16**(2), 310–320 (2011)
2. Kanako, M., Mitsuharu, M., Fumio, K., Shuuji, K., Kenji, K., Kazuhito, Y.: Human-like walking with toe supporting for humanoids. In: International Conference on Intelligent Robots and Systems, San Francisco, CA, USA (2011)
3. Kim, J.Y., Park, I.W., Lee, J., Kim, M.S., Cho, B.K., Oh, J.H.: System design and dynamic walking of humanoid robot khr-2. In: International Conference on Robotics and Automation Barcelona, Spain (2005)
4. Matthieu, L., et al.: The poppy humanoid robot: leg design for biped locomotion. In: International Conference on Intelligent Robots and Systems, Tokyo, Japan (2013)
5. Fumiya, L., Yohei, M., Jürgen, R., André, S.: Toward a human-like biped robot with compliant legs. Robot. Auton. Syst. **57**, 139–144 (2009)
6. Muro-de-la-Herran, A., et al.: Gait analysis methods: an overview of wearable and non-wearable systems highlighting clinical applications. Sensors **14**, 3362–3394 (2014)
7. Shull, P.B., Jirattigalachote, W., Hunt, M.A., Cutkosky, M.R., et al.: Quantified self and human movement: a review on the clinical impact of wearable sensing and feedback for gait analysis and intervention. Gait Posture **40**, 11–19 (2014)
8. Tao, W., et al.: Gait analysis using wearable sensors. Sensors **12**, 2255–2283 (2012)
9. Abdul, R.A.H., Zayegh, A., Begg, R.K., Wahab, Y.: Foot plantar pressure measurement system a review. Sensors **12**, 9884–9912 (2012)
10. Tarnita, D., Marghitu, D.: Analysis of a hand arm system. Robot. Comp. Integr. Manuf. **29**(6), 493–501 (2013)

11. Tarnita, D., Catana, M., Tarnita, D.N.: Nonlinear analysis of normal human gait for different activities with application to bipedal locomotion. Ro. J. Tech. Sci. Appl. Mech. **58**(1–2), 177–192 (2013)
12. Mohamed, A.A., Baba, J., Beyea, J., Landry, J., Sexton, A., McGibbon, C.A.: Comparison of strain-gage and fiber-optic goniometry for measuring knee kinematics during activities of daily living and exercise. J. Biomech. Eng. **134**, 084502 (2012)
13. Van der Linden, M.L., Rowe, P.J., Nutton, R.W.: Between-day repeatability of knee kinematics during functional tasks recorded using flexible electrogoniometry. Gait Posture **28**, 292–296 (2008)
14. Tarnita, D., Catana, M., et al.: Experimental measurement of flexion-extension movement in normal and osteoarthritic human knee. Rom. J. Morphol. Embryol. **54**(2), 309–313 (2013)
15. Tarnita, D.: Wearable sensors used for human gait analysis. Rom. J. Morphol. Embryol. **57** (2), 373–382 (2016)
16. Sutherland, D.H.: The evolution of clinical gait analysis Part III—kinetics and energy assessment. Gait Posture **21**, 447–461 (2005)
17. Leusmann, P., Mollering, C., Klack, L., et al.: Your floor knows where you are: sensing and acquisition of movement data. In: Proceedings of 2011 12th IEEE International Conference on Mobile Data Management (MDM), Luleå, Sweden, pp. 61–66 (2011)
18. Lincoln, L. S., et al.: An elastomeric insole for 3-axis ground reaction force measurement. In: Proceedings of 2012 4th IEEE RAS EMBS International Conference on Biomedical Robotics and Biomechatronics (BioRob), Rome, Italy, pp. 1512–1517 (2012)
19. http://www.biometricsltd.com
20. Moriguchi, C.S., Sato, T.O., Gil Coury, H.J.C.: Ankle movements during normal gait evaluated by flexible electrogoniometer. Rev. bras. Fisioter. **11**(3) (2007)
21. Hirakawa, Y., Hara, M., Fujiwara, A., Hanada, H., Morioka, S.: The relationship among psychological factors, neglect-like symptoms and postoperative pain after total knee arthroplasty. Pain Res. Manag. **19**(5), 251–256 (2014)
22. Alexandru, C.: Software platform for analyzing and optimizing the mechanical systems. In: Proceedings of the 10th IFToMM International Symposium on Science of Mechanisms and Machines—SYROM, 665–677 (2009)
23. Alexandru, C.: Optimal design of the mechanical systems using parametric technique & MBS (Multi-Body Systems) software. Adv. Mater. Res. **463–464**, 1129–1132 (2012)
24. Wojtyra, M.: Dynamical analysis of human walking. 15th European ADAMS Users, Conference Technical Papers, Rome, Italy (2000)
25. Lu, T.W., Chang, C.F.: Biomechanics of human movement and its clinical applications. Kaohsiung J. Med. Sci. **28**, 13–25 (2012)
26. Kecskemethy, A.: Integrating efficient kinematics in biomechanics of human motions. Procedia IUTAM **2**, 86–92 (2011)
27. Chowdhury, S., Kumar, N.: Estimation of forces and moments of lower limb joints from kinematics data and inertial properties of the body by using inverse dynamics technique. J. Rehabil. Robot. **1**, 93–98 (2013)
28. MSC.ADAMS 2013 User Manual
29. Stansfield, B.W., Hillman, S.J., et al.: Regression analysis of gait parameters with speed in normal children walking at self-selected speeds. Gait Posture **23**, 288–294 (2006)
30. Fregly, B. J., Reinbolt, J. A., et al.: Design of Patient-specific gait modifications for knee osteoarthritis rehabilitation. IEEE Trans. Biomed. Eng. **54** (9) (2007)
31. Calafeteanu, D., Tarnita, D., et al.: Influences of varus tilt on the stresses in human prosthetic knee joint. Appl. Mech. Mater. **823**, 143–148 (2016)
32. Tarnita, D., Catana, M., Dumitru, N., Tarnita, D.N.: Design and simulation of an orthotic device for patients with osteoarthritis, In: New Trends in Medical and Service Robots, Mechanisms and Machine Science, vol. 38, pp. 61–77, Springer Publishing House (2016)
33. Catana, M.: Tarnita, D., Tarnita, D.N.: Modeling, simulation and optimization of a human knee orthotic device. Appl. Mech. Mater. **371**, 549–553 (2013)

34. Bolcu, D., Stanescu, M.M., et al.: Study about the nonuniformity from composite materials reinforced with fiber glass fabric. Mater. Plast. **51**(1), 97–100 (2014)
35. Stănescu, M.M., Bolcu, D., et al.: Determination of damping factor, to vibrations of composite bars, reinforced with carbon and kevlar texture. Mater. Plast. **47**(4), 492–496 (2010)
36. Tarnita, D., Tarnita, D.N., et al.: Numerical simulations of human tibia osteosynthesis using modular plates based on Nitinol staples. Rom. J. Morphol embryol **51**(1), 145–150 (2010)
37. Tarnita, D., Catana, M., Tarnita, D.N.: Contributions on the modeling and simulation of the human knee joint with applications to the robotic structures, In: New Trends on Medical and Service Robotics, Mechanisms and Machine Science vol. 20, pp. 283–297, Springer (2014)
38. Pisla, D., et al.: Kinematics and workspace modeling of a new hybrid robot used in minimally invasive surgery. Robot. Comp. Integr. Manuf. **29**(2), 463–474 (2013)
39. Vaida, C., et al.: Orientation module for surgical instruments-a systematical approach. Meccanica **48**(1), 145–158 (2013)

Motion Control Algorithm for a Lower Limb Exoskeleton Based on Iterative LQR and ZMP Method for Trajectory Generation

S. Jatsun, S. Savin and A. Yatsun

Abstract In this paper a problem of controlling a lower limb exoskeleton during sit-to-stand motion (verticalization) in sagittal plane is studied. It is assumed that left and right sides of the exoskeleton are moving symmetrically. The main challenge in performing this motion is to maintain balance of the system. In this paper we use the zero-moment point (ZMP) methodology to produce desired trajectories for the generalized coordinates that would allow the system to remain vertically balanced. The limitations of this approach is that, it requires relatively accurate work of the feedback controller that ensures that the exoskeleton follows generated trajectories. In this work we use Iterative Linear Quadratic Regulator (ILQR) as a feedback controller in order to obtained the required accuracy. In the paper a way of trajectory generation that uses ZMP methodology is discussed, the results of the numerical simulation of the exoskeleton motion are presented and analyzed. A comparison between a natural human motion (for a human not wearing an exoskeleton) and the simulated motion of an exoskeleton using the proposed algorithm is presented.

Keywords Lower limb exoskeleton · Sit-to-stand motion · ZMP trajectory generation · Iterative linear quadratic regulator · Control system design

1 Introduction

Exoskeleton development is an important research topic in robotics with a wide range of practical applications. Exoskeletons have been used for providing assistance to elderly and disabled people, rehabilitation, and for enhancing the performance of industrial workers and combatants. There are different challenges

S. Jatsun · S. Savin (✉) · A. Yatsun
Department of Mechanics, Mechatronics and Robotics, Southwest State University, Kursk, Russia
e-mail: savin@swsu.ru

S. Jatsun
e-mail: teormeh@inbox.ru

M. Husty and M. Hofbaur (eds.), *New Trends in Medical and Service Robots*, Mechanisms and Machine Science 48, DOI 10.1007/978-3-319-59972-4_22

associated with those applications. The main problem is the necessity to guarantee the safety of the human [1, 2].

There are many aspects of safety problem for exoskeleton wearers, many of them are discussed in article [2]. One of the most crucial safety problems is maintaining vertical balance of the exoskeleton. A popular approach to solving this problem for walking robots is the use of zero-moment point (ZMP) control [3]. The methodology of ZMP control as applied to bipedal robot and exoskeleton is discussed in papers [4–8]. Publication [9] presents the use of ZMP control to a lower limb exoskeleton during sit-to-stand motion. As stated in paper [5] some realizations of ZMP control can be criticized for lack of adaptive properties; and as mentioned in [10], the fact that ZMP method is often implemented using a simplified model of the system can lead to additional control errors. We note that solutions to both of these problems are proposed in the same papers. Paper [11] describes the implementation of optimization-based control that uses information about the ZMP position, which was used on the Atlas robot during the DARPA Robotics Challenge. While this approach is computationally intensive for an on-board system, it can provide a way to further improve the safety of lower-limb exoskeletons, especially in the case of assistive exoskeletons for paraplegic patients.

In this paper we focus on sit-to-stand motion. The execution of this motion puts high demands on the exoskeleton's control system, making the problems discussed above more challenging. For medical and assistive exoskeletons the task of standing up has additional importance, because its automation removes the need of human assistance for exoskeleton users [12, 13]. Publications [12–17] discuss different aspects of sit-to-stand motion, including problems of control. Adaptive feedback controllers for exoskeletons performing sit-to-stand motion are studied in papers [18, 19].

The goal of this paper is to study a control strategy uses ZMP trajectory generator and Iterative Linear Quadratic Regulator (ILQR).

2 Description of the Exoskeleton

An exoskeleton consists of the following basic elements: 1—a corset that fixes the exoskeleton to the patient's body by means of straps, 2—thigh links installed on the corset by means of two two-axes hinges, one of which is equipped with an electric drive, 3—shin link fixed onto the hips by means of actuated rotary joint, 4—feet links attached to the shin by means of a three-axes hinge, two of which are equipped with rotary electric drives. All the electric drives have current sensors, which allow us to control the values of torques generated by these electric drives (Fig. 1).

All the hinges of the exoskeleton are equipped with rotation angle sensors (absolute encoders), and each motor's rotor is additionally equipped with an incremental encoder. The feet contain pressure sensors that measure normal reactions. Information from the sensors is preprocessed using onboard microcontrollers and then the data is send to the onboard PC that realizes the control system.

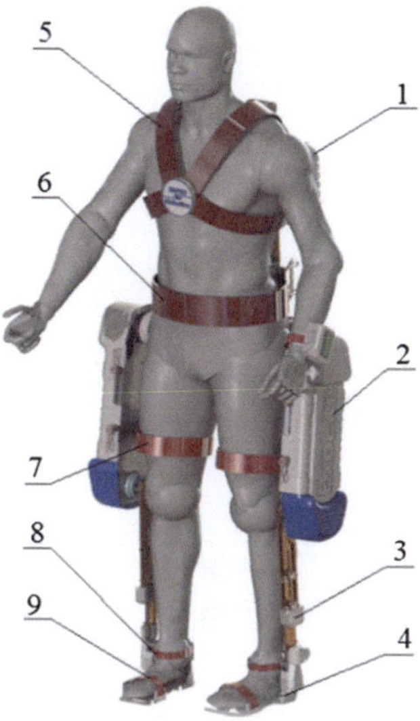

Fig. 1 General view of the exoskeleton (3D model); *1* exoskeleton torso, *2* thigh link, *3* shin link, *4* foot link, *5–9* connecting belts

3 Mathematical Model of the Exoskeleton

In this chapter, we consider a mathematical model of the lower limb exoskeleton performing sit-to-stand motion in the sagittal plane. We make an assumption that during the sit-to-stand motion both leg links, as well as all the thigh links move parallel to each other. We assume that the feet remain motionless for the whole duration of verticalization. This allows us to model the exoskeleton as a four link serial mechanism, as shown in Fig. 2.

On the diagram in Fig. 2 points O_2-O_4 are rotational joints that connect the links, points C_1-C_4 are the centers of mass of the corresponding links, φ_2-φ_4 are the angles that determine the orientation of the corresponding links. The *i*-th link has mass m_i, length l_i and inertia I_i. The mass of the whole mechanism is denoted as $m = \sum_{i=1}^{4} m_i$.

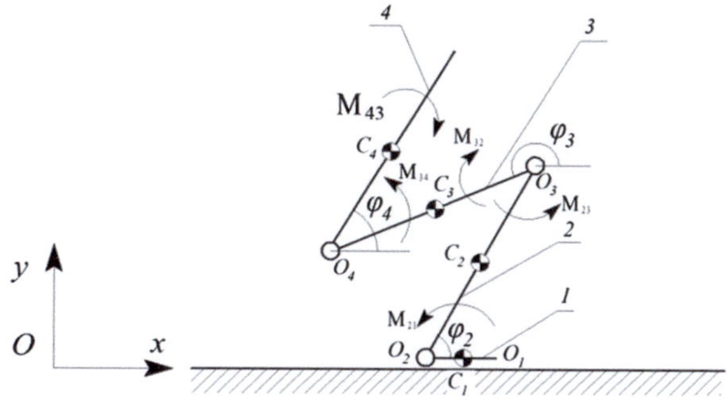

Fig. 2 Analytical diagram of the exoskeleton; *1–4* first–fourth links

Using the introduced notations we can write the equation that describes the position of the center of mass of the mechanism:

$$\begin{cases} x_C = x_{O1} + \sum_{i=1}^{4} (K_i \cos(\varphi_i)) \\ y_C = y_{O1} + \sum_{i=1}^{4} (K_i \sin(\varphi_i)) \end{cases} \quad (1)$$

where x_C, y_C are the Cartesian coordinates of the robot's center of mass, x_{O1}, y_{O1} are the coordinates of point O_1 (the tip of the foot). Coefficients K_i are given as follows:

$$K_1 = l_1(M - 0.5m_1)/m, \quad (2)$$

$$K_2 = l_2(0.5m_2 + m_3 + m_4)/m, \quad (3)$$

$$K_3 = l_3(0.5m_3 + m_4)/m, \quad (4)$$

$$K_4 = 0.5l_4 m_4/m. \quad (5)$$

To write the equations of motion we introduce a vector of generalized coordinates $\vec{q}$:

$$\vec{q} = [\varphi_2 \quad \varphi_3 \quad \varphi_4]^{\mathrm{T}}. \quad (6)$$

The dynamics of the robot then can be described by the following equations:

$$\mathbf{\Lambda}(\vec{q})\ddot{\vec{q}} + \vec{C}\left(\vec{q}, \dot{\vec{q}}\right) + \vec{G}(\vec{q}) + \Phi(\vec{q}) = \mathbf{H}\vec{M}, \quad (7)$$

where $\dot{\vec{q}} = [\dot{\varphi}_2 \quad \dot{\varphi}_3 \quad \dot{\varphi}_4]^{\mathrm{T}}$ is a vector of generalized velocities, $\ddot{\vec{q}} = [\ddot{\varphi}_2 \quad \ddot{\varphi}_3 \quad \ddot{\varphi}_4]^{\mathrm{T}}$ is a vector of generalized accelerations, $\mathbf{\Lambda}(\vec{q})$ is a joint space inertia matrix, $\vec{C}\left(\vec{q}, \dot{\vec{q}}\right)$ is a vector of generalized forces of inertia, $\vec{G}(\vec{q})$ is a vector of generalized gravitational forces, $\Phi(\vec{q})$—vector of generalized dissipative forces, $\vec{M} = [M_{21} \quad M_{32} \quad M_{43}]^{\mathrm{T}}$ is a vector whose components are the torques of the motors, H is a matrix connecting the torques of the motors with generalised forces they generate. The joint space inertia matrix $\mathbf{\Lambda}(\vec{q})$ can be found as the matrix of the quadratic form of kinetic energy $\mathbf{\Lambda}(\vec{q}) = \frac{\partial^2 T(\vec{q}, \dot{\vec{q}})}{\partial \dot{\vec{q}}^2}$, where T is the kinetic energy of the system (see [20] for a complete treatment of these equations, and [21] for notation). The scalar form of the presented equations can be found in paper [22].

In the following chapters we will be considering the case when vector $\vec{M}$ is a function of control error.

For some of the formulations in the next chapter we need to write the dynamics in the state-space form. To do that we introduce a state vector $\vec{s}$:

$$\vec{s} = \begin{bmatrix} \dot{\varphi}_2 & \dot{\varphi}_3 & \dot{\varphi}_4 & \varphi_2 & \varphi_3 & \varphi_4 \end{bmatrix}^{\mathrm{T}}. \quad (8)$$

Using this notation we can write the following equations of motion in vector form:

$$\dot{\vec{s}} = f(\vec{s}) = \begin{bmatrix} \mathbf{\Lambda}^{-1}\left(\mathbf{H}\vec{M} - \vec{C} - \vec{G} - \Phi\right) \\ s_1 \\ s_2 \\ s_3 \end{bmatrix} \quad (9)$$

The system of first-order ordinary differential equations (ODE) (9) can be used to simulate motion of the exoskeleton for given $\vec{M}$. In Sect. 4.2 this system of equations will be used to derive Iterative Linear Quadratic Regulator (ILQR).

4 Control System Design

In this chapter we discuss the proposed control system design. In the first part we the method of trajectory generation for the center of mass (CoM) during sit-to-stand motion. The method allows us to move zero moment point (from here onwards we denote it as point P) towards the center of the support polygon. In the second part we look at the augmented ZMP Control strategy.

4.1 ZMP Trajectory Generation

Establishing the desired trajectory of the CoM of the mechanism can be used as a step in formulating verticalization control task [18, 19, 23]. The ZMP methodology presents tools to find the CoM's trajectory that allows the zero moment point P to stay within the support polygon. For the model described in the previous chapter the position of point P can be found from the following expression:

$$x_P = x_C - (mg + m\ddot{y}_C)^{-1}\left(m\ddot{x}_C y_C - \sum_{i=2}^{4} J_i \ddot{\varphi}_i\right) \quad (10)$$

where g is the gravitational acceleration.

Point P should stay within the support polygon in order to maintain the mechanism's balance, which means that the following inequalities should hold:

$$(x_{O1} - l_1) < x_P(t) < x_{O1}, \quad t \in [0 \quad t_f] \tag{11}$$

where t_f is the duration of sit-to-stand motion.

We define the desired trajectory for point P in the following way:

$$x_P^*(t) = \begin{cases} \sum_{k=0}^{3} z_k \cdot t^k & if \quad t < t_1 \\ 0.5 \cdot l_1 & if \quad t \geq t_1 \end{cases} \tag{12}$$

where z_k are polynomial coefficients given by the following expressions:

$$z_0 = x_P(0), z_1 = 0, z_2 = \frac{3}{t_f^2}\left(x_{O1} - \frac{1}{2}l_1 - x_P(0)\right), \tag{13}$$

$$z_3 = \frac{2}{t_f^3}\left(x_P(0) - x_{O1} + \frac{1}{2}l_1\right), \tag{14}$$

where $x_P(0)$ is the initial position of point P.

Assuming that the desired motion of the CoM in the vertical direction $y_C^*(t)$ is given, for example as a polynomial function as was done in [18], we can use (10) and (12) to write an equation that can be solved for the CoM acceleration in the horizontal direction:

$$m y_C^* \ddot{x}_C^* - m(g + \ddot{y}_C^*)(x_C^* - x_P) - \sum_{i=2}^{4} I_i \ddot{\varphi}_i^* = 0. \tag{15}$$

To find $\ddot{\varphi}_i^*$ we can use the following derivation:

$$\ddot{q}^* = \begin{bmatrix} \ddot{\varphi}_2^* \\ \ddot{\varphi}_3^* \\ \ddot{\varphi}_4^* \end{bmatrix} = \left(\frac{\partial \dot{r}_t}{\partial \dot{q}}\right)^{-1} \left(\ddot{r}_t^* - \frac{\partial \dot{r}_t}{\partial q} \dot{q}^*\right), \tag{16}$$

$$\dot{q}^* = \left(\frac{\partial r_t}{\partial q}\right)^{-1} \dot{r}_t^*, \tag{17}$$

where $r_t = [x_C \quad y_C \quad \varphi_4]^{\mathrm{T}}, \ddot{r}_t^* = [\ddot{x}_C^* \quad \ddot{y}_C^* \quad \ddot{\varphi}_4^*]^{\mathrm{T}}$ and $\dot{r}_t^* = [\dot{x}_C^* \quad \dot{y}_C^* \quad \dot{\varphi}_4^*]^{\mathrm{T}}$.

After substituting (16) into (15), we obtain a second order linear ODE that can be solved numerically or analytically to obtain the desired trajectory $x_C^*(t)$. In practice it might be beneficial to add a damping term to the equation to decrease the oscillations in the solution.

4.2 Iterative Linear Quadratic Regulator

Using the method of trajectory generation for the CoM described above it is possible to build a control system that drives the CoM along that trajectory. Figure 3 shows a design of such a control system.

The CoM Trajectory Generator module determines $x_C^*(t)$ and its derivatives by solving (15); the Inverse Kinematics module finds values of generalized coordinates that cause the CoM to move along the desired trajectory. The analytical solution of this problem can be found in [18]. The Robot module represents the dynamics of the mechanism as described by (7). The ZMP Finder module uses (10) to find the ZMP's current position. Vector $\vec{e}$ is the control error, and it is determined as $\vec{e} = \vec{s}^* - \vec{s}$.

The work of the ILQR module is described below. ILQR is an iterative control algorithm that requires local linearization of the system model (for detailed description see [23]). Here we consider the case when the new linearization is made on every iteration. The linearized model of the system has form:

$$\dot{\vec{s}} = \mathbf{A}\vec{s} + \mathbf{B}\vec{M} + \vec{b}, \tag{18}$$

where $\mathbf{A} = \partial\vec{f}/\partial\vec{s}, \mathbf{B} = \partial\vec{f}/\partial\vec{M}$ (both evaluated at the point $\vec{s} = \vec{s}^*(t)$), $\vec{b}$ is the vector that describes the difference between the actual model of the system and its linearized version. Vector $\vec{b}$ can be found using the following expression:

$$\vec{b} = \vec{f}(\vec{s}) - \mathbf{A}\vec{s} - \mathbf{B}\vec{M}, \tag{19}$$

Vector function $\vec{s}^*(t)$ denotes the desired position of the system and it has form:

$$\vec{s}^*(t) = \left[\vec{q}^*(t) \quad \dot{\vec{q}}^*(t)\right]^{\mathrm{T}}. \tag{20}$$

We define quadratic cost function J:

$$J = \int \left[(\vec{s} - \vec{s}^*)^{\mathrm{T}}\mathbf{Q}(\vec{s} - \vec{s}^*) + (\vec{M} - \vec{M}^*)^{\mathrm{T}}\mathbf{R}(\vec{M} - \vec{M}^*)\right] dt, \tag{21}$$

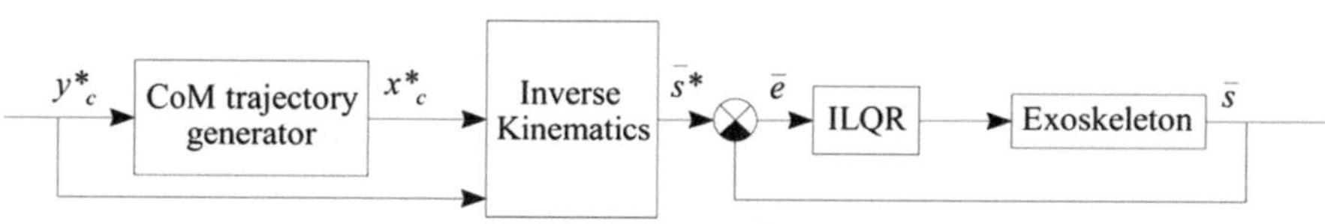

Fig. 3 ZMP control design

where **Q** and **R** are quadratic positive-definite matrices of proper dimensions. Using the standard procedure we can find the gain matrix **K** (see for complete treatment of the LQR problem see [24]). The control action then takes the following form:

$$\vec{M} = -\mathbf{K}(\vec{s} - \vec{s}^{\,*}) + \vec{M}^{*}. \tag{22}$$

where $\vec{M}^{*} = \vec{M}^{*}(\vec{q}^{\,*}, \dot{\vec{q}}^{\,*}, \ddot{\vec{q}}^{\,*})$ is the compensating control action that depends on the desired position of the system. It can be found by substituting desired values for generalized coordinates and their first two derivatives into (7), and then solving for $\vec{M}^{*}$:

$$\vec{M}^{*} = \mathbf{H}^{-1}\left[\mathbf{\Lambda}(\vec{q}^{\,*})\ddot{\vec{q}}^{\,*} + \vec{C}(\vec{q}^{\,*}, \dot{\vec{q}}^{\,*}) + \vec{G}(\vec{q}^{\,*}) + \Phi(\dot{\vec{q}}^{\,*})\right], \tag{23}$$

We cab observe that substituting (22) into (21) gives us another form of the cost function J:

$$J = \int (\vec{s} - \vec{s}^{\,*})^{\mathrm{T}}(\mathbf{Q} + \mathbf{K}^{\mathrm{T}}\mathbf{R}\mathbf{K})(\vec{s} - \vec{s}^{\,*})dt, \tag{24}$$

The Eq. (22) describes the work of the ILQR module on the diagram on the Fig. 3.

5 Numerical Simulation Results

Let us first consider the case when the zero moment point P lies within the support polygon at the beginning of the motion. In that case only normal ZMP trajectory generation and ILQR controller are working during the motion. In the Fig. 4 the time functions of actual and desired position of P, as well as horizontal displacement of the center of mass, are shown.

We should note that the actual position of the point P is different from its desired position because of control error and. The graphs in Fig. 4 show that both desired and actual position of point P lies within interval $[0 \quad 0.2]$, which represents robot's support polygon in this planar case. As we can see the center of mass and the point P are moving in the same manner and their graphs are relatively similar. It suggests this case it would be possible to control position of the center of mass instead of point P (as it was done in [25, 26]).

To review the influence of the verticalization time on the performance of the controller let us consider the case when the sit-to-stand motion takes 2 s. In the Fig. 5 the same graphs are shown for this case.

Graphs in the Fig. 5 show that the center of mass and the point P are now moving in different way; the center of mass still monotonically moves towards the center of the support polygon, but the point P moves away from it for the first 0.8 s

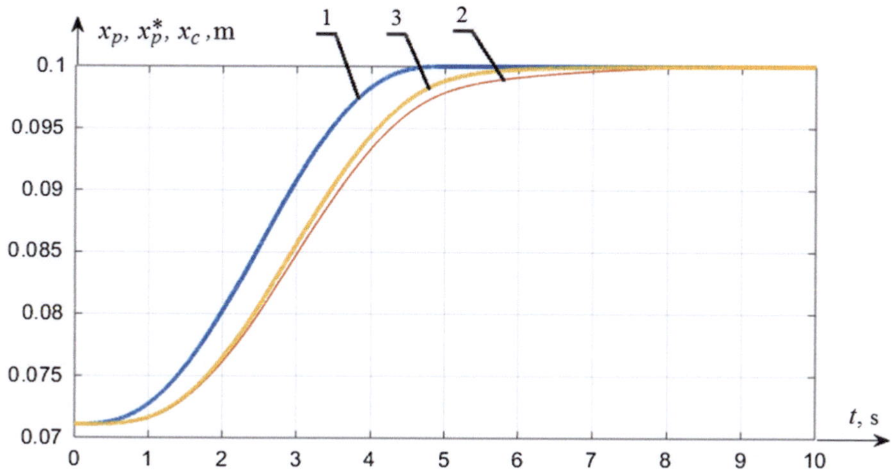

Fig. 4 Graphs of desired and actual position of point P for the case when verticalization; *1* desired position of point P, *2* actual position of point P, *3* horizontal displacement of the center of mass

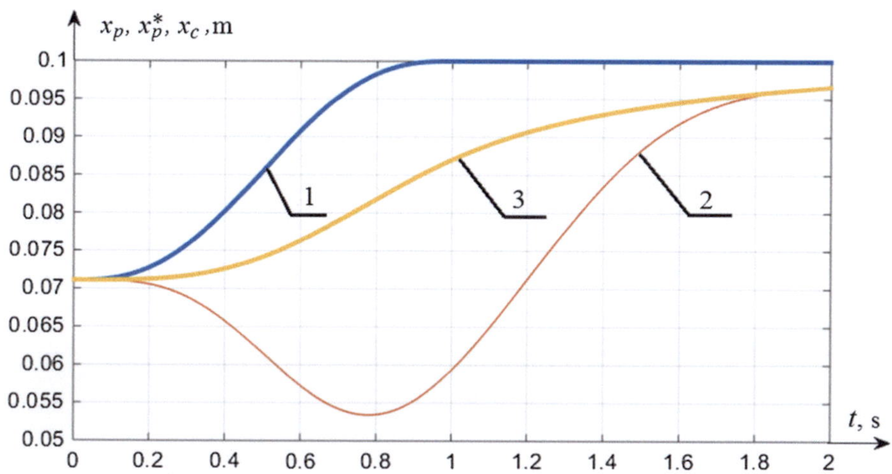

Fig. 5 Graphs of desired and actual position of point P for the case when verticalization; *1* desired position of point P, *2* actual position of point P, *3* horizontal displacement of the center of mass

(40% of the duration of the motion). The fact that changing duration of the sit-to-stand process has this influence on the performance of the control system is explained by the fact that faster raise requires bigger accelerations of the joints, leading to bigger inertial forces.

We can note that the center of mass moves towards the center of the support polygon without oscillations. The fact that the generated desired value for the center of mass position has no oscillations allows the control system to generate desired time dependencies for generalized coordinates demonstrate relatively slow rate of change, which makes the feedback control easier.

6 Comparison with Natural Human Motion

In this section we compare the motion of the system that uses ZMP controller with the natural human motion during verticalization. For the experimental studies a sensor system "ExoMeasurer" build in Southwest State University was used. ExoMeasurer is an exoskeleton that can be fixed to a human with straps and belts. The links have variable lengths, which allows to use the sensor system on individuals of different height. The system includes rotation sensors, accelerometers and pressure sensors, which allows to calculate the orientation and motion parameters of the exoskeleton, determine whether or not the feet have are in contact with the ground.

The questions of determining the positions of the centers of mass of different parts of human body are discussed in medical literature, here [27] was used as a reference.

On the Fig. 6 the trajectory of the center of mass of a human during sit-to-stand motion is shown.

As we can see, the control system attempts to move the center of mass of the mechanism the same way as a human does during verticalization. The human's motion is characterized by wider motion of the center of mass, with visible oscillations. The center of mass trajectory produced by the ZMP based control system is more conservative and does not show oscillation.

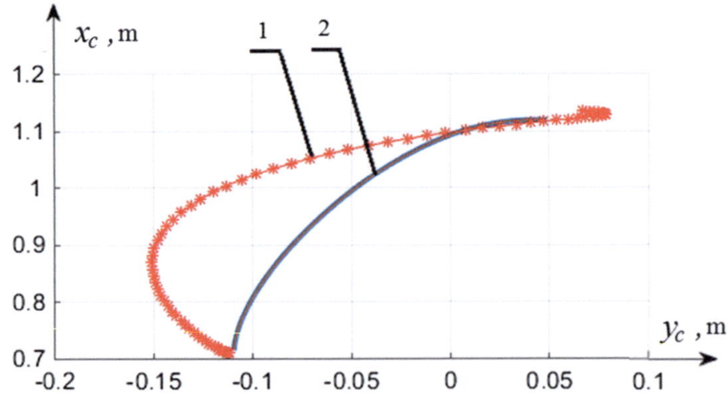

Fig. 6 Center of mass's trajectory; *1* experimental results, *2* motion of the exoskeleton obtained through simulation

7 Conclusion

In this paper a control system design for a lower limb exoskeleton was considered. To generate the trajectory of the center of mass of the exoskeleton ZMP methodology was used. Using the obtained desired trajectory for the center of mass the trajectories for joint angles were produced using inverse kinematics. The feedback control was implemented with iterative linear quadratic regulator. Use of that regulator allowed to maintain small control error which made it possible to realize motion along the trajectory obtained from ZMP method. A drawback of the ILQR is the high computational intensity, which makes it necessary to use an onboard computer to do the computations.

In the paper the results of the numerical simulation of the exoskeleton motion are presented and analyzed. It is shown that the duration of the verticalization has significant influence of the behavior of the control system. Obtained results suggest that for a slower verticalization time it may not be necessary to control the position of the zero-moment point and that controlling horizontal displacement of the center of mass instead might be sufficient for maintaining vertical balance, because the two values behave in a similar manner. For faster sit-to-stand motion it is shown that the trajectory of the horizontal displacement of the center of mass significantly differs from the position of the zero moment point.

A comparison between natural human motion (for a human not wearing an exoskeleton) and the motion of a human in an exoskeleton is presented. It is shown that the trajectory of the center of mass of a human (without exoskeleton) during verticalization is similar to the same trajectory exoskeleton model that uses ZMP trajectory generation. At the same time natural human motion shows more oscillatory and less conservative behavior.

We should note that this study did not take into account inaccuracy of the sensors. This may limit the application of the obtained results for the cases when an exoskeleton is equipped with sensors that introduce significant disturbance in the feedback channel.

The future work includes studying the influence the update rate of ILQR has on the behavior of the control system and applying the proposed method to control a physical model of a lower limb exoskeleton.

Acknowledgements Work is supported by RSF, Project № 14-39-00008.

References

1. Anam, K., Al-Jumaily, A.A.: Active exoskeleton control systems: state of the art. Proc. Eng. **41**, 988–994 (2012)
2. Contreras-Vidal, J.L., Grossman, R.G.: NeuroRex: a clinical neural interface roadmap for EEG-based brain machine interfaces to a lower body robotic exoskeleton. In: 2013 35th

Annual International Conference of the IEEE Engineering in Medicine and Biology Society (EMBC), pp. 1579–1582. IEEE (2013)
3. Barbareschi, G., Richards, R., Thornton, M., Carlson, T., Holloway, C.: Statically vs dynamically balanced gait: analysis of a robotic exoskeleton compared with a human. In: 2015 37th Annual International Conference of the IEEE Engineering in Medicine and Biology Society (EMBC), pp. 6728–6731. IEEE (2015)
4. Vukobratović, M., Borovac, B.: Zero-moment point—thirty five years of its life. Int. J. Hum. Rob. **1**(01), 157–173 (2004)
5. Kajita, S., Morisawa, M., Harada, K., Kaneko, K., Kanehiro, F., Fujiwara, K., Hirukawa, H.: Biped walking pattern generator allowing auxiliary zmp control. In: 2006 IEEE/RSJ International Conference on Intelligent Robots and Systems, pp. 2993–2999. IEEE (2006)
6. Mitobe, K., Capi, G., Nasu, Y.: Control of walking robots based on manipulation of the zero moment point. Robotica **18**(06), 651–657 (2000)
7. Choi, Y., You, B.J., Oh, S.R.: On the stability of indirect ZMP controller for biped robot systems. In 2004 IEEE/RSJ International Conference on Intelligent Robots and Systems, 2004. (IROS 2004). Proceedings, vol. 2, pp. 1966–1971. IEEE (2004)
8. Low, K.H., Liu, X., Goh, C.H., Yu, H.: Locomotive control of a wearable lower exoskeleton for walking enhancement. J. Vib. Control **12**(12), 1311–1336 (2006)
9. Panovko, G., Savin, S., Jatsun, S., Yatsun, A.: Simulation of controlled motion of an exoskeleton in verticalization process. J. Mach. Manuf. Reliab. (2016) (in publishing)
10. Kajita, S., Kanehiro, F., Kaneko, K., Fujiwara, K., Harada, K., Yokoi, K., Hirukawa, H.: Biped walking pattern generation by using preview control of zero-moment point. In: IEEE International Conference on Robotics and Automation, 2003. Proceedings. ICRA'03, vol. 2, pp. 1620–1626. IEEE (2003)
11. Feng, S., Whitman, E., Xinjilefu, X., Atkeson, C.G.: Optimization-based full body control for the DARPA robotics challenge. J. Field Robot. **32**(2), 293–312 (2015)
12. Tsukahara, A., Hasegawa, Y., Sankai, Y.: Standing-up motion support for paraplegic patient with robot suit HAL. In: IEEE International Conference on Rehabilitation Robotics, 2009. ICORR 2009, pp. 211–217. IEEE (2009)
13. Tsukahara, A., Kawanishi, R., Hasegawa, Y., Sankai, Y.: Sit-to-stand and stand-to-sit transfer support for complete paraplegic patients with robot suit HAL. Adv. Robot. **24**(11), 1615–1638 (2010)
14. Jun, H.G., Chang, Y.Y., Dan, B.J., Jo, B.R., Min, B.H., Yang, H., Kim, J.: Walking and sit-to-stand support system for elderly and disabled. In: 2011 IEEE International Conference on Rehabilitation Robotics (ICORR), pp. 1–5. IEEE (2011)
15. Taslim Reza, S.M., Ahmad, N., Choudhury, I.A., Ghazilla, R.A.R.: A fuzzy controller for lower limb exoskeletons during sit-to-stand and stand-to-sit movement using wearable sensors. Sensors **14**(3), 4342–4363 (2014)
16. Salah, O., Ramadan, A.A., Sessa, S., Ismail, A.A., Fujie, M., Takanishi, A.: Anfis-based sensor fusion system of sit-to-stand for elderly people assistive device protocols. Int. J. Autom. Comput. **10**(5), 405–413 (2013)
17. Mughal, A.M., Iqbal, K.: 3D bipedal model for biomechanical sit-to-stand movement with coupled torque optimization and experimental analysis. In: 2010 IEEE International Conference on Systems Man and Cybernetics (SMC), pp. 568–573. IEEE (2010)
18. Jatsun, S., Savin, S., Yatsun, A., Malchikov, A.: Study of controlled motion of exoskeleton moving from sitting to standing position. In: Advances in Robot Design and Intelligent Control, pp. 165–172. Springer International Publishing (2016)
19. Jatsun, S., Savin, S., Yatsun, A., Turlapov, R.: Adaptive control system for exoskeleton performing sit-to-stand motion. In 10th International Symposium on Mechatronics and its Applications (ISMA), pp. 1–6. IEEE (2015)
20. Jatsun, S., Savin, S., Yatsun, A., Postolnyi, A.: Control system parameter optimization for lower limb exoskeleton with integrated elastic elements. In: Proceedings of the International Conference on CLAWAR (2016) (in publishing)
21. Featherstone, R.: Rigid Body Dynamics Algorithms. Springer (2014)

22. Jatsun, S.F., Vorochaeva, A., Yu, L., Yatsun, A.S., Savin, S.I.: The modelling of the standing-up process of the anthropomorphic mechanism. In: Proceedings of the International Conference on CLAWAR, pp. 175–182 (2015)
23. Li, W., Todorov, E.: Iterative linear quadratic regulator design for nonlinear biological movement systems. In: ICINCO, vol. 1, pp. 222–229 (2004)
24. Anderson, B.D., Moore, J.B.: Optimal Control: Linear Quadratic Methods. Courier Corporation (2007)
25. Jatsun, S., Savin, S., Lushnikov, B., Yatsun, A.: Algorithm for motion control of an exoskeleton during verticalization. In ITM Web of Conferences, vol. 6. EDP Sciences (2016)
26. Jatsun, S., Savin, S., Yatsun, A.: Parameter optimization for exoskeleton control system using sobol sequences. In: Proceedings of 21st CISM-IFToMM Symposium on Robot Design (2016) (in publishing)
27. Plagenhoef, S., Evans, F.G., Abdelnour, T.: Anatomical data for analyzing human motion. Res. Q. Exerc. Sport **54**(2), 169–178 (1983)

FSTT Algorithm: Can Tides Assist Bio-Inspired Gradient Taxis?

J.Ch. Varughese, R. Thenius, F. Wotawa and Th. Schmickl

Abstract In this article we introduce a variation of the Firefly-Slime mold-Taxis (FSTaxis) algorithm, which is an emergent gradient ascent solution using external environmental influences such as tides, wind among others. Such external environmental influences are useful sources of energy for movement. If utilized, this results in substantial energy saving compared to robots relying solely on propulsion. Assistance using external factors can be adopted by various types of service robots depending on their environment of operation (for example, rescue robots, robotic underwater exploration). The variant of the FSTaxis algorithm we present in this paper combines bio-inspired communication strategies to achieve gradient taxis purely based on neighbor-to-neighbor interaction and tidal movements for mobility. In this article, we discuss the modified algorithm in detail and further introduce first simulation results obtained using a multiagent simulation environment.

Keywords Gradient taxis · Tides · Self organization · Swarm robotics · Bio-inspiration

1 Introduction

In swarm robotics, a set of rules are employed in a swarm of robots to solve complex problems. Much research has been done in the recent past on swarm robotics to show how complex problems can be solved by a swarm of simple robots [2, 10, 12]. Swarm robotics has drawn inspiration from nature to mimic complex behaviors by using simple rules. Swarm intelligence has found applications in optimization problems in various fields [8, 9]. For example, multi-modal optimization [17] has taken inspiration from fireflies and such efforts have shown promising results. In

J.Ch. Varughese (✉) · R. Thenius · Th. Schmickl
Artificial Life Lab, Department of Zoology, Karl-Franzens-Universität Graz, Graz, Austria
e-mail: joshua.varughese@uni-graz.at

J.Ch. Varughese · F. Wotawa
Institute for Software Technology, Techische Universität Graz, Graz, Austria

M. Husty and M. Hofbaur (eds.), *New Trends in Medical and Service Robots*, Mechanisms and Machine Science 48, DOI 10.1007/978-3-319-59972-4_23

project subCULTron [14], the vision is to develop an underwater society of learning, adapting, self-sustaining robots which can be used for various applications. Given the challenges of robotic systems underwater such as limited availability of classical communication systems, limited mobility etc., there need to be stable but simple solutions. Swarm robotics is an especially attractive solution for subCULTron and similar projects as it imposes minimum economic and computational resource demands while yielding solutions to complex problems [7].

Many algorithms have been presented in the past about possible emergent gradient taxis algorithms based on swarm behavior [2, 11]. Since swarm intelligent solutions present a gradient taxis solution based on simple rules, the robots executing these tasks can be inexpensive and simple. Such algorithms are excellent solutions for robotics where mobility is independent and recharging does not pose an issue. However, for robots that need to explore inaccessible niches autonomously, (for example, rescue robots, robots in nuclear reactors, underwater robots where payload should be low) saving energy by any means is of paramount significance. With the context of such application areas, we will explore whether robots can use environmental influences for mobility.

In the past, a gradient taxis solution has been presented called the FSTaxis algorithm. This algorithm is a feasible bio-inspired solution for gradient taxis based on swarm behavior for underwater robotics. The FSTaxis algorithm is applicable to robots that have a means for independent movement. In this paper, we will formulate a variant of the FSTaxis algorithm which will enable the robots to utilize an external influence for movement. The following sections will explain the algorithm, the method used for testing the algorithm and corresponding results. This algorithm is an example of how emergent solutions can be made possible using an external assistance without using complex computation, large amount of memory and with minimum power consumption.
The objectives of this paper are as follows:

1. Describe a variant of the FSTaxis algorithm.
2. Test the algorithm in a gradient to show its gradient taxis capability.
3. Discuss strengths and weaknesses of the algorithm.

2 Inspiration

As mentioned in the introduction, the FSTaxis algorithm and its variant presented in this paper draws inspiration from nature. Before presenting the algorithm, we will discuss briefly the bio-inspiration for the parent algorithm. This section briefly discusses bio-inspired communication strategies used by slime mold and fireflies and also the motion strategy using an external environmental influence.

2.1 Biological Inspiration

Communication strategy of the FSTaxis algorithm draws inspiration from the aggregation phase of slime mold. Aggregation in slime molds occur in case of scarcity of food. During the aggregation phase, some slime mold cells (centers) release Cyclic Adenosine Mono Phosphate (cAMP) into the environment thus creating a temporary chemical concentration spike around them [13]. Concentration of cAMP diffuses rapidly into the environment and therefore the chemical spike is transitory. This chemical spike attracts other slime mold cells towards the centers. When surrounding cells perceive this chemical signal, they release cAMP themselves, thereby relaying the signal and then move towards the "recruiting centers". This will start a cumulative process of the centers attracting slime mold cells far removed from the recruiting centers. The periodicity of the release of cAMP by the cells is 12–15 s [1]; in between releases, individual cells are insensitive to cAMP pulses in the environment. This interval can be understood as the refractory phase of the amoeba and forms the basis for refraction time in the FSTaxis algorithm. The signal relaying mechanism described above forms the basis for spatiotemporal patterns known as scroll waves [13]. The emergence of scroll waves enable the amoeba to move towards the recruiting centers for successful aggregation.

Another source of inspiration for the FSTaxis algorithm is fireflies. Fireflies have been a subject of elaborate studies in the past [3] for their spectacular bioluminescence and cooperative behavior for attracting mate or prey. Fireflies cooperatively blink in unison in order for the swarm to have a higher chance of attracting mates or prey [3]. A simple physical mechanism known as phase coupled oscillation synchronization is responsible for the cooperative blinking in fireflies. Initially, the individual fireflies blink randomly; when it perceives a blink in its surrounding, it blinks again and then resets its own frequency to match the other [4]. Eventually, the fireflies achieve complete synchronization.

2.2 External Environmental Influence

Forces naturally present in the environment like tides, wind, waves etc. have been utilized by humans in different ways to harvest energy [15]. Many animals and plants also utilize such external influences for migration, reproduction etc. [5, 6]. If utilized, the external influences can save massive amounts of energy. Since this paper is written as part of research in aquatic robotics, focus will be on tides as the external influence. Tides produce complex water movement depending on several factors such as shape and composition of the shoreline, depth, etc. Water movement can be as simple as bidirectional to complex swiveling movements. For the sake of simplicity, we will model the tides to be bidirectional with a constant speed, v_t with heading changing periodically, p_t. Randomness in the heading of the tides is applied to simulate a scenario closer to the actual water movement.

3 The FSTaxis and Tide Algorithm

The Firefly-Slime mold-Taxis and Tides (FSTT) algorithm makes use of the bio-inspired communication strategy of the FSTaxis algorithm. The behavior of agents in the FSTT algorithm can be broadly classified into *Ping behavior* and *Motion behavior*. The ping behavior of the FSTT algorithm corresponds exactly with that of the FSTaxis algorithm. Motion behavior, on the other hand, will differ considerably from the FSTaxis algorithm since FSTT algorithm uses only tidal movements for mobility. The only difference between the FSTaxis algorithm and its variant, the FSTT algorithm, is in its procedure for movement as seen in the Algorithm 1. In the FSTaxis algorithm, an agent is self propelled and in the FSTT algorithm, the agent relies solely on external influences such as tides.

3.1 Ping Behavior

Each agent has three communication states: "active", "refractory" and "inactive" as shown in the state transition diagram Fig. 1. Initially, all agents are in the inactive mode and have an internal countdown timer. The timer value is associated with its position in the environmental gradient. In the inactive mode, the agent monitors incoming pings. If the agent receives a ping, it itself goes into the pinging state where it broadcasts a ping for a period of time, t_p. During t_p, the agent is said to be pinging and after t_p, the agent enters the refractory mode for a period of time, t_r. In the refractory state, the agent ignores all incoming pings. After the refractory time, the agent sets itself back to inactive mode.

Each agent has an inherent cycle time determined by the environmental gradient at its position. If the internal timer (value associated with the environmental value at its physical position) of any agent counts to zero before a ping is received, the agent enters pinging mode and broadcast a ping. The agent sets its own ping frequency, f_p, by associating it with the gradient value at its position, g_p. This ping ("original ping") is further relayed by the neighboring agents as per the ping behavior explained above. The agent that triggers the original ping (the agent whose f_p counted to zero) is referred to as the "leader" hereafter in this paper.

In order to scale ping frequencies to meaningful values, two preset maximum and minimum are selected for the gradient under consideration. Let these values be g_{max} and g_{min}. Equation 1 demonstrates the relation between ping frequency of agents and the environmental value under consideration. In Eq. 1, α and ω are constants that can be modified to achieve meaningful values of ping frequency.

$$f_p = \alpha + \frac{(g_p - g_{min})}{(g_{max} - g_{min})} * \omega \quad (1)$$

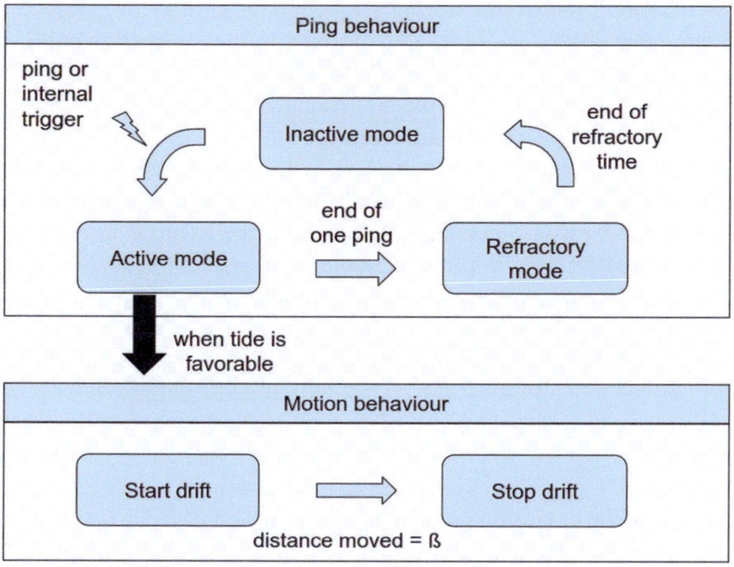

Fig. 1 The state transition diagram of the FSTT algorithm is shown here. The algorithm has two behaviors—ping behavior and motion behavior. There are three states in ping behavior: active, refractory and inactive. An agent transitions from inactive to active state when it receives a ping from another agent or when its own internal clock triggers. After the ping duration, the agent transitions into a refractory mode. After the refractory time, the agent transitions back into the inactive mode. While in active mode, if the tide is favourable, motion behavior is triggered and the agent moves a preset distance in the direction of the tide at tide speed

3.2 Motion Behavior

Motion behavior in FSTT algorithm is dependent on the ping mode of the agent. An agent in inactive mode does not move. As shown in Fig. 1, motion is initiated in the active mode. When any agent receives a ping it sets itself to active mode, sets its own heading towards the received ping and checks if the direction of external influence such as the tide is favorable. In order to check if the tide is favorable, the agent compares the direction of the incoming ping and the tide direction. If the tide has a component in this direction, the agent releases itself and moves with the tide at tide speed v_t for fixed distance β. A ping can only be perceived within the limited sensor range, s_r, of the robot, therefore it limits the number of agents that are able to affect any particular agent. In the scenario described above, it is possible that each agent receives multiple pings from different directions, h_n, where n is the number of agents pinging. In such as case, the agent will calculate the mean heading, h_{mean}, and set its heading towards this mean. Another scenario which will occur is that the agent finds that the tide is not suitable for movement. In this case, the agent remains fixed to the water body bed (by fixing itself on the ground) and continues to monitor incoming pings and storing their incoming direction. Once the tide is favorable, the agent will release itself and move in the mean direction of all incoming pings received while monitoring. If an agents internal clock triggers, an "original" ping based on the environmental value is broadcast; then, this agent labels itself the leader and does not move in that particular cycle.

When a swarm of agents execute the FSTT algorithm as per description above, scroll waves of pings similar to that in slime mold (as mentioned in Sect. 2.1) propagates through the swarm. Since the swarm is not free to move in every direction, the agents will move as close as possible to the most frequently received ping, which is the agent at the maximum environmental gradient value. This is due to the fact that the internal timer of the robot at highest gradient value will count to zero first, the direction of the wave will be from the higher to lower gradients. Therefore, the agents will want to move towards the agents with highest ping frequency but has to wait till the tide is favorable. Since a bi-directional tide model in Sect. 2.2 is considered, the agents will use the forward and backward movement to get as close as possible to "leader". When the agents are in their new position, their internal clock takes the values of the environmental factor (gradient value). Whichever agents internal clock triggers first becomes the leader and the swarm then gathers around this agent. This repeated choosing of leaders and gathering around the leader will draw the swarm towards areas with higher gradient value and in essence emerges into a gradient ascent.

4 Method

To demonstrate the gradient ascent capability by using tides, we choose a gradient with one maxima at the center. The equation of the test gradient is shown in Eq. 2 and here, γ representing the radius of the gradient circle. Figure 2 shows the initial

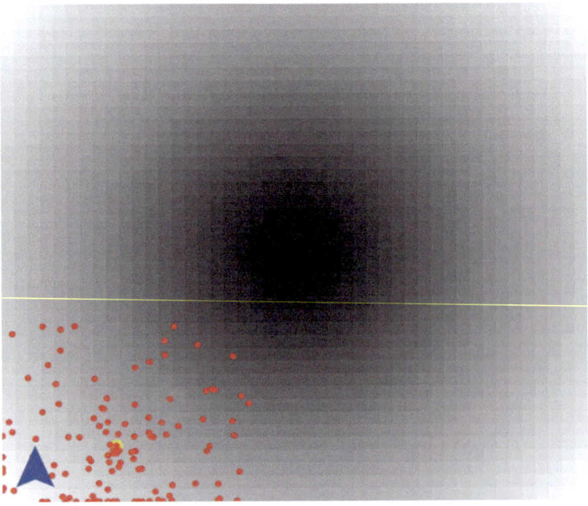

Fig. 2 Figure shows the initial formation with 120 agents in the simulation environment, netlogo. Here, the *dark dots* are agents and the gradient shown to the center of the arena represents the depth gradient. The *bright circle* shows the mean position of the entire swarm. The *blue arrow* on the *bottom left corner* represents the tide direction

Algorithm 1 The FSTaxis algorithm

```
repeat
    procedure PING BEHAVIOR(t_p, t_r, v_a, t_f)
        for all agents do
            if pingmode = refractory mode then
                count down t_r
                if t_r = 0 then
                    set state ← inactive mode
                    set t_f ← 1/f_p - Equation 1
                    set leader status ← "OFF"
                end if
            end if
            if pingmode = active state then
                count down t_p
                if t_p = 0 then
                    set state ← refractory mode
                end if
            end if
            if pingmode = inactive mode then
                if any ping received? then
                    set state ← active mode
                    set move agent ← "ON"
                end if
            end if
            count down t_f
            if t_f = 0 then
                set state ← active mode
                set leader status ← "ON"
            end if
        end for
    end procedure
until forever


repeat
    procedure MOVEMENT(move agent, leader status)
        for all agents with movement = "ON" and leader status ! = "ON" do
            while distancecovered < β do
                Create empty list, l
                for i ← 1, no : ofpingsreceived do
                    append list l ← h_i
                end for
                calculate h_mean of list, l
                set agent heading h_a ← h_mean
                if h_mean - heading of current < 90 then
                    dive up
                    drift with the tide at speed v_t for distance β
                    dive down
                end if
            end while
            set move agent ← "OFF"
        end for
    end procedure
until forever
```

Table 1 Table showing all parameters used for demonstrating the FSTT algorithm

Parameters							
Variable	ω	g_{max}	g_{min}	s_r	β	α	γ
Value	0.1	150	5	3	4	0.008	29.06
Units	–	m	m	patches	m	–	–

formation with 120 agents in netlogo. As previously mentioned, randomness has been added to the motion of both the heading and speed of tides in order to make the simulation as close to the real scenario as feasible. A circular gradient has been used to demonstrate the gradient (depth) ascent capability of the FSTT algorithm. In Fig. 2, shades of black has been used to depict the local depth value. Dark colored areas are deeper and the light colored areas are shoallower.

As mentioned before, the frequencies are scaled according to Eq. 1 and Table 1 shows all the constants used in this experiment. The simulation environment used is Netlogo 4.3.1 [16]. In Netlogo, the test area is divided into "patches" (spatial units) and the agents are called "turtles". For the purpose of this experiment, depth is the physical quantity associated with each patch. The sensor radius of each agent is measured in patches and in this experiment it is taken to be three patches.

It is of merit at this point to describe the characteristics of turtles used for simulation. Each turtle is capable of choosing whether to move with the tide or not. In underwater robotics, this will mean that the robots have a mechanism to restrict themselves from moving with the water, for example, by fixing themselves to the water body bed. Each agent has a sensor to detect direction of tides in simulation. In a real scenario, this will translate to the underwater robots having a flow sensor. In addition to these capabilites, the turtles are able to sense the value of the gradient at its location, a sensor to detect incoming pings and also the ability to broadcast pings.

$$f(x) = \sqrt{x^2 + y^2} - \gamma \tag{2}$$

5 Results

Initially, as shown in Fig. 3, the swarm displays a linear formation purely by drift. Figure 4 shows how the robots further aggregate into small sub-swarms. Each of these sub-swarms is then able to navigate individually to the goal as seen in Fig. 4. The stages in aggregation and navigation towards the goal is shown in Figs. 2, 3, 4. After 50,000 iterations, the swarm reaches the deepest point of the environment (converges) to the goal and then oscillates around the goal as shown in Fig. 5. The bright marking shows the trajectory of the mean of all 120 agents. The back and forth motion is seen in the trajectory due to the bidirectional nature of the tide.

It is also worth mentioning the effect on formation in case of the total absence of randomness in the tide. If tides were purely bidirectional without any randomness, it would mean that the agents have only two directions to move which are: forward

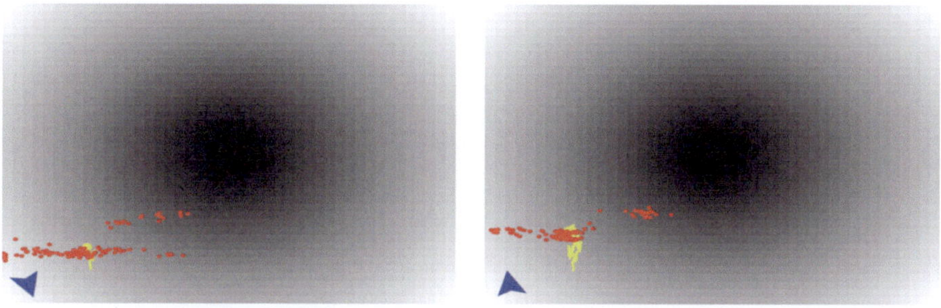

Fig. 3 The figures show intermediate formations by agents executing the FSTT algorithm in simulation. Initially, the agents form a linear formation. Here, the *dark dots* are agents and the gradient shown to the *center* of the arena represents the depth gradient. The *bright marking* shows the mean trajectory of the entire swarm. The *blue arrow* on the *bottom left corner* represents the tide direction. The *dark areas* shows the deeper zones and the *light colored areas* depict low depth

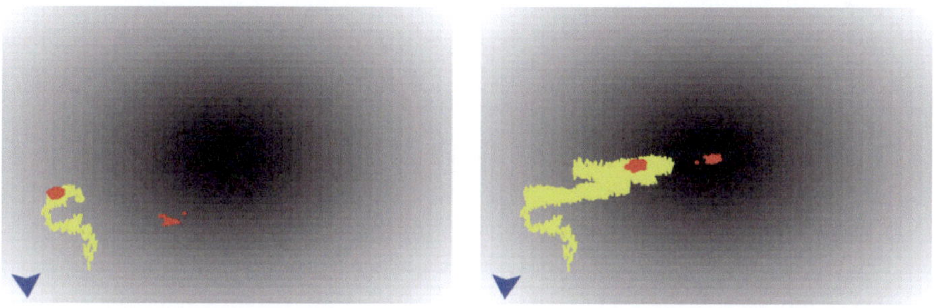

Fig. 4 The figures show intermediate formations by agents executing the FSTT algorithm in simulation. After the initial linear formation, the agents split into aggregates of smaller swarms. Here, the *dark dots* are agents and the gradient shown to the *center* of the arena represents the depth gradient. The *bright marking* shows the mean trajectory of the entire swarm. The *blue arrow* on the *bottom left corner* represents the tide direction. The *dark areas* shows the deeper zones and the *light colored areas* depict low depth

Fig. 5 This figure shows the final formation of agents executing the FSTT algorithm with all the agents having converged to the goal

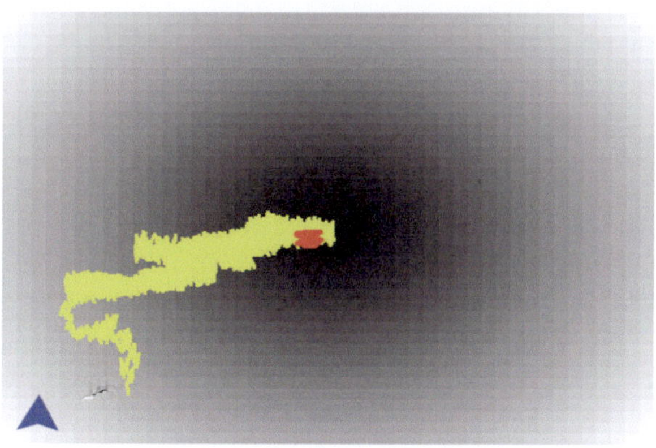

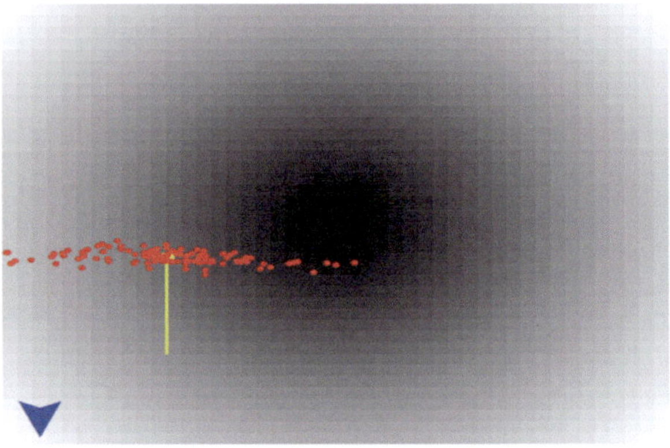

Fig. 6 This figure shows the formation of agents executing the FSTT algorithm with purely bidirectional tide. The agents form a line in the middle of the arena

and backward. In such as case, the expectation is that tides will bring the agents as close as possible to the goal. In this scenario, the agents will move from the initial position and form a line as shown in Fig. 6. The trajectory of the swarm in this case is a straight line due to absence of any sidewards movement by the agents.

6 Discussion

As seen in the Sect. 5, the FSTT algorithm is able to successfully navigate a swarm of agents to the goal (highest environmental gradient value) by repeatedly using the water movement due to tides. It is also important to note that the FSTT algorithm uses no global knowledge for navigation. While being significantly slower than the FSTaxis algorithm, the energy saved is massive since it depends solely on tides for movement. This approach is valuable in salvaging all possible ways of saving energy.

Since the ping behavior requires the agents to move towards the mean ping, the swarm splits into sub-swarms. After splitting into sub-swarms, each sub-swarm is able to navigate individually to the goal and reunite with the there with the other sub swarms as per Figs. 4 and 5.

Although tides in the real world are more complicated than a bidirectional tide, this simple tide model enables the demonstration of the idea presented in this paper. The assumption that tides are bidirectional does not hinder the implementation of the algorithm in more complicated scenarios. In case of more complicated water movements, the agents will still be capable of determining if the tides are favorable by determining the difference between the direction of the incoming ping and the direction of water movement.

As per Fig. 6, we see that randomness in water movement enables the agents to have more degrees of freedom than purely bidrectional freedom. Even though such a case is idealistic, results associated with purely bidirectional tides show that the agents are able to inch closer to the goal.

7 Conclusion

The FSTaxis algorithm forms the basis for the FSTT algorithm by taking advantage of tide movement. It is evident that FSTT algorithm is able to guide a swarm of robots to the highest point in a gradient with a single maxima. In the future, there is opportunity to validate the algorithm by adding noise to the gradient and investigating boundary conditions. Multi-modal gradients can be used to observe the behavior of the FSTT algorithms in presence of multiple maxima. It is expected that FSTT algorithm will perform similar to the FSTaxis algorithm.

It is also worth mentioning that the tide model assumes a period of 50 iterations. In reality, tides reverse only twice in a day. Convergence at around 50,000 iterations mean that the convergence time we are looking at runs into several months. This long convergence time is possibly the result of overly strict simulation environment of tides. While the basic capability of the algorithm for gradient ascent is evident from simulation, the test of feasibility of the hardware requirements such as ping broadcasting technology and water current measurement are still a focus of ongoing research. In the future, feasibility tests of this algorithm will be done with real world hardware. Nevertheless, the FSTT algorithm based on the results presented in Fig. 5 is a novel, innovative and energy saving solution for underwater robots.

By learning the nature of tides or other external influences present in the environment, agents will be able to move closer to the goal. If such a capability is combined with independent motion capability, it will result in massive energy savings and enable long term autonomy of robots in difficult environments. FSTT algorithm implementation can be also considered as a partial solution for independent mobility instead of a sole mobility solution.

Acknowledgements This work was supported by EU-H2020 Project no. 640967, subCULTron, funded by the European Unions Horizon 2020 research and innovation programme under grant agreement No. 640967.

References

1. Alcantara, F., Monk, M.: Signal propagation during aggregation in the slime mould dictyostelium discoideum. Microbiology **85**(2), 321–334 (1974)
2. Bjerknes, J.D., Winfield, A., Melhuish, C.: An analysis of emergent taxis in a wireless connected swarm of mobile robots. In: IEEE Swarm Intelligence Symposium, pp. 45–52. IEEE Press, Los Alamitos, CA (2007)
3. Buck, J., Buck, E.: Biology of synchronous flashing of fireflies. Nature **211**, 562–564 (1966)
4. Camazine, S., Denenbourg, J.L., Franks, N.R., Sneyd, J., Theraulaz, G., Bonabeau, E.: Synchronized flashing among fireflies. pp. 143–166. Princton University Press, Princton (2001)
5. Chapman, J.W., Nesbit, R.L., Burgin, L.E., Reynolds, D.R., Smith, A.D., Middleton, D.R., Hill, J.K.: Flight orientation behaviors promote optimal migration trajectories in high-flying insects. Science **327**(5966), 682–685 (2010). doi:10.1126/science.1182990, http://science.sciencemag.org/content/327/5966/682

6. Friedman, J., Barrett, S.C.: Wind of change: new insights on the ecology and evolution of pollination and mating in wind-pollinated plants. Ann. Bot. (2009)
7. Kennedy, J., Eberhart, R.C.: Particle swarm optimization. In: IEEE International Conference on Neural Networks. IEEE Press, Los Alamitos, CA (1995)
8. Nakagaki, T.: Smart behavior of true slime mold in a labyrinth. Res. Microbiol. **152**, 767–770 (2001)
9. Schmickl, T., Crailsheim, K.: A navigation algorithm for swarm robotics inspired by slime mold aggregation. In: Şahin, E., Spears, W.M., Winfield, A.F.T. (eds.) Swarm Robotics—Second SAB 2006 International Workshop. Lecture Notes of Computer Science, pp. 1–13. Springer, Berlin, Heidelberg, New York (2007)
10. Schmickl, T., Hamann, H.: BEECLUST: A swarm algorithm derived from honeybees. In: Y. Xiao (ed.) Bio-inspired Computing and Communication Networks. CRC Press (2011)
11. Schmickl, T., Hamann, H., Stradner, J., Mayet, R., Crailsheim, K.: Complex taxis-behaviour in a novel bio-inspired robot controller. In: H. Fellermann, M. Dörr, M.M. Hanczyc, L.L. Laursen, S. Maurer, D. Merkle, P.A. Monnard, K. Støy, S. Rasmussen (eds.) Proceedings of the ALife XII Conference, pp. 648–655. MIT Press (2010)
12. Schmickl, T., Thenius, R., Möslinger, C., Radspieler, G., Kernbach, S., Crailsheim, K.: Get in touch: cooperative decision making based on robot-to-robot collisions. Auton. Agents Multi-Agent Syst. **18**(1), 133–155 (2008)
13. Siegert, F., Weijer, C.J.: Three-dimensional scroll waves organize dictyostelium slugs. PNAS **89**(14), 6433–6437 (1992)
14. subCULTron: Submarine cultures perform long-term robotic exploration of unconventional environmental niches. http://www.subcultron.eu/ (2015)
15. Turner, J.A.: A realizable renewable energy future. Science **285**(5428), 687–689 (1999). doi:10.1126/science.285.5428.687, http://science.sciencemag.org/content/285/5428/687
16. Wilensky, U.: Netlogo. Center for Connected Learning and Computer-Based Modeling, Northwestern University, Evanston, IL. http://ccl.northwestern.edu/netlogo/ (1999)
17. Yang, X.S.: Firefly algorithms for multimodal optimization. In: Stochastic Algorithms: Foundations and Applications, pp. 169–178. Springer (2009)

Erratum to: Inter-individual Differences in Conscious and Unconscious Processes During Robot-Child Interaction

I. Giannopulu and T. Watanabe

Erratum to:
Chapter "Inter-individual Differences in Conscious and Unconscious Processes During Robot-Child Interaction" in: M. Husty and M. Hofbaur (eds.), *New Trends in Medical and Service Robots*, Mechanisms and Machine Science 48, DOI 10.1007/978-3-319-59972-4_11

In the original version of the book, Figures 4–6 in Chapter 11 have to be updated with new figures. The erratum chapter and the book have been updated with the change.

The updated original online version of this chapter can be found at https://doi.org/10.1007/978-3-319-59972-4_11

M. Husty and M. Hofbaur (eds.), *New Trends in Medical and Service Robots*,
Mechanisms and Machine Science 48, DOI 10.1007/978-3-319-59972-4_24

MIX
Papier aus verantwortungsvollen Quellen
Paper from responsible sources
FSC® C105338

If you have any concerns about our products,
you can contact us on
ProductSafety@springernature.com

In case Publisher is established outside the EU,
the EU authorized representative is:
Springer Nature Customer Service Center GmbH
Europaplatz 3, 69115 Heidelberg, Germany

Printed by Libri Plureos GmbH
in Hamburg, Germany